# Diverse roles for Occupational Therapists

*Full the full range of M&K Publishing books please visit our website:*
www.mkupdate.co.uk

# Diverse roles for Occupational Therapists

Jane Clewes
Robert Kirkwood

**Diverse roles for Occupational Therapists**
Jane Clewes
Robert Kirkwood

ISBN: 978-1-910451-06-9

First published published 2016

British Library Cataloguing in Publication Data

A catalogue record for this book is available from the British Library

**Notice**

Clinical practice and medical knowledge constantly evolve. Standard safety precautions must be followed, but, as knowledge is broadened by research, changes in practice, treatment and drug therapy may become necessary or appropriate. Readers must check the most current product information provided by the manufacturer of each drug to be administered and verify the dosages and correct administration, as well as contraindications. It is the responsibility of the practitioner, utilising the experience and knowledge of the patient, to determine dosages and the best treatment for each individual patient. Any brands mentioned in this book are as examples only and are not endorsed by the publisher. Neither the publisher nor the authors assume any liability for any injury and/or damage to persons or property arising from this publication.

To contact M&K Publishing write to:

M&K Update Ltd · The Old Bakery · St. John's Street

Keswick · Cumbria CA12 5AS

Tel: 01768 773030 · Fax: 01768 781099

publishing@mkupdate.co.uk

www.mkupdate.co.uk

Designed and typeset by Mary Blood

Printed in Scotland by Bell & Bain, Glasgow

# Contents

# List of boxes

## A note about the case studies

*All people quoted (including service users and colleagues) have given their appropriate permissions. Unless otherwise shown, all case examples have been anonymised as appropriate. Some of the case study examples are composites built up from general experience.*

# List of figures

# About the authors

**Kim Atkinson** MSc, DipCOT

Kim Atkinson graduated from the Wolverhampton School of Occupational Therapy in 1988; she worked for Occupational Therapy services in Southampton District before embarking on a full-time MSc in Rehabilitation Studies at the University of Southampton. Kim went on to take up a post as Lecturer in Occupational Therapy at the University of East Anglia. It was here that she consolidated her interest in fostering professional development throughout the career structure, having an opportunity to be involved in developing and delivering both under-graduate and post-graduate programmes of study for a range of healthcare professions. On moving to Wales, Kim returned to practice in mental health with what is now Abertawe Bro Morgannwg University Health Board (ABMUHB). She maintained her link with education by working with the academic team at Swansea University in its development of the MSc in Advanced Practice and delivering the programme to the early cohorts of students. Kim continues to work for ABMUHB as the Lead Occupational Therapist for Adult, Rehabilitation and Forensic Mental Health Services. Her role is embedded within the mental health service and she has responsibilities for nursing and dietetic staff as well as for occupational therapists. In addition to her work with ABMUHB, Kim is a Specialist Member for the Mental Health Review Tribunal (England).

**Karen Bradshaw** MA-HRM

Karen has worked for the past 25 years in the charity field, including substance misuse, domestic violence, older people and people with hearing impairments, more recently working across three local authorities in health and social care arenas. She is an experienced project manager involved in developing national services utilising telephony, digital equipment and devices. She has been involved in the telecare and telehealth arena for nine years, sits on the executive board for UKTelehealthcare and has been actively involved in shaping the telecare world by embracing innovative equipment and quality services. Karen is a qualified Life Coach which helps inform her approach to client work.

**Hazel Bryce** MA, BSc (Hons)

Hazel has a background working in mental health; she has spent a period of time working abroad in Nigeria as an Occupational Therapist. She is interested in how the arts can be used to enrich our understanding of people's lives. One of her passions is acting as a watch leader, whilst tall ship sailing with a mixed ability crew.

**Julie Carr** PgDip, BSc (Hons)

Julie is the Clinical Legislation Manager at South West Yorkshire Partnership NHS Foundation Trust. She originally trained as an Occupational Therapist and has contributed to the profession in roles including chairing the College of Occupational Therapists' Mental Health NEC, and the

Education, Practice and Publications group; as Mental Health Officer of the COT Council, which involved advising through parliamentary processes for mental health-related legislation; and as a member of the Recovering Ordinary Lives' steering group. She has worked with the NIT regarding the implementation of the amended Mental Health Act. She is currently venturing into the clinical negligence arena.

**Hannah Chapman** PgDip, MA, BSc Econ

Hannah manages a project supporting asylum seekers and refugees in Swansea to access their chosen occupations. Her occupational therapy related roles include coordinating a mental health service, private practice, social services and sitting on the BAOT Welsh board. Prior to this she was a project manager in the third sector and still retains a number of trustee roles. She is currently undertaking a Diploma in Solution-Focused Practice and has a passion for the therapeutic benefits of keeping chickens. She graduated as an occupational therapist from Cardiff in 2011.

**Jane Clewes** MClinRes, MA, PgDip, CertMHS, DipCOT, FHEA

Jane has practised as an Occupational Therapist for over 30 years, working in a variety of mental health clinical settings, different roles and organisations. She edited the *Mental Health Occupational Therapy* newsletter for some years, has worked as a lecturer, and is a Valued Friend of the College of Occupational Therapists. She recently worked as a 'Mental Health Professional', a generic post, in liaison psychiatry, and currently is employed full-time as a Best Interests Assessor.

**Paula Conneely** PgDip, BSc (Hons)

Paula works as a Clinical Specialist with the Meriden Family Programme, part of the Birmingham and Solihull Mental Health Foundation Trust. She qualified with a BSc (Hons) in Occupational Therapy in 1994 and has since worked in a variety of roles including inpatient rehabilitation, community and assertive outreach services. Paula trained in Behavioural Family Therapy (BFT) with the Meriden Family Programme in early 1998 and trained as a Trainer later that year. She joined the Meriden Programme team in 2004. Since that time she has continued to be actively involved in working with families and providing clinical supervision, while developing and delivering staff training in the UK, Ireland and Canada.

**Nick Dutton** PgDip, DipCOT

Nick has worked in the NHS since 1989, first as an Occupational Therapist in acute and community mental health centre settings, then as a care coordinator and most recently as a Cognitive Behavioural Therapist.

**Lesley Haley** MA (Hons), BSc (Hons)

Lesley Haley has worked since 2011 as a Clinical Studies Officer with the Clinical Research Network in England (North East and North Cumbria) and Tees, Esk and Wear Valleys (TEWV) NHS

Foundation Trust. Her current Clinical Studies Officer role includes facilitating staff, service users and carers to participate in National Institute Health Research (NIHR) funded research, across mental health and learning disabilities services. Since qualifying in 1997, she has worked as an Occupational Therapist in physical health, and moved in 1999 into acute adult mental health and adult learning disabilities services in TEWV NHS Foundation Trust.

### Keir Harding BSc (Hons)

Keir qualified as an Occupational Therapist in 1999 and has worked in mental health ever since. Keir became interested in working with personality disorder in 2008 after struggling to be effective in working with this client group. He has been an intrinsic part of teams setting up day therapeutic communities and one of these won an NHS Wales award in 2010. Keir delivered a symposium at the British and Irish Group for the Study of Personality Disorder Conference in 2016 and has been shortlisted for another NHS award for the service he presented. Keir is currently the lead therapist in the East Cheshire Personality Disorder Hub.

### Rachel Hickey MSc, PgDip, BA

Rachel has worked in a variety of mental health and learning disability settings as an Occupational Therapist. She has a special interest in creativity and has completed research in creativity within Psychiatric Intensive Care Units. Rachel has a passion for working with clients with a learning disability who also have mental health needs. Rachel is currently working in a community learning disability team in Rhondda Cynon Taf within Abertawe Bro Morgannwg University Health Board.

### Anne-Marie Jerman BSc (Hons)

Since gaining her degree at the University of Wales College of Medicine Cardiff in 2003, Anne-Marie's career has consisted of a variety of posts throughout South and West Wales and has included both the private sector and NHS. Rotational band 5 posts in trauma and orthopaedics, general surgery and elderly mental health preceded a band 6 post in trauma and orthopaedics at the Princess of Wales Hospital, Bridgend. Her next post was working for a Condition Management Programme, and this is where her passion for extended and emerging roles for Occupational Therapists in mental health began. Her role consisted of delivering group and individual CBT-based sessions with the aim of enabling people to gain or return to employment. She then worked in two different private low secure hospitals with people with serious mental illness and significant forensic histories. In 2009 she embarked on a career in Crisis Resolution and Home Treatment Team (CRHT). She worked for four years as the Occupational Therapist in the North Cwm Taff CRHT before moving to Pembrokeshire CRHT in 2014 to assume her current post where she continues to be a lone Occupational Therapist, an 'Unscheduled Care Practitioner', Pembrokeshire CRHT, Hywel Dda University Health Board.

**Lucy Johnson** BSc (Hons)

Lucy has a background in learning disability and mental health inpatient units. She has worked in eating disorders for three years and this is very much an area she enjoys. Lucy presented a workshop on recovery in 2016 at the International Eating Disorders Conference in London, and a workshop on rehearsed spontaneity around meals in 2015 at the BEAT Eating Disorders Conference, with the team at Newmarket House. She presented on the use of a creative motivational scrapbooking group in eating disorders at the East Anglian Eating Disorders Network Conference, and authored an article for OT News (2014) on the group. She gives presentations to local child and adolescent community mental health teams and schools about the role of Newmarket House and how to support people with eating disorders. She is involved with the training and assessment of student occupational therapists at the University of East Anglia for non-fieldwork modules. Lucy is also a Royal College of Psychiatry AIMS-QED (Quality Network for Eating Disorders) trained peer reviewer. She enjoys scuba diving in the UK and abroad as well as travelling/backpacking.

**Robert Kirkwood** D.OccT, MSc, PgDipOT, BA (Hons)

Rob has worked in the NHS since qualifying as an Occupational Therapist in 2002. Following time within an Occupational Therapist rotation post, Rob worked initially in adult mental health before moving to Child and Adolescent Mental Health (CAMHS) where he has worked as both a clinical specialist occupational therapist and a Primary Mental Health Worker (PMHW) for the past eight years. During this time, Rob has also completed a professional doctorate in occupational therapy at the University of Brighton, utilising participatory action research methods to develop cooperative inquiries with young people with hearing impairment. Rob has presented findings from his research at conferences and workshops both nationally and internationally.

**Gill Knott** PgDip, BHSc (Hons)

Gill has worked in a variety of mental health settings over a number of years, including Assertive Outreach and Community Rehab. She has an ongoing interest in mental health research which started in 2013 with a collaboration exploring the value base of occupational therapy and how this fits with occupational therapists carrying out the AMHP role. Gill currently works as a Community Occupational Therapist in the Disability Services Team in west Leeds for Leeds City Council and is a practising AMHP.

**Carmen Lewis** MSc, BSc (Hons)

Carmen qualified as an Occupational Therapist in 2003 and completed a Master's degree in mental health in 2009. She has extensive experience of working in the forensic mental health field, having spent a number of years working in a medium secure unit, prior to working in a low secure and community forensics team. She then went on to spend over seven years working firstly in Swansea and then Cardiff prison, setting up and developing occupational therapy services. She always had a special interest in working with complex cases and clients with a diagnosis of personality disorder and has recently taken up a new challenge, leaving the prison setting to join the Cynnwys Therapy Service to work with clients with Borderline Personality Disorder in Cardiff and Vale UHB.

**Sarah Mead** MA, MSc, PgDip, BA, FHEA

Sarah is an independent occupational therapy supervisor and senior lecturer in occupational therapy at the University of Brighton, specialising in occupational therapy in diverse settings, vocational rehabilitation and bariatric care.

**Katja Michel** MEd, BSc (Hons)

Katja has worked in child and adolescent mental health services in the West Midlands for over 11 years. Her experiences working in the changing world of child and adolescent mental healthcare have influenced her commitment and desire to enable users of services to make their experiences heard and, through this, influence how services are delivered.

**Karen Newberry** MA, PgCert, BSc (Hons), FHEA

Karen has had a keen interest in mental health occupational therapy for over 20 years. She has worked clinically within a cross-section of mental health services, including the development of assertive outreach services. Throughout her clinical work, and in her current role as a Senior Lecturer in Occupational Therapy at the University of Derby, she has continued to be interested in new and emerging roles for occupational therapists, not only in terms of profession-specific skills, but also in terms of building therapeutic relationships and the therapeutic use of self to facilitate occupational engagement.

**Rachel Nias** PgDip, BSc (Hons)

Rachel qualified as an Occupational Therapist in 2013 with prior experience in social care and forensic settings. She takes an active interest in evidence-based practice and is passionate about incorporating occupational therapy philosophy into daily practice. She currently works as an Occupational Therapist in Cardiff.

**Clare O'Reilly** MSc, BSc

Clare is an Occupational Therapist with a passion for mental health and wellbeing. She qualified with an honours degree in Occupational Therapy from Trinity College Dublin in 2002 and completed an MSc in Occupational Therapy at Queen Margaret University, Edinburgh, in 2007. She has a keen interest in eating disorders and has worked in an adult eating disorders inpatient service before undertaking her current role as a specialist clinician in the Service for High-Risk Eating Disorders (SHED) community team in South Wales. Clare has received training in Dialectical Behaviour Therapy (DBT) and has participated in a full DBT team for the past five years, using these skills alongside her core Occupational Therapy interventions to support people to achieve their full potential. She has also established a 'contemplation' group to support those individuals who have become 'stuck' and are struggling to make further changes. Clare completed the Royal College of Nursing Clinical Leadership Programme in 2014 during which she promoted staff health and wellbeing by encouraging health staff to take scheduled breaks. Clare is originally from Ireland.

**Jackie Parsonage** MResCP, BSc (Hons)

Jackie has worked as a clinician in a variety of mental health settings over the last 15 years and has latterly specialised in early intervention in psychosis. She has an ongoing interest in mental health research which started in 1997, with collaboration between academics, service users and clinicians, exploring users' experience of recovery from psychosis. Most recently she has applied the skills from the NIHR Master's of Research in Clinical Practice awarded by St George's University which she completed in 2012. Latterly Jackie worked as Acting Team Leader, Occupational Therapist and Care Coordinator for H&H EIS, CNWL NHS Foundation Trust until moving to her new role as a Disabled Student Allowance Assessor (DSA) in September 2016.

**Nick Pollard** PhD, MSc, MA, DipCOT, FHEA

Nick worked in psychiatric settings for 12 years before joining Sheffield Hallam University as a senior lecturer and research coordinator. He has written widely on occupational therapy and has coedited several key texts. These include: Sakellariou, D. & Pollard, N. (eds) (2016–17 in progress) *Occupational Therapies Without Borders: Integrating justice with practice*, 2nd edn. Edinburgh: Elsevier Science; *Occupying Disability* (2015, with Pamela Block, Devva Kasnitz and Akemi Nishida); and *Meaningful Living Through Occupation* (2015, with Moses Ikiugu).

**Annoula Raptis** BSc (Hons)

Annoula's interest in psychological therapies was fostered following a lecture on Cognitive Behavioural Therapy (CBT) at university. It inspired her to undertake a research study investigating the use of CBT and Mindfulness-Based Cognitive Therapy (MBCT) for hypochondriasis. She has now taken up the opportunity to work as a Psychological Mental Health Professional which has affirmed her enthusiasm for psychological therapies and is keen to build her knowledge and skill base within this field of practice. She is currently exploring 'third wave' therapies such as Acceptance and Commitment Therapy (ACT), compassion-focused therapy and mindfulness to find out how they can augment or provide an alternative to CBT.

**Carol Savage** MSc, BSc (Hons)

Carol has worked in adult mental healthcare services across England and Wales for almost 30 years. For the past two years she has worked as a Recovery Lead implementing Recovery services within her locality for individuals with severe and enduring mental illness, their families, friends and carers. She has a particular interest in finding the right combination of services, treatments and support systems to empower individuals to build a satisfying, meaningful life for themselves, beyond their illness. This interest continues to fuel her desire to assume a leadership role in the area of Recovery-related research and practice, and investigate the issues that may arise from doing so. Carol currently works as a specialist Occupational Therapist.

**Claire Terrington** BSc (Hons)

Claire has worked in assertive outreach in inner city Birmingham for 14 years, setting up the occupational therapy service for assertive outreach within the locality. She has a passion for working with those experiencing severe and enduring mental illness and works across the Trust to further develop these services. Her interests lie in developing services that integrate the use of self to build therapeutic relationships, and the use of meaningful occupation. She is currently employed as a senior Occupational Therapist.

**Clare Weale** MSc (Hons), BSc (Hons)

Clare qualified as an Occupational Therapist from Brunel University. She also has a degree in Psychology and a Master's in Gender Politics and Culture from Birkbeck. She was drawn to becoming an Occupational Therapist because her analytical personality and pragmatic nature is suited to clinical practice. She has specialist interests in community mobility and assistive technology/telecare and experience working in these areas with different client groups in local authority and third sector settings.

**Amie Witherspoon** BSc (Hons)

Amie qualified as a Sports Therapist from the University of Central Lancashire. She has since gained experience of working in NHS, local authority and third sector settings. She has several years of experience working as an Occupational Therapy Assistant in an acute hospital Trust and as the Assistive Technology Coordinator for a local authority in London. She is currently working as the Integrated Community Equipment Service Coordinator for a local authority in the North West.

# Acknowledgements

The editors and authors wish to thank everyone who has contributed to the production of this book, whether through giving permission to use quotations or case studies, giving practical assistance (e.g. proofreading or making comments), giving encouragement or support, or making contributions such as agreeing to be interviewed. These include:

Margot Akeroyd, David Atkinson, Veronica Ball, Katrina Bannigan, Miranda Barber, Rachel Barker, Jina Barrett, Jane Bradley, Helen Bucke, Cathy Clarke, Katie Elliot, Alison Fear, Lucy Gameson, Neil Gordon, Debbie Green, Wendy Griffiths, the Haley family, Alan Hirons, Zoe Hughes, Di Hurley, Susanne Leeson, Katie McDonald, Gerard McFeely, Julia McHugh, Helen Mosley, Caroline O'Haire, Mr & Mrs Parsonage, Nick Pollard, Jean Ruddle Mendieta, Carol Savage, Donna Smart, Genevieve Smyth, Susan Steer, Gill Strong, Marie-Clare Trevett, A. Wadden, Carolyn Wilkes, and Caroline Young. Also, colleagues from: the Clinical Research Network, the College of Occupational Therapists, the Health Research Authority, and the Tees Esk and Wear Valleys NHS Foundation Trust.

# Abbreviations

**ACCT** Assessment, Care in Custody and Teamwork
**ACT** Assertive Community Treatment
**ACT** Acceptance and Commitment Therapy
**ADHD** Attention Deficit Hyperactivity Disorder
**ADL** Activities of Daily Living
**AfC** Agenda for Change
**AHP** Allied Health Professions
**AIMS** Accreditation for Inpatient Mental Health Services
**AKI** Acute Kidney Injury
**AMCP/AMCaP** Approved Mental Capacity Professional
**AMHP** Approved Mental Health Professional
**AMPS** Assessment of Motor and Process Skills
**AO** Assertive Outreach
**AOT** Assertive Outreach Team
**ARFID** Avoidant/Restrictive Food Intake Disorder
**ASW** Approved Social Worker
**AT** Assistive Technology
**AWOL** Absent WithOut Leave
**BA** Behavioural Activation
**BABCP** British Association for Behavioural and Cognitive Psychotherapies
**BAOT** British Association of Occupational Therapists
**BED** Binge Eating Disorder
**BFT** Behavioural Family Therapy
**BIA** Best Interests Assessor
**BJOT** *British Journal of Occupational Therapy*
**BMI** Body Mass Index
**BPD** Borderline Personality Disorder
**CAB** Citizens' Advice Bureau
**CAHPR** Council of Health Professions Research
**CAMHS** Child and Adolescent Mental Health Services
**CAOT** Canadian Association of Occupational Therapists
**CAST** Creative Arts Steering Team
**CBT** Cognitive Behavioural Therapy
**CBT-E** Enhanced Cognitive Behaviour Therapy for eating disorders
**CCG** Clinical Commissioning Group
**CCOPII** Client-centred Community Occupational Performance Initial Interview
**CHAIN** Contact, Help, Advice and Information Network
**CHD** Coronary Heart Disease
**CIWA** Clinical Institute Withdrawal Assessment for Alcohol
**CMHT** Community Mental Health Team
**CMOP** Canadian Measure of Occupational Performance
**COPD** Chronic Obstructive Pulmonary Disease
**COPM** Canadian Occupational Performance Measure
**COT** College of Occupational Therapists
**CPA** Care Programme Approach
**CPD** Continuing Professional Development
**CPN** Community Psychiatric Nurse
**CR** Cognitive Restructuring

**CRHT** Crisis Resolution and Home Treatment

**CRN** Clinical Research Network

**CTIMP** Clinical Trials of Investigative Medicinal Products

**CTO** Community Treatment Order

**CV** Curriculum Vitae

**CYP-IAPT** Children and Young People Improving Access to Psychological Therapies

**DAF** Deprived Areas Fund

**DBS** Disclosure and Barring Service

**DBT** Dialectical Behaviour Therapy

**DCSF** Department for Children, Schools and Families

**DGH** District General Hospital

**DIT** Dynamic Interpersonal Therapy

**DLF** Disabled Living Foundation

**DNA** Did Not Attend

**DoH** Department of Health

**DoL/DoLS** Deprivation of Liberty/Deprivation of Liberty Safeguards

**DSH** Deliberate Self-Harm

**DSA** Disabled Student Allowance Assessor

**DST** Decision Support Tool

**DUP** duration of untreated psychosis

**DWP** Department of Work and Pensions

**ECHR** European Convention for Human Rights

**EI** Early Intervention

**EIP** Early Intervention in Psychosis

**EMI** Elderly Mentally Ill

**EMPSA** Eating and Meal Preparation Skills Assessment

**EPPIC** Early Psychosis Prevention and Intervention Centre

**ERP** Exposure Response Prevention

**FACT** Flexible Assertive Community Treatment

**FCE** Functional Capacity Evaluation

**GAD** Generalised Anxiety Disorder

**GAD-7** Generalised Anxiety Disorder measure, version 7

**GAS** Goal Attainment Scale

**GCP** Good Clinical Practice

**GP** General Practitioner

**GPS** Global Positioning System

**HADS** Hospital Anxiety and Depression Scale

**HAI** Health Anxiety Inventory

**HAS** Health Advisory Service

**HCPC** Health and Care Professions Council

**HMP** Her Majesty's Prison

**HRA** Health Research Authority

**HSE** Health & Safety Executive

**IAPT** Increasing Access to Psychological Therapies

**IEPA** International Early Psychosis Association

**IES-R** Impact of Events Scale – Revised

**IMCA** Independent Mental Capacity Advocate

**ImROC** Implementing Recovery through Organisational Change

**IOM** Integrated Offender Management

**IPP** Indeterminate sentence for Public Protection

**IPS** Individual Placement and Support model

**IPT** Interpersonal Therapy

**IQ** Intelligence Quotient

**IRM** Intentional Relationship Model

**IV** Intra-venous

**IVR** Institute for Volunteering Research

**KPI** Key Performance Indicator

**KSF** Knowledge Skills Framework

**KUF** Knowledge and Understanding Framework

**LA** Local Authority

**LD** Learning Disability/Difficulty

**LGBT** Lesbian, Gay, Bisexual and Transgender

**LRAS** Local Resource Allocation Systems

**LTHC** long-term health conditions

**MA** Managing Authority

**MAPPA** Multi Agency Public Protection Arrangements

**MBCT** Mindfulness Based Cognitive Therapy

**MCA** Mental Capacity Act

**MDT** multi-disciplinary team

**MHRS** Mental Health Recovery Star

**MI** Motivational Interviewing

**MOCA** Model of Creative Ability

**MoD** Ministry of Defence

**MOHO** Model of Human Occupation

**MOHOST** Model of Human Occupation Screening Tool

**NAPICU** National Association of Psychiatric Intensive Care and Low Secure Units

**NHS** National Health Service

**NICE** National Institute for Health and Care Excellence

**NIHR** National Institute for Health Research

**NIT** National Implementation Team

**NLIAH** National Leadership and Innovation Agency for Healthcare

**NLP** Neuro-Linguistic Programming

**NOMS** National Offender Management Service

**NR** Nearest Relative

**NSF** National Service Framework

**OCAIRS** Occupational Circumstances Assessment Interview and Rating Scale

**OCD** Obsessive Compulsive Disorder

**OCI** Obsessive Compulsive Inventory

**OCN** Open College Network

**OPHI** Occupational Performance History Interview

**OSA** Occupational Self-Assessment

**OSFED** Other Specified Feeding and Eating Disorders

**PDG** Professional Development Group

**PDSS** Panic Disorder Severity Scale

**PHQ-9** Patient Health Questionnaire (version 9)

**PICU** Psychiatric Intensive Care Unit

**PMHP** Psychological Mental Health Practitioner

**PMHW** Primary Mental Health Worker

**PONI** Prisoner Ombudsman for Northern Ireland

**PPO** Prolific and Priority Offender

**PROMS** Patient Reported Outcome Measures

**PSW** Penn State Worry questionnaire

**PTSD** Post Traumatic Stress Disorder

**PWP** Psychological Wellbeing Practitioners

**R&D** Research & Development

**RAID** Rapid Assessment, Interface and Discharge

**RCP** Royal College of Psychiatrists

**RCT** Randomised Controlled Trial

**RMN** Registered Mental Nurse

**RP** Relevant Person

**RPR** Relevant Person's Representative

**SB** Supervisory Body

**SCT** Supervised Community Treatment

**SCVR** Safer Custody and Violence Reduction

**SE-AN** Severe and Enduring Anorexia Nervosa

**SENCo** Special Educational Needs Coordinator

**SEED** Severe and Enduring Eating Disorder

**SFT** Solution-Focused Therapy

**SI** Sensory Integration

**SMART** (specific, measurable, achievable, realistic and timed)

**SMI** serious mental illness

**SOC** Selection Optimisation with Compensation

**SORT** Sheffield Outreach Team

**SPA** Single Point of Access

**SPIN** Social Phobia Inventory

**SSCM** Specialised Supportive Clinical Management

**SW** Social Worker

**TC** Therapeutic Community

**TCSE** Triangle Consulting Social Enterprise Limited

**TECS** Technology Enabled Care Services

**TSA** Transferable Skills Analysis

**TTC** Time to Change

**UK** United Kingdom

**UKCC** United Kingdom Central Council for Nursing, Midwifery and Health Visiting

**UKOTRF** UK Occupational Therapy Research Foundation

**UNCRPD** United Nations Convention on the Rights of Persons with Disabilities

**UTI** Urinary Tract Infection

**VR** Vocational Rehabilitation

**W&ASAS** Work and Social Adjustment Scale

**WHO** World Health Organisation

**WRAP** Wellness & Recovery Action Plan

**WRI** Worker Role Interview Tool

**wte** whole time equivalent

# Foreword

This refreshing and direct book is written by practitioners about practice. It is based in the day to day experience of what occupational therapists working in mental health do with change, and if there is one word that characterises that work, it is 'change'. The practitioner has a continual pressure of change, from the macro level of policy all the way through to the need to accommodate changes in the plan outlined for the next few hours of work. It is a potentially very confusing and challenging working environment, in which all practitioners have to think quickly, juggle conflicting demands, reassess priorities and respond rapidly to emerging situations. The practitioner is at the same time continuously learning, from colleagues, from clients and their families or carers, acquiring new details of changing legislation, benefits or policy, new service configurations, new approaches to problems, new issues to negotiate. It can become very difficult in these circumstances to hold on to a core of practice, the elements of the profession which make it occupation-centred, rather than so focused on the other priorities and demands that identity is lost.

This book reads like a series of conversations with good supervisors who can help the newly qualified therapist, the practitioner trying to reconnect with their bearings or the plainly flummoxed to gain a perspective on their objectives. It sets out clear strategies and objectives for people who are managing their practices through extended roles or in emerging situations which may take them beyond the traditional positions for which they may have trained. It is about how people really cope with multiple demands and contains honest accounts of experiences as well as reflective challenges. Throughout the text there are the voices of practitioners and service users talking about their experiences and dilemmas, and there is a strong focus on navigating and asserting occupation-based practices through changes in delivery with arguments to support the inclusion of occupational therapists through the key contributions they can make to intervention processes. There are many useful case examples and a lot of suggestions for further reading.

When I qualified as an occupational therapist in 1991 and began working in psychiatry, occupational therapy practice was very different. Two key differences were that there was more time to reflect, and therapists were more able to lead or participate in group activities. Occupational therapists were arguing to be included in the care coordinator role as outlined by Hannah Chapman in Chapter 1, and while there were certainly arguments about boundaries between professional groups the problems of genericism had not yet emerged. My first role was as a basic grade in a former asylum in the last throes of its existence. Some of the people who lived there had been first admitted before the Second World War, one of them had been a patient from the time the asylum had briefly taken patients in the post-First World War influenza outbreak, but had never been discharged. New drugs such as clozapine seemed to have dramatic effects on people who had been unable to make improvements on the traditional neuroleptics, and this meant that some people were able to achieve stability and make the move into community settings. Others, however, could not benefit.

Some of the asylum staff were very resistant to the idea that these last patients, those who had been most institutionalised, should be moved into the community at all. They felt from their long experience that the community was unsafe and unsympathetic to the needs of these people. There were antagonisms between professional groups as people were sent up to the occupational therapy department too heavily medicated to function, or else were very agitated and unable to tolerate being with others, so would have to be brought back to the wards. When this happened, often the response would be 'Can't you cope with him/her, love? Only *we* have to work with them all the time'.

On the wards many people did not have their own private space and found it hard to keep personal possessions, while their clothes were bundled up and washed together, so that everyone wore shapeless items that were lifeless and often shrunken. The institutional behaviours were recognisable from Goffman's *Asylums* (1968), Solzhenitsyn's *One day in the life of Ivan Denisovitch* (1962/2000) or even the dystopian explorations of what society as a total institution might be like, such as Zamyatin's *We* (1921/1993). People traded in cigarette ends, chocolate, coffee, tea and sex, and many were withdrawn and either challenging to engage or at least would find it difficult to tolerate much interaction.

At this time, the terms 'occupational deprivation' and 'client-centred practice' had not been developed. The Recovery approach had not been adopted in mental health. I found myself questioning the value of psychiatric practice and became interested in the work of Foucault and in the psychiatric survivors' movement. I could not decide whether psychiatric care was oppressive or whether its shortcomings were due to wider socio-economic and political factors, and yet it was obvious that people needed safe therapeutic environments and the possibility of regaining their equilibrium. As a couple of my acquaintances had been admitted to acute wards while I was in training it was clear to me that mental health was a field were one could easily arrive at a situation where you yourself could become a service user. When eventually I had my own experiences of depression and anxiety, although it may have been an excessive fear, I was very concerned to avoid crossing the threshold into attending services myself.

Later I worked in an assertive outreach service, which gave me many rewarding opportunities to work with people in similar ways to those described in the chapters by Jackie Parsonage, Hazel Bryce, Karen Newberry and Clare Terrington, though at this point, in the late 1990s, assertive outreach was evolving from a community-based mental health team approach. Mental health services had not developed the wide range of specialisations set out here and they had not acquired the level of understanding that we now have concerning conditions such as personality disorders, which were only just beginning to be recognised as treatable. On the other hand, it was very evident that the concerns of my previous asylum colleagues were not unfounded. The community was a harsh and difficult environment for those with mental health issues, and many of the situations which affected the people I was working with originated, at least partly, in the attitudes of other community members. The oppression of those experiencing mental distress contained both structural elements (in the sense that authorities were not always as sympathetic to needs as they could be) and strong social elements (due to the lack of wider awareness, or purely predatory behaviours). These issues had significant occupational effects in terms of freedom to access the community at large, or even to attend services using public transport, which often interacted with the symptoms that people experienced. These challenges are recognised by occupational therapists and other team members as part of the holistic aspect of mental health, and there are plenty of examples here of ways to tackle such complex issues.

Now as an educator, as someone regularly visiting students on placement and in communication with practitioners, I often reflect on what it would be like to return to practice myself. Perhaps the first port of call would be to read this excellent and practical book, cover to cover.

*Nick Pollard*

# References

Goffman, E. (1968). *Asylums*. Harmondsworth: Pelican.

Solzhenitsyn, A. (1962/2000). *One Day in the Life of Ivan Denisovitch,* Translated by Ralph Parker. London: Penguin.

Zamyatin, Y. (1921/1993). *We*. Translated by Clarence Brown. London: Penguin.

# Introduction

Occupational therapists get everywhere, it would seem, and this book is testament to the breadth of roles being undertaken by occupational therapists in the UK today. The diversity of practice settings that appear to be available to occupational therapists was certainly a strong factor that drew me, and no doubt countless others, to the profession. It will undoubtedly be a key reason why you are reading this book as well.

The idea for this book arose out of a desire to collect the knowledge and experience of practitioners within diverse and extended roles and present them in a way that would be easily accessible and help occupational therapists at any stage of their career better understand and explore a wide range of professional roles to which the tenets of occupational therapy may be applied. The reader may wish to turn straight to a specific chapter describing an area they themselves work in or have thought about, or browse the chapters to find practical guidance that may fuel their inspiration for future career prospects. Reading how other occupational therapists are applying their knowledge and skills in different settings allows us to reflect upon our own situation and evaluate to what extent we are maintaining the core competencies of our profession within our own practice. I would urge you, the reader, to explore the chapters that you may not have otherwise felt were relevant to your own situations. Even if we are perfectly comfortable in our existing roles and have no desire to move elsewhere or take on additional responsibilities, the chapters in this book offer a rich context from which to reflect upon our own experience, broaden our understanding and triangulate our knowledge.

Whilst championing some less well-worn career paths that occupational therapists have taken, this book gives honest accounts that combine practical descriptions with a range of occupational therapy theory and models set against a backdrop of differing service structures. Some authors shine a light upon underlying challenges, such as staying connected with the profession and difficulty maintaining professional identity, while others describe often turbulent theoretical meeting points as different disciplines come together within their services. However, throughout the book, chapter after chapter, authors emphasise our profession's core skills, as the key tenets of occupational therapy are reaffirmed through their work. Grounded in practice-based knowledge and peppered with case studies to help us get beneath the surface of the roles, each chapter gives the reader an opportunity to apply these rich descriptions of different practice settings to their own roles. For example, doing with, not for, our client group is touched upon in several chapters. We are also challenged to consider why certain attitudes exist within diverse roles and how an occupational lens may help to bring about change. One example of this is our response when clients 'DNA', in terms of moving towards case closure; from a holistic perspective, this should speak to us about the client's wider difficulties with engagement. In another chapter the concept of independence is challenged when, from a systemic perspective, interdependence is felt to be the best goal for the client and their family.

Several authors grapple with how the therapeutic use of self to enhance client-centred practice is borne out in difficult practice contexts such as Assertive Outreach and working with personality disorder. The challenge of managing generic roles for occupational therapists is highlighted by practitioners working in roles from intensive care units to cognitive behavioural therapy-based services. Other chapters celebrate the synergy that clearly exists between the values of occupational therapy and those that underpin existing service models such as recovery or rehabilitation teams, early intervention services, creative arts-based group work and client-centred participation focused roles. The call for further research to underpin the value that occupational therapy adds to these roles is echoed in many of these chapters and serves as a clear reminder of our professional duty to contribute to the research base in all areas and at all levels.

Laced through this book are clear processes of clinical reasoning that underpin the array of interventions described within diverse roles. Essentially, such clinical reasoning must stem from the core training and central tenets of occupational therapy. For if we, in our various roles, are still regulated by the Health & Care Professions Council (HCPC), then we are still maintaining our registration as occupational therapists. By so doing, we align ourselves to those central tenets. This book provides robust evidence from practitioners in the field who are endeavouring to do just that in diverse, extended and often challenging roles. We should take heart from the examples these occupational therapists have given us, applying their training, knowledge and experience in such diverse ways, and allow their stories to bolster our own professional confidence to do the same.

*Robert Kirkwood*

# Chapter 1

# Occupational therapists as care coordinators

*Hannah Chapman*

## Introduction

This chapter explores the role of the occupational therapist within care coordination. To begin with, the history and purpose of care coordination is explored. Care coordination is then considered through three perspectives: occupational therapists', referral agencies' and service users'. These perspectives draw upon literature and conversations with service users and professionals, as well as on personal experience.

A number of narratives are drawn together: the author does not intend to provide exhaustive coverage of all the many opinions and issues surrounding care coordination, but aims to offer a taster of the roles and some of the benefits and challenges involved. The chapter goes on to explore how occupational therapists can think about working most effectively within a care coordination culture, working either as care coordinators themselves or in partnership with care coordinators; it concludes by looking at future directions in this area.

## Key points

- Occupational therapists working in mental health are likely to encounter the care coordination process.
- The care coordination role involves a complex skill set which, arguably, occupational therapists are well placed to meet, but equally may push them into generic work.
- It is down to each individual occupational therapist whether they feel a generic role such as care coordination is suitable to them; there is space both for 'core' roles which deepen the knowledge base and more generic roles which widen the knowledge base of the profession.

- Physical health fields may well adopt a care coordination approach in the future.
- Care plans can potentially be used as an audit tool to demonstrate the importance of occupation to recovery.
- Service users are calling for a more holistic and less medically focused approach to care coordination.

# What is a care coordinator?
## Legislation and background

The role of the care coordinator was born out of legislation and key events dating back to the early 1990s. For a number of decades prior to this there had been increasing movements towards 'de-institutionalisation' by closing down large 'asylums' and shifting the focus to supporting people in the community or local hospitals instead (Great Britain 1990). However, during this time, high profile cases in the media (such as that of a seemingly unprovoked murder carried out by a man with a diagnosis of schizophrenia in the community) led to public concern about discharged patients losing contact with mental health services (Killaspy 2006, pp. 249–250). In the light of these events it was felt that more support was needed for people during the shift from living in institutions to living in the community. Thus the care coordination process came about.

Originally outlined in a government document in 1990 (DoH 1990), the Care Programme Approach (CPA) was introduced in England as 'a framework for effective mental healthcare for people with severe mental health problems' (DoH 2006, p. 4) and aimed to support people living in the community to access the support they needed. It aimed to be a 'joined up' service for people using mental health services as Goodwin & Lawton-Smith (2010) state:

> At its inception, it required Health Authorities, in collaboration with local authority Social Services Departments, to put in place specified arrangements for the care and treatment of mentally ill people in the community. It provided a framework for hospital discharge planning and aftercare, and it was intended that those on CPA should be able to access services 24 hours a day, 365 days a year.
>
> (Goodwin & Lawton-Smith 2010, p. 4)

The CPA was then introduced in Scotland in 1992 and Wales in 2004 (Sainsbury Centre for Mental Health 2005). This legislation has now grown and evolved in differing ways throughout the UK. Since the late 1990s, Wales, Northern Ireland and Scotland have had devolved powers to develop their own mental health legislation (Lawton-Smith & McCullough 2013). This has affected how mental health services are delivered in each country.

Despite the regional variations and shifts over time it has been recognised (Goodwin and Lawton-Smith 2010) that there are key elements involved which have remained as standard within the approach.

These are:

- A systematic assessment of each patient's health and social care needs.

- The drawing up of a care plan to address those needs.

- The appointment of a 'key worker' to oversee the delivery of the care plan.

- Regular review of the patient's needs and care plan.

(Goodwin & Lawton-Smith 2010, p. 5)

These elements outline the broad principles of the approach, and the description of a 'key worker' refers to the role we now know and recognise as Care Coordinator. In this sense the care coordinator is the person who is responsible for holding together a person's care plan within the CPA.

Eligibility for a care coordinator also varies from country to country. For instance, in Wales, under the *Mental Health Measure* (Welsh Government 2010), anyone under secondary mental health services is entitled to a care plan and care coordinator. In England the criteria for eligibility are laid out ißn government documentation (DoH 2008, pp. 13–14). This guidance states that services should continue to use their own criteria for assessing people for secondary mental health services and then use the criteria in the guidance to assess whether people could benefit from using the CPA. However, in Northern Ireland the processes in some care trusts have shifted from a care management approach to a case management approach. This means a range of professionals are responsible, not just one care manager as before.

Throughout the UK many care coordinators are based within Community Mental Health Teams (CMHTs), but may also be based in assertive outreach teams and other similar services. Care coordination is not linked to one profession; social workers, nurses, psychologists, occupational therapists or other relevant mental health professionals can take on the role. It is, however, understood that a care coordinator should be the person best suited to support the client to meet his/her needs, or the professional who has the most involvement with the client.

When researching for this chapter, it was evident that clear consistent guidance and legislation on the Care Programme Approach can be difficult to come by – particularly the variations within each country and geographical location. Many local health boards, trusts or areas may have their own guidance and policies; however, this may not be publicly available. As will be explored later, one criticism of the CPA is that clients do not feel actively involved in the process. A key response to this might be clearer information on the background and legislation in an easy to understand format.

To summarise, the clear message from the available resources is that the CPA is intended to be an approach that links the client with a key professional who can support them to navigate the health and social care systems to put in place a plan that the client feels is most conducive to their own recovery in the community.

## Purpose of care coordination

The CPA exists so that people have increased control and input into the direction of their support as well as ensuring they do not 'slip through the net'. It also aims to encourage integration of care between services so that a service user has one single point of reference regarding support for their mental and physical health and wellbeing. As it aims to be holistic, it does not focus on one specific area of a person's life, but looks at all areas to see where support is needed.

The purpose of a care coordinator is to involve the person and bring together all the different areas of his/her Recovery into a single document, and to ensure that the complete Recovery approach is being carried out. In this sense care coordinators 'require the skills and competencies to act both as care managers to individual patients … as well as have the power to exert the authority to ensure that care plans are implemented' (Goodwin & Lawton-Smith 2010, p. I). Therefore, the care coordinator often acts not only as a therapist, but also as a 'contract manager'.

Often the care coordination process may start when someone is discharged from hospital. It has been recognised that crisis often occurs very soon after hospital discharge (DoH 2012, p. 5). Therefore, another crucial role of the care coordinator is to ensure that a post-discharge appointment is carried out at the earliest possible time (usually within one week) if supporting someone who has just left hospital. Although, this initial contact is vital, as we shall see through the following chapter, it is also deemed essential to continue this ongoing level of contact and support throughout the process. These appointments should be arranged prior to discharge from hospital and are often known as a 'face to face'.

## Care plans

The driving document within care coordination is the care plan (also known as 'care programme approach plan' or 'care and treatment plan'). This document should be a holistic plan which is guided by the client, outlining the support needed to aid them on their Recovery journey.

The plan will take different formats in different locations. In Wales (Welsh Government 2010), there is a set format based on eight areas of a person's life related to Recovery:

- Physical wellbeing
- Finance and money
- Accommodation
- Work and occupation
- Medical and other treatments
- Social, cultural and spiritual
- Education and training
- Caring and parenting relationships.

In other countries, content of care plans will be guided by the employer locally in line with government guidance (DoH 2008). However, Goodwin and Lawton-Smith (2010) summarise generally what may need to be in a care plan:

> The complexity of the role of the care co-ordinator is reflected in the complexity of care plans. A comprehensive care plan will include both mental health needs, including any clinical care, and physical health needs. It should cover daily living skills, daytime activities including employment, education and training, social and family relationships including the needs of carers and families, finances/welfare benefits, and risk behaviour such as self-neglect or misuse of drugs and alcohol. It should also take into account any needs associated with gender, sexuality, ethnicity and spirituality. Having identified all needs, it then sets out the services that will be provided to meet them, such as a day centre or an employment advice service, and what services they might be able to call on when unwell.
>
> (Goodwin & Lawton-Smith 2010, p. 5)

Care plans are legal documents and practitioners should be competent to answer questions on their content (Robdale 2012). In addition to care plans, care coordinators are also required to conduct risk assessments as part of the process.

In all countries and settings, the aim is that the care plan should be an empowering document: written in the first person from the client's point of view and being led by that client's needs and wants.

# The role of occupational therapists in care coordination

Whether or not occupational therapists are working as care coordinators themselves, their work in mental health and other services may lead to encounters with care coordination at some point.

There have been a number of debates on whether occupational therapists should take on generic roles such as care coordination. Although these opinions will be summarised briefly, the purpose of this chapter is not to continue the generic versus specialist debate. This is because it could be argued that this decision is down to the individual occupational therapist personally and it may be dependent on their beliefs, priorities and capacities as to whether they wish this route to be part of their career path.

The chapter does, however, give us an opportunity to consider the experiences of individuals and organisations who have had an occupational therapist as a care coordinator, as well as those of occupational therapist care coordinators themselves. It is hoped that reviewing these experiences in the context of current and future legislation can give us some guidance on how to move forward as a profession within the context of a care coordination culture.

## The generic versus specialist debate

The debates mentioned above have included discussions regarding whether the role of care coordinator dilutes the core skills of an occupational therapist or enhances them. Occupational therapists are not the only professionals questioning the generic nature of care coordination. Nurses (Simpson 2005) as well as social workers (Clifton & Thorley 2014) also feel that they have unique specialist training which risks being diluted in generic work.

Within the field of occupational therapy there appear to be broadly two schools of thought. The first is that occupational therapists have a unique skill and area of expertise, and that this can be jeopardised, and sometimes even negatively affected, by taking on generic roles such as care coordination. The second is that generic roles such as care coordination offer an opportunity to use skills in a new way and contribute to the development of the systems. Many authors, and individual therapists, naturally meet somewhere in between the two.

Culverhouse and Bibby (2008) argue that acting as a care coordinator not only takes up additional time for the professional, but can also be detrimental to the therapeutic relationship because the professional needs to focus on areas of a person's care plan that are not always conducive to a strengths-based approach, e.g. medication management.

Hughes and Parker (2014), however, suggest that occupational therapists as care coordinators can bring additional enhancement to the role by use of specialist techniques within a generic role. Petican and Bryant (2007) build upon the debate by exploring the role of the care coordinator within the context of occupational science theory, and draw upon theories of occupational justice to demonstrate the unique role and duty that occupational therapists have in CMHTs. They suggest that 'in the case of generic working, occupational therapists should create strategies to allow for an occupational focus or abandon it altogether' (p. 144).

Other authors have explored the role within the context of professional identity. Dige (2009) argues that 'professional practitioners with a strong professional identity will be more inclined to collaborate than those with a weaker identity, who will be more likely to cling to a narrow understanding of their own professionalism' (p. 97). This reflects the fact that professional identity can cause anxiety for occupational therapists in particular because the profession can often be misunderstood by the general public. It is understandable that many occupational therapists wish to stay in traditional roles where their identity is clear.

Considering all aspects of the literature it could be thought best to respect both schools of thought. Arguably, as a profession we need both types of practitioner: those sticking to 'core' work and deepening the knowledge base in traditional roles as well as practitioners widening the scope of the profession by exploring new roles and opportunities. Both of these areas can be seen to support the profession, and more importantly the experience of the client.

It may therefore be suggested that employers of care coordinators have a role to play in this area. Typically, CMHTs continue to employ one or two occupational therapists in the team and the care coordinator role is then shared out amongst all team members. If jobs were to be advertised as 'care coordinator', open to any relevant professional, then there would be the option for occupational therapists (and other professionals) to choose which route they wish to follow, rather than feeling as if care coordination is something that has been forced upon them.

Occupational therapists can, and do, make excellent care coordinators. However, they are only likely to be successful if they are comfortable in the role. Therefore, occupational therapists working in either way should be respected for the decision they have taken and encouraged to work to their optimum in the area they feel is right for them. For this reason, it is important to look beyond the literature and consider the opinions of those occupational therapists who are linked with care coordination roles.

## Occupational therapists' experiences as care coordinators

As mentioned, it is inevitable that the experience of care coordination will vary for individual therapists depending on their background, their style of working, the stage of their career, and their practice setting. In theory, a care coordination role should be allocated to the person who is most suitable, i.e. someone who is already involved with the client, or has a suitable skill set. Professionals may also be called upon to use skills unique to their profession in addition to their care coordinator roles.

One senior occupational therapist working in a community mental health setting commented that the allocated headings for the Welsh template for care and treatment plans resonate clearly with key areas which are covered in occupational therapy. She felt that using the care and treatment plan merely boiled down to using a different format to record much of the work they were already doing with clients. She used the care plan in addition to her own assessments and interventions and found that the plan could be kept consistent within both sets of documentation.

Another occupational therapist agrees that care coordination is an opportunity to 'show people how occupational therapists are so well suited to undertake this role'. She expands on this by saying that with the changing job market many more occupational therapists are working in the community. She states that 'learning about care coordination at university is so important. Particular skills are needed when you first come into this job, such as how to prioritise and manage your time, assessing and managing risk, understanding the therapeutic use of self and being an independent practitioner'.

Other occupational therapists, however, have found that the administrative tasks associated with being a care coordinator can be burdensome. One personality disorder specialist commented that:

> Care coordination can be seen as a largely administrative role. It involves ensuring that the needs identified by an assessment (which need not have been done by the care coordinator) are met with a care plan that identifies who takes responsibility for the different interventions. A risk assessment and crisis plan need to be

completed and it could be argued that much of this is done to show that it has been done, rather than any therapeutic benefit is produced. I often felt that the documentation was something that had to be 'got out of the way' before the real work could be done.

The mixture of opinions above demonstrates how individuals as well as their settings, and possibly even their countries of operation, can influence their experience of care coordination.

In addition, because services are increasingly 'contracted out', the care coordinator role can often involve coordinating other service provision. This could be seen to offer an opportunity to make contact with other organisations and groups, e.g. supported housing and third sector organisations, that might not necessarily be encountered through a purely occupational therapy role. In another sense, however, it could be seen as a move away from the therapeutic work and more towards contract management and bureaucratic processes.

## The referral agencies' perspective

Although care plans usually originate in health and social care, they aim to promote integrated working by ensuring that there is one guiding document relating to all the other agencies and services with which people are involved during their journey of recovery. This includes groups, agencies and services across a range of sectors.

Often if agencies or services are being 'commissioned' to support somebody they will wish to see copies of the care plan and risk assessment before carrying out their own assessments or work. Services may wish to know on which exact aim or goal in a person's plan they are being requested to work. A clear care plan would be essential for these services as it dictates the work they are expected to carry out.

Often service providers have a very different relationship to service users than that of care coordinators – particularly in housing settings where support staff spend a large amount of time with service users. As a consequence, they often, though unintentionally, become informal advocates for the service user and may get to know the client a lot better than the care coordinator does. For this reason their views on care coordination make up an important part of the picture. See Box 1.1 for an illustrative case study.

### Box 1.1: First case study

A housing association has a scheme to support tenants experiencing mental ill health. Tenants who are deemed to have additional support needs with regards to their mental health live in accommodation which has 24-hour support from staff. The aim is to support them to manage their tenancy, with a view to moving on to more permanent accommodation. All of their referrals come from the statutory sector and all potential tenants must have a care plan and associated risk assessment. In this way the housing association is contracted to carry out a specific part of a person's care plan. The housing association will also have their own assessments, plans and evaluations which they use with tenants, with their main focus being on supporting a person to maintain his/her tenancy. As a service, the staff provide support with activities of daily living, socialisation, confidence building and 'move-on'.

## Experiences of care coordinators

Housing association staff are used to working with care coordinators from a range of professional backgrounds. Such staff state that the most important difference that they notice between individual care coordinators is how involved each one is with a person's ongoing support. Some care coordinators visit regularly and involve other staff in care plan review meetings. Others are rarely seen. This has a particular impact when guidance is needed. For example, in some instances where they feel a client is becoming unsafe or in a situation that makes other tenants unsafe, it is often the case that the care coordinator will be 'called in' to assess the situation.

Staff describe how, in some cases, they get the impression that once a person is engaged with them, the care coordinator moves the client's file to the bottom of a pile; this coordinator then seems to forget about the particular client who is perceived as being in a 'safe' place. In these instances, other professionals say they feel as if they have to become the care coordinators themselves, pushing for the client to be able to access the things that he/she wants and needs. Or in some cases, when they feel the client is ready to move on to accommodation that gives them more independence, they are having to prompt the care coordinator to action this.

## Experience of care plans

Staff outside the CMHT also state that they notice a difference in the way care plans are written. They feel that it is useful when a care plan is broken down into component parts and goals and they can have an overview of what other services are carrying out. This makes it easier to ensure they are working on the area they are meant to, and not overlapping or conflicting with any other services. Staff also stated that clear information about the client as a person and their preferences, needs and also their relapse indicators, is very useful.

Staff did also state, however, that sometimes the care plans themselves can prove to be a barrier to progressing. This is because staff feel they cannot initiate certain actions until they have been 'approved' by the care coordinator and written into the care plan. For a team of staff who get to know a client well and may have conversations with them regularly about their hopes and aspirations this may well prove to be frustrating. For this reason, staff felt that care plans outlining goals that were not 'set in stone' and were open and flexible were far more useful as working documents. They said that they also had feedback from clients that they did not worry about 'failing' or not reaching goals if the goals were more flexible and broad – for instance, statements about their aspirations, strengths and preferred future, rather than set goals that they feel under pressure to achieve.

## Experiences of different professions

When asked about different professionals being care coordinators, many staff answered that it was more about the care coordinator as an individual rather than their professional background. They did, however, state that they have observed the following trends between the professions they encountered:

> With regard to community psychiatric nurses, staff felt that the main difference was that they were able to come and administer medication such as depot injections in the home environment if needed. This made it easier if service users were finding it difficult to get out and about for any reason. They also felt that nurses were able to advise on medication and side effects.

> With regard to social workers, staff stated that they noticed that there was often an understanding of benefit entitlements and legal rights. However, more often than not, the client was advised to contact neutral welfare rights advice services anyway. Staff also felt that social workers were more able to support where there were issues around safeguarding.

> With regard to occupational therapists, staff stated that they often noticed that the specific goals were broken down and the focus was often more in line with their own work as a staff team, e.g. community exposure, life skills. They felt that the occupational therapists that they did encounter as care coordinators tended to take an interest in their opinions on how clients were functioning. They did highlight, however, that they did not encounter many occupational therapists as care coordinators.

The case study in Box 1.1 can be shown to highlight the important skill set that is needed to be a care coordinator, perhaps supporting the previously stated opinion that the care coordination role should be taught at university level. As an essential skill of some occupational therapists is that of checking the safety and effectiveness of equipment, perhaps another essential skill is also ensuring that the service which people use, in order to engage in their chosen occupations, is safe and effective (as is done through the care coordination role). The exploration of different professions suggests that occupational therapists are not always commonly associated with the care coordinator role, but that where they are, their skills around occupational analysis and setting meaningful goals are useful for partner organisations.

# The service users' perspective

The care coordination process aims to put the client at the centre of his/her own care, and service users' experiences should be at the forefront when considering developments within the area. These views may include opinions on whether or not occupational therapists give added value to the care coordination role. For 'from a service user's point of view it does not seem to matter necessarily what professional background the person comes from, but more important is the level of rapport with that professional' (Robdale 2012, p. 57).

Gould (2012) carried out a study aiming to capture the views of service users regarding the care programme approach. A combination of questionnaires and focus groups was used and it was found that:

> **All respondents wanted a focus on whole-person (holistic) approaches, not on medication alone. They mentioned support with everyday life issues, access to a wide range of therapies and remedies, befriending schemes, support from other service users and self-management approaches, for example.**
>
> (Gould 2012, p. 9)

This shows that occupational issues and self-management can be a clear priority for people using the CPA. In addition, 'this research clearly shows that a system which too often defines people by their diagnosis and medication finds it difficult to recognise the whole person and the unique individual' (Gould 2012, p. 4). Therefore, although people may not necessarily specify from which profession they would like their care coordinator to be, they do show a desire to be treated in a way that sees them beyond their illness.

The case study in Box 1.2 talks through a client's varying experiences of care coordination from different people in different geographical areas and settings and how occupational therapy interacted with this process. It is outlined in her own words (below) and then drawn upon for discussion in the next section of this chapter. It is felt pertinent to draw the perspectives of this chapter together using the words of the service user themselves.

## Box 1.2: Second case study

Having experienced about five care coordinators, I shall at certain times, contrast the most effective (A) with the downright detrimental (Z).

### Active participation

Although any care coordinator (within their remit) can offer the following, an occupational therapist is an asset to the care coordination process as their skills can be used as follows to strengthen both client confidence (in the community setting) and therapeutic relationship.

Care coordinator A greatly increased my independence by taking the time/initiative to offer support with the following and luckily when she was not available, my occupational therapist took the lead:

- Taking me out for lunch when I was too unwell to cook for myself and was having a hard time coping with eating out.

- Bringing me sandwiches (she even asked my favourite) when too unwell to leave the house. As I had an eating disorder this prevented my weight from dropping, kept me at university and negated the need for return to hospital.

- Meeting me after my therapy sessions for a calming pot of tea. I had no family nearby so this enabled me to better cope with the acute anxiety (side effect of psychotherapy).

## Coordination

My occupational therapist's knowledge of multiple mental health conditions, coupled with her broad expertise in rehabilitation enhanced the tasks and produced greater results when combined with the support of the social worker (care coordinator A) who was coordinating the process. They worked closely together meaning that neither duplicated any task. Instead, they drew up a comprehensive care plan encompassing goals for each area of my life. In this way I felt less demoralised as they were more like a source of coaching and support than therapists.

Where a skill set was missing (such as with Obsessive Compulsive Disorder (OCD) making kitchen work unbearable), they allocated an hour a week to supporting me with this. The occupational therapist would predominate here, then meet the social worker later that week to discuss with her, then with myself, how I felt it was going and to problem solve further. I feel it helped that they were based within the same building as each other. It felt like a seamless, effortless manner of efficiency and it worked excellently.

My care coordinator shared my case so closely (having obtained my permission) with my occupational therapist that if one were unavailable the other booked me in. Again, an excellent strategy for care coordination and the perfect example of good practice in my lay view.

## Drawing on client's passions and strengths and getting to know the whole person

Care coordinator A would engage me in a discussion about my passions which included photography and volunteering my time to support others in their own mental health recovery. This led to my gaining a degree when I would otherwise have been too unwell to attend university.

Care coordinator Z considered this a waste of time, something to be held onto for the future when I became well enough to pursue these things. She simply had no time and did not bother getting to know me as a person. As a result, she saw a cluster of symptoms and felt overwhelmed. She allowed me to drop activity after activity offering no encouragement or support in continuing my passions. As a result, my world shrank as my illness expanded proportionately.

Care coordinator A meanwhile, learned all she could about me and shared common interests. This meant we learned to like one another, it broke the ice (which had been frozen solid by a previous CMHT) and strengthened my trust so that by our third or fourth session we could commence very difficult tasks such as cooking. The occupational therapist followed her lead and when conducting exposure for OCD I would get so caught up in our discussions about an exciting life ahead that I would forget to be so afraid. In time I managed to do things previously unthinkable because the conversations had enabled me to try them on numerous occasions and get through okay. This is not the conventional way of conducting exposure work (usually you must feel the anxiety) but it worked for me. This brings us to a final element of well initiated care coordination:

## Individualised care plans

Care coordinator A found out not just what was wrong with me, but focused more on what my goals were, what I loved and how my illness prevented me from achieving these aims. She broke each goal down into a therapeutic one which inspired me to tackle the painful treatment tasks, because they were made personalised and meaningful.

The plan and its content was discussed with me, written by the care coordinator then reviewed and signed by myself. It was then reviewed at regular intervals. It was assessed together on monthly intervals or more frequently where increased input required.

In contrast, care coordinator Z felt 'overwhelmed and at a loss as to how to help' so she asked me to write my own care plan and she would sign it. I was too unwell to do this but fought my way through without support, making myself more unwell. Care coordinator Z did not amend the plan or sign it and I went 12 months without a copy, without any therapy at all, until one by one my activities were dropped and I was unable to leave the house alone.

## Summary

From my experiences, I feel that the five Cs for care coordinators should include:

- Communication
- Care
- Coordination
- Commitment
- Compassion.

# Discussion

We have seen that care coordination is embedded in policy and that occupational therapists working in mental health in a range of settings may need to work alongside care coordinators or become care coordinators themselves. As services become increasingly integrated it is also likely that physical health fields will need to have an increased understanding of the systems used in mental health settings. So maybe the question is: how can we best link occupational therapy into the systems of care coordination?

Increasingly, occupational therapists may be termed to be 'providers' as part of a person's care and treatment plan. This can be through CMHTs, but as occupational therapists move into more and more diverse settings, it may also be through work in the private, housing or third sector. Our client case study has shown us that even if occupational therapists are not care coordinators themselves, in order to act effectively within this system they need to have a good knowledge of the process and be prepared to be actively engaged in it.

## Capturing the value of occupation

Shifts towards prudent healthcare mean that therapists need to demonstrate that what they are doing is cost-effective, and that they are making the minimum intervention possible to produce the maximum health benefits. Occupational therapists are increasingly likely to find themselves having to demonstrate their value. In order for this value to be seen, they may need to demonstrate that the need for occupational fulfilment is there in the first place as a route to Recovery. As care plans hold so much information about how people are 'doing' things in order to aid their Recovery, such plans (written by a range of professionals) may be useful as a tool to demonstrate that occupation influences health and wellbeing. One advantage of the care programme approach is that it can easily be audited in order to determine local health needs – arguably many of these health needs will be occupationally-focused.

If occupational therapists want to influence the future development of the CPA, then they need to be involved. This may mean ensuring that the importance of occupations themselves is recognised on key/core documentation that is shared with a number of agencies. This could be achieved through writing care plans themselves, or by being closely involved in them (as was the occupational therapist in the client case study). Although this could lead to a short-term focus on the importance of occupations, rather than occupational therapy, it may be hoped that the importance of occupational therapy as an intervention would naturally follow.

## Showing the value of occupation

We have seen from our exploration of the opinions of occupational therapists acting as care coordinators that there can be frustration regarding the role. We have also seen from the client case study that the role of care coordination, carried out correctly, can be successful and can draw upon the natural alliances with occupational therapy. This potentially puts occupational therapists in a good position to contribute to the evidence base of best practice in care coordination, by being used as examples. In the client case study we saw a social worker operating in an occupationally-focused way in partnership with the occupational therapist. Research evidence shows that clients are calling for a more holistic approach to care planning (Gould 2012) which includes physical health and wellbeing. It seems there is potential for occupational therapists to become the 'experts' in holistic, occupation-focused care coordination and to guide the process of transformation of the system.

It is likely that there will be a shift towards personalisation and personal budgets in mental health, as has happened in the physical health field, and the idea of Local Resource Allocation Systems (LRAS) has been proposed (Mind 2009). Currently there is no set way of offering this to service users, and it still leads to confusion amongst service users and professionals. Therefore, the onus is on care coordinators as they have a crucial role in making this happen (Mind 2009). This could be an opportunity for occupational therapists to use their natural skills around empowerment and enablement to lead in this cultural shift: for instance, proposed accredited training for service users in 'how to get a great care and treatment plan'. Occupational therapists could be in a good position to support people to attend, and become facilitators in, this training as part of their Recovery.

Again, audit offers a potentially good opportunity for promotion of occupationally-focused care plans. If people are beginning to have increased say over how their personal budgets are spent, are they choosing to invest in occupationally-focused services? Mind (2015) outlines a list of proposed ways in which clients may wish to spend their budget. Virtually all the ideas on the list are occupational in nature – so if this is anything to go by then the answer is yes!

## Sharing the value of occupation

The importance of occupation in Recovery has the potential to be clearly demonstrated through the use of care plans and the potential use of the personalisation agenda. However, in terms of recognising the importance of occupational therapists in this setting, our challenges may be more varied. The College of Occupational Therapists (2006) has called upon services to challenge the practice of retaining a post for a single discipline when any of a range might be able to fill it. In some ways, within care coordination we have now moved to the other side of the debate. Occupational therapists have been fighting for years to have our skills recognised as equal to other professions. This is now happening through areas such as care coordination, but we are still a minority profession within this area, and many clients and service providers interact more regularly with social workers and nurses. Increasing our visibility through roles such as care coordination may in turn increase understanding of occupations in the communities where work is carried out. On the flip side, there is a risk that occupational therapists could become associated with a care coordination role only.

Through the referral agency case study, we have seen that other professions are valued for the skills that they can bring to care coordination and that, although occupational therapists' skills are valued, they are not so frequently seen by outside agencies and client groups. Occupational therapy could potentially add value to the Recovery of many more people than it does at present. If we are to be an effective multi-disciplinary team, then we may need to share our good ideas that provide value for the client.

If personal budgets become a reality then it is likely that the care coordination role may become more varied: more creativity may be needed in setting up new groups, classes and activities if the client group calls for them and they do not already exist. There is further potential here for occupational therapists to research and promote the value of occupation.

# Conclusion

In this chapter we have explored the many opinions and experiences surrounding care coordination and occupational therapy within a care coordination context. We have seen that the roles can present in a number of ways. However, the prominent theme seems to be that people are calling for a more holistic, and less medically-focused, system of care coordination.

Recent discussions on how the field of physical health can learn from mental health (Gilburt & Peck 2014) could potentially lead to a care coordination model being used in physical health fields. If this were the case then arguably the 'dual' training of occupational therapists puts them in a good position to take the lead in this area.

It has already been acknowledged within the national media that occupational therapists are key in leading the way to transforming healthcare (e.g. *Guardian* 2015). The subsequent challenge will be to ensure that occupational therapists are placed in the roles and settings that best allow them to support this transformation, and, more importantly, are enabled, through occupation-based empowerment, to support their clients to take the lead in making these changes happen.

# Useful resources

- Department of Health (2008). *Refocusing the Care Programme Approach: Policy and Positive Practice Guidance.* London: TSO.
- Welsh Government (2010). *Mental Health Measure* (Wales). Cardiff: Welsh Government.
- Goodwin, N. & Lawton-Smith, S. (2010). Integrating care for people with mental illness: the care programme approach in England and its implications for long-term conditions management. *International Journal of Integrated Care* **10**, http://www.ijic.org (last accessed: 12.1.2016).
- Rethink website: https://www.rethink.org/diagnosis-treatment/treatment-and-support/cpa
- Hafal CPA guide: http://www.hafal.org/pdf/CPA_English.pdf
- Mind (2009). *Personalisation in Mental Health: Breaking Down the Barriers: A Guide for Care Coordinators.* London: Mind. http://www.together-uk.org/wp-content/uploads/downloads/2011/11/putting_us_first_overcoming.pdf

# References

Clifton, J. & Thorley, C. (2014). *Think Ahead: Meeting the Workforce Challenges in Mental Health Social Work.* London: Institute for Public Policy Research.

College of Occupational Therapists (2006). *Recovering Ordinary Lives: The Strategy for Occupational Therapy in Mental Health Services: A Strategy for the Next Ten Years.* London: COT.

Culverhouse, J. & Bibby, P.F. (2008). Occupational therapy and care coordination: the challenges faced by occupational therapists in community mental health settings. *British Journal of Occupational Therapy* **71** (11), 496–498.

Department of Health (1990) *The Care Programme Approach for People with a Mental Illness Referred to the Specialist Psychiatric Services.* London: TSO.

Department of Health (2006). *Reviewing the Care Programme Approach 2006: A Consultation Document.* London: TSO.

Department of Health (2008). *Refocussing the Care Programme Approach: Policy and Positive Practice Guidance.* London: TSO.

Department of Health (2012). *Preventing Suicide in England. A Cross-Government Outcomes strategy to Save Lives.* London: TSO.

Dige, M. (2009). Occupational therapy, professional development and ethics. *Scandinavian Journal of Occupational Therapy* **16** (2), 88–98.

Gilburt, H. & Peck, E. (2014). *Service Transformation Lessons from Mental Health.* London: The King's Fund.

Goodwin, N. & Lawton-Smith, S. (2010). Integrating care for people with mental illness: the care programme approach in England and its implications for long-term conditions management. *International Journal of Integrated Care* **10**, http://www.ijic.org (last accessed: 12.1.2016).

Gould, D. (2012). *Service Users' Experiences of Recovery under the 2008 Care Programme Approach.* London: Mental Health Foundation.

Great Britain. (1990). *The National Health Service and Community Care Act.* London: HMSO.

*Guardian* (2015). 'Punching above their weight': the impact of occupational therapists. *Guardian*, 27 January. http://www.theguardian.com/social-care-network/2015/jan/27/impact-of-occupational-therapists (last accessed: 26.5.2015).

Hughes, S. & Parker, H. (2014). 'Community practice' in *Creek's Occupational Therapy and Mental Health,* eds. W. Bryant, J. Fieldhouse & K. Bannigan, 5th edn. London: Churchill Livingstone Elsevier.

Killaspy, H. (2006). From the asylum to community care: learning from experience. *British Medical Bulletin* **79–80** (1), 245–258.

Lawton-Smith, S. & McCullough, A. (2013). A brief history of specialist mental health services: mental health foundation. *International Journal of Integrated Care* **10**, http://www.ijic.org (last accessed: 12.1.2016).

Mind (2009). *Personalisation in Mental Health: Breaking Down the Barriers: A Guide for Care Coordinators.* London: Mind.

Mind (2015). *Personal budgets for social care.* http://www.mind.org.uk (last accessed 26.5.2015).

Petican, A. & Bryant, W. (2007). Sustaining a focus on occupation in community mental health practice. *British Journal of Occupational Therapy* **70** (4), 140–146.

Robdale, N. (2012). 'Care planning in the community' in *Practical Care Planning for Personalised Mental Health Care,* ed. M. Lloyd. Maidenhead: Open University Press.

Sainsbury Centre for Mental Health (2005). *The Care Programme Approach – Back on Track?* London: Sainsbury Centre for Mental Health.

Simpson, A. (2005). Community psychiatric nurses and the care coordinator role: squeezed to provide limited nursing. *Journal of Advanced Nursing* **52** (6), 689–699.

# Chapter 2

# Occupational therapists and assertive outreach

*Karen Newberry and Claire Terrington*

## Introduction

This chapter outlines the fundamental principles of Assertive Outreach (AO), within the ever changing health and social care landscape, and considers the valuable, yet under-researched contribution occupational therapy can make. Whilst the name given to the work may change, the need for skills in engaging individuals with complex mental health needs, often coupled with chaotic lifestyles, who have struggled to effectively benefit from standard community treatments, remains.

Consideration is given to how the profession's core skills, through an innovative and flexible approach, can be used to meet the needs of referred individuals. A case study illustrates how occupational therapy can both facilitate service engagement and enable achievement of occupational goals. Challenges are not just presented by individuals' complex situations, but by fellow professionals, who can struggle to understand this specialist area of work. Points for reflection are identified; as relatively few occupational therapists currently work in this area, the ability to reflect and self-evaluate is essential to maintain resilience, and to offer a service that is truly to meaningful to the individuals referred.

## Key points

- Engagement in a sound therapeutic relationship is essential prior to commencing any further aspects of occupational therapy. Occupational engagement can be a useful tool within this, however developing this relationship can be exceptionally time consuming and complex.

- It may be necessary to undertake some aspects of activity/occupation for the individual until they are able to undertake the activity/occupation with you, prior to becoming independent. Other professionals may question this labour intensive approach.

- Innovative use of profession-specific skills such as activity analysis, grading and adaptation are subjectively highly valuable, but lack robust evidence for effectiveness with this group of individuals.

- Personal and professional challenges include non-engagement, undertaking assessments that can be used as outcome measures, maintaining professional boundaries, issues of relapse and readmission, complex financial, personal and social situations, supporting someone who repeatedly makes what appear to be unwise lifestyle choices and avoiding over-dependency.

# What is Assertive Outreach?

Assertive Outreach teams, also known as Assertive Community Treatment (ACT) teams, provide a community-based service for individuals with severe and enduring mental health problems. Individuals are typically high users of inpatient care, and have difficulty engaging with mental health services. They receive regular input from the team, which could be daily or at least weekly, and there is a high emphasis on working with individuals' needs and strengths to engage them in a therapeutic relationship. To enable this, caseloads are relatively small, and the case manager has a significant key worker role, which includes many generic psychosocial interventions and involvement in practical tasks, as well as undertaking roles more traditionally associated with the worker's job title. Teams are multi-disciplinary in nature, usually predominantly mental health nurses with a combination of social workers, psychiatrists, psychologists, support workers and occupational therapists. There is a shared team approach alongside case management, hence the individual's needs are, wherever possible, met by the team as opposed to referring on. The assertive outreach service is not time limited; however if an individual's mental health becomes stable and they are able to engage in services, they are gradually transferred to a traditional Community Mental Health Team (CMHT).

The assertive outreach model has been implemented within specific drug and alcohol, learning disability and self-harm teams. Whilst some aspects of this chapter may be helpful in those settings, the focus of this chapter is on individuals with severe and enduring mental illness, the most common diagnoses being psychosis, schizophrenia and bipolar disorder. In assertive outreach, individuals tend to have relatively unstable mental health, are particularly vulnerable and often have chaotic lifestyles. Issues of insecure accommodation, stigma and discrimination, social isolation, self-neglect, financial instability/debt, exploitation from others, reluctance to take medication, use of non-prescribed drugs, lack of insight, family breakdown and poor physical health are commonplace.

# The assertive outreach evidence base

In the UK assertive outreach teams were established from around 1996. A Cochrane review (Marshall & Lockwood 1998) indicated that assertive community treatment was a clinically effective approach, particularly around the reduction of inpatient care and overall costs. Despite the rigorous nature of the Cochrane review, the transferability of the mainly US and Australian-based research into UK healthcare practice has more recently been questioned. Longitudinal studies have compared assertive community treatment with standard CMHTs at 18 months (Killaspy et al. 2006), 36 months (Killaspy et al. 2009) and 10 years (Killaspy et al. 2014). Despite highlighting the success of assertive outreach in engagement, no clinical advantage of assertive community treatment over CMHTs emerged. In the 10-year follow up study, around a third of the assertive community treatment caseload with psychosis had not stabilised enough to move to a CMHT, and a quarter of those originally allocated to a CMHT had transferred to assertive community treatment, questioning what would have happened to these individuals had there not been the option of assertive community treatment. These longitudinal studies highlight several limitations, including being based in a large inner city area; also of note is a lack of clarity on whether occupational therapists were part of the teams involved in the sample.

Resulting from the debate around the effectiveness of assertive outreach, new models of working have been launched, using principles originating from the Netherlands (Bond & Drake 2007, Van-Veldhuizen 2007), broadly referred to as the Flexible Assertive Community Treatment (FACT) model. The assertive outreach function is fulfilled by the standard CMHT, approximately 90 per cent of the caseload receives standard CMHT input and a flexible 10 per cent receive a more intensive assertive outreach style service, using the principles of a shared caseload, high frequency of visits and daily planning to meet diverse needs. The main advantage being advocated is that individuals can move between the two types of service according to need, reducing long and expensive assertive outreach treatment when need is low, the latter being a primary criticism of traditional assertive outreach in the UK (Firn et al. 2013). Again, based on existing FACT studies, it is unclear how occupational therapists are involved. Limitations of the studies, including a lack of UK-based longitudinal research into FACT, continue to raise questions regarding the best way to deliver an effective assertive outreach style of service.

## The role of occupational therapy

As the needs of individuals accessing assertive outreach tend to be complex and multi-faceted, occupational deprivation is a common phenomenon, as is occupational injustice arising from stigma and social exclusion. There is undoubtedly a significant role in assertive outreach services for occupational therapists' skills, both profession-specific and generic.

## Service engagement and occupational engagement

Engagement issues are a common reason for referral to assertive outreach services. Individuals are reluctant to engage in traditional services for various reasons including previous negative experiences, poor mental health, side effects of medication, lack of insight or a fear of hospital admission. Definitions of engagement conceptualise it as attracting someone's interest or attention, and emphasise the desire of the now engaged individual to participate, be involved or connect (Hitch 2009). Two key aspects arise from this: that of the individual being engaged with the assertive outreach service as a whole, and a separate but related concept of occupational engagement. The whole-team approach tasks occupational therapists with both these aspects.

## Box 2.1: Reflection 1

How would *you* feel about engaging in the standard mental health services offered in the locality you live in? Which aspects would promote and which would inhibit your engagement?

Addis and Gamble (2004) suggest how service engagement might be achieved. Five assertive outreach nurses identified the importance of spending time with people, being persistent in returning to visit even when the individual previously declined to see you, and the need for professionalism to be subservient to relating to individuals on an interpersonal level. A caring attitude of working and learning together was additionally identified; this requires a high level of genuineness on the part of the worker. The emphasis of all initial contacts is on service engagement and therapeutic use of self to facilitate the interpersonal relationship. This labour intensive generic engagement can initially feel alien, and can be challenged by occupational therapy colleagues and managers who lack any assertive outreach experience. However, Burns (2004) sees structured and reflective thinking around therapeutic use of self as a strength of occupational therapy within assertive outreach.

Taylor and Melton (2009) provide a valuable underpinning of therapeutic use of self in their Intentional Relationship Model (IRM) which stresses the importance of a deep understanding of the individual's interpersonal skills and preferences, and proactively varying interpersonal responses according to these. As an assertive outreach practitioner this ability to vary therapeutic approach is an essential aspect of engagement.

## Box 2.2: Reflection 2

How flexible are you in your approach to individuals you are working with? Think of examples when you have consciously altered your approach according to the individual's interpersonal preferences.

In addition to the findings of Addis and Gamble (2004), Hitch (2009), from an occupational therapy perspective, advocated the benefits of occupational engagement to facilitate overall assertive outreach service engagement. The IRM (Taylor & Melton 2009) allies the therapeutic relationship and occupational engagement, arguably supporting the notion that enabling people to do the things they want and need to do through occupational engagement can also support the more generic service engagement.

# Engagement moving into active occupational therapy

Many assertive outreach clients have very practical needs; hence the need for the provision of practical resources to be part of service engagement as stressed by Hitch (2009). A pragmatic and flexible approach to the occupational therapy role is essential. Practical needs may revolve around shopping, preparing food, managing bills and doing laundry or cleaning. All are familiar occupations that form the basis of many occupational therapy interventions in wider CMHTs. However, traditionally occupational therapists would not be involved in directly meeting these needs by 'doing for' the individual. Instead, they would focus immediately on promoting independence in occupational performance.

## Box 2.3: Reflection 3

How do you feel about 'doing for' an individual, especially when the task may be time consuming, such as cleaning someone's kitchen, bathroom and toilet and often when they are experiencing significant self-neglect, so the task is not particularly pleasant?

This 'doing for' in assertive outreach can be both a personal challenge and professional challenge; critics of assertive outreach may suggest 'doing for' is both costly and promotes dependency, whereas Hitch (2009) identified that in assertive outreach the structure of occupations being organised for individuals was an important component of engagement. Without such engagement there will be no opportunity to move to the next step of 'doing with' and finally to 'doing independently'. What would appear to be an initial cheaper solution of a generic support worker 'doing for' has two significant concerns for occupational therapy in assertive outreach:

- Most individuals have been offered standard care packages prior to referral to assertive outreach which include being 'done for' by community support workers; however these have usually resulted in disengagement and ultimately relapse. Seminal author Wilcock (1997) identified the need to 'do' is an integral part of human life as occupational beings; if the being 'done for' has no essence of leading to 'doing with' or 'doing independently' it is unsurprising that disengagement occurs.

- Whilst an assertive outreach support worker, rather than an assertive outreach occupational therapist, could 'do for', if the specialist occupational therapy skills of activity analysis, grading, adaptation and occupational goal setting are not being employed to move into 'doing with' and then facilitate 'doing independently', long-term dependency on the assertive outreach support worker to 'do for' could arise. Again this could increase both the risk of disengagement and overall costs. In line with the whole-team approach in assertive outreach, although the interventions may not always be directly delivered by the occupational therapist, it is worth considering whether specialist occupational therapy skills could be utilised by others in the assertive outreach team through supervision and intervention planning by the occupational therapist.

# Assessment

Whilst some informal narrative and observational assessment occurs during the initial engagement process, when and how to commence more structured occupational therapy assessment can be much less clear cut. These initial informal assessment methods have significant advantages, as many individuals have been subjected to numerous, more structured assessments which they may have experienced negatively. Also low concentration and reduced cognitive functioning associated with symptomatology can make more formal paper-based assessments difficult to complete in a meaningful way. A narrative approach enables the individual to take the lead in both pace and what they choose to discuss or share, enabling person-centredness and avoiding potentially problematic paperwork.

These less formal assessment methods also present challenges, such as not providing an objective baseline from which to measure progress in terms of outcome measures. This can be demotivating for the individual and the therapist, particularly as progress can be relatively slow within assertive outreach. With little research on the effectiveness of occupational therapy in assertive outreach, if this is difficult to demonstrate on a local level through outcome measures, then there is little evidence on which to continue commissioning further assertive outreach occupational therapy services at all.

A useful assessment tool that provides such an outcome measure is the Model of Human Occupation Screening Tool (MOHOST) (Parkinson *et al.* 2006). The narrative information and observation obtained by the occupational therapist, alongside information from the rest of the team and any relatives or carers, can be included in this assessment, thus formalising the information initially collected and complementing the concept of the whole-team approach. The MOHOST enables an accurate record of current occupational functioning to be made, and can be repeated at a later date to provide evidence of progress. It is advisable to complete something like a MOHOST early in the engagement process, often at the point of 'doing for' and certainly by the stage of 'doing with', to ensure progress is accurately recorded. Roberts-Jones' (2009) Concise Occupational Assessment, designed to record past, present and future occupational performance and related goals, can also be useful as it is in a format that is easily and quickly completed. Use of this tool is, however, more challenging as an outcome measure and is yet to develop a rigorous evidence base.

Similarly to occupational therapy-specific assessments, whole-team assessments are used to both inform treatment plans and provide outcome measures. One such tool is the Mental Health Recovery Star (MHRS) (MacKeith & Burns 2008), covering 10 dimensions: managing mental health, physical health and self-care, living skills, social networks, work, relationships, addictive behaviour, responsibilities, identity and self-esteem, and trust and hope. Clearly occupational therapy makes a profession-specific contribution in many dimensions such as living skills, work, self-care and social networks, as well as more generic contributions to areas such as self-esteem and managing mental health. The MHRS has advantages of being visual, collaboratively completed with the individual and developed within practice through service user and staff partnership; however, its psychometric properties are still under debate in terms of its appropriateness as an outcome measure (Killaspy et al. 2012).

# Goal setting and treatment planning

Goal setting within assertive outreach requires careful consideration. Whilst some individuals may benefit from a traditional approach of negotiating detailed formal goals, for many a more informal agreement tends to be more successful. Informal frequent reiteration of these goals and discussion around whether they are still priorities is essential as an individual's circumstances can quickly change. The reality of this is that longer-term goals may have to be reprioritised or put on hold, however, it is important to ensure these goals are not lost in the long term.

Occupational therapists have long claimed to be person-centred, especially with regards to goal setting, mirroring the philosophy of the whole assertive outreach team. In addition to this being one of the most professionally rewarding aspects of assertive outreach, helping the individual identify things they really want to do is complex. A range of symptoms impacting on motivation and decision making, paired with lengthy or distressing histories of mental ill health, have often resulted in attempts to do the things individuals want to do being abandoned by the individual or actively discouraged by others. The Recovery model has heightened the awareness of the need for hope for the future and that others may need to be the holders of this hope (Fieldhouse 2008). This is of particular relevance in supporting the individual to rediscover their goals; a sense of optimism as well as realism is essential.

Aspirations are diverse, spanning what could seem relatively inconsequential goals, such as preparing a simple meal, to those some would discount as unrealistic, such as international travel, through to aspirations some would consider outside the realms of mental health service provision, such as going to a nightclub. As an assertive outreach occupational therapist, being non-judgemental is paramount to remaining person-centred, and the importance of being able to actively look for creative solutions cannot be underestimated.

## Box 2.4: Reflection 4

An individual can only identify one goal but it is significantly above their current level of occupational performance. How would you feel about this in relation to client-centred practice, and what aspects of specialist or occupational therapy-specific skills might you be able to use to guide your practice?

## Activity analysis

A detailed analysis of the occupational form of the seemingly unrealistic goal is essential to determine if there is a 'fit' with the individual. Keilhofner and Forsyth (2009) identify activity analysis as finding the 'fit' between the characteristics and needs of the individual and the occupation, to allow them to engage in a new or former occupation. Often the individual's goal is very long-term, and can be broken down into several more achievable short-term goals, where a 'fit' is more apparent.

## Grading and adaptation

A graded approach (Creek & Bullock 2008) to each of the short-term goals is usually essential; again it may begin with some 'doing for' and 'doing with' prior to 'doing independently'. Vygotsky (1978) equates this grading to providing scaffolding; working towards the goal is facilitated by temporarily constructed support. The scaffolding is gradually dismantled as the individual's independence is increased. Fieldhouse (2012) identifies an aspect of this scaffolding as being a travel companion on the recovery journey ('doing with'), rather than a travel agent who would provide information and let the individual go alone. Within this journey there may be a point when the individual reaches their full potential, but the scaffolding support is still required so fairly permanent adaptation of the occupation is needed in terms of finding a new way to achieve the same or similar outcome. Adaptation, for example by the permanent support of a friend, relative, volunteer, or paid support worker, may mean the end goal can be achieved in a slightly different way, but graded introduction of this adapted way of meeting the end goal is likely to be essential.

## Therapeutic risk taking

Risk averse behaviour on the part of traditional services, partnered with real or perceived previous high risk behaviours, has historically led to individuals not being supported to meet their goals. However, due to the more intensive and flexible nature of assertive outreach service delivery, positive therapeutic risk taking can be embraced through a person-centred approach to risk management, while acknowledging that some degree of risk is essential to self-esteem, skill acquisition and most importantly progress (COT 2006). The risk must be assessed and a meaningful plan established with the individual's fullest possible involvement, taking into account their capacity. Many individuals are aware of risks or can be supported to develop an understanding of them, and thus can take an active role. As an occupational therapist the whole-team approach is an important aspect of positive therapeutic risk taking and careful, accurate documentation is required.

## The environment

Occupational therapists in assertive outreach need the ability to efficiently and effectively locate community resources and build relationships with the people in the individual's normal environment, who provide opportunities directly linked to the individual's aspirations. Sustainable opportunities can be secured by aiming for genuine long-term occupational engagement, independent of mental health service provision. Time invested in developing an understanding of the social capital (Cameron *et al.* 2003) within an individual's local community is time well spent. Fieldhouse (2012) identified increased community participation as a significant beneficial outcome of occupational therapy in assertive outreach, and reintegration of the individual into their community to enhance their quality of life is a key aim of assertive outreach services. Resources might include colleges, employment agencies, leisure centres, charities, food banks, physical health clinics, sexual health clinics and faith groups. Locating resources can be challenging; looking at notices in local shops, contacting community faith leaders, getting local community newsletters or asking at places like the local post office or corner shop are helpful additions to scoping via the Internet. Face-to-face or phone approaches are often most successful, with smaller community resources often being willing to share knowledge, especially about other local resources, and to offer significant practical input. Issues of maintaining confidentiality of individuals as they are supported to integrate into community resources require careful consideration, with initial discussions with the individual being of paramount importance.

## Box 2.5: Reflection 5

> Will those staffing the community resource know who you work for? Will you tell them? Will other people using the community resource know by the way you dress (including your diary and badge) that the individual has mental health needs? If you need to ask for a receipt to gain reimbursement from your employer for the cost of your involvement in the community resource, will those running the resource have heightened awareness of your role, and realise the individual has mental health needs? How will you address this with the individual you are working with?

## Maintaining motivation and volition

Maintaining motivation and volition for occupational goals is a significant challenge for individuals accessing assertive outreach services. This may be due to symptomatology, side effects of medication, chaotic lifestyles, and limited social support and encouragement from others. As part of a graded programme, conscious use of external positive reinforcement is valuable – for example the IRM therapeutic modes of encouraging and instructing. By providing verbal positive reinforcement alongside direction, positive elements of occupational performance can be reinforced with an aim of them being repeated (Taylor & Melton 2009). Fieldhouse (2012) extends the concept of providing external motivation to the role of creating an affirming environment in which graded empathetic and non-judgemental support is provided by the occupational therapist until the individual gains independence.

Ultimately it is vital the individual experiences internal reinforcement if they are going to maintain an occupation independently in the longer term. Theoretically if the goal is person-centred, working towards it would usually include gaining some internal reinforcement; however, symptoms or side effects of medication, such as blunting of emotional responses, may negate this. The individual may need active support to develop self-awareness of the pleasure, satisfaction, enjoyment, self-esteem or the many other positively reinforcing feelings associated with goal accomplishment, the aim being that this would lead to long-term motivation to undertake the task again. It is valuable to use backward chaining techniques to ensure that the individual experiences a sense of accomplishment by completing the final and usually most rewarding part of the activity themselves. Aspects of the occupational form leading up to this latter stage may again depend on the occupational therapist 'doing for'.

# Unpicking complex challenges

The reality of working as an occupational therapist in assertive outreach is that complex challenges occur at many levels. Reflecting, gaining support from other assertive outreach team members, clinical supervision from someone who has an understanding of assertive outreach and occupational therapy, and networking with other occupational therapists working in assertive outreach are all good practice. On a personal level, self-management in terms of ensuring a good work–life balance, adhering to the hours you are contracted to, and being proactive in seeking and maintaining the aforementioned support are vital to maintain resilience and avoid burnout.

In many assertive outreach teams there may only be one occupational therapist so gaining appropriate support and supervision from an occupational therapist who understands the nature of the service can be difficult. Also in some services challenges can arise around adhering to wider organisational occupational therapy policies, procedures and areas of custom and practice. Issues highlighted earlier (like 'doing for', undertaking generic tasks, having a less formal approach, not discharging people who miss appointments, and not being able to undertake extensive standardised assessments and outcome measures) can create additional pressures. Many fellow occupational therapists without assertive outreach experience may find it difficult to understand why you are undertaking generic work when you frequently identify the need for more occupational therapists. The lack of an assertive outreach occupational therapy evidence base alongside this means it is common for new assertive outreach occupational therapists to struggle not only to know what to do, but also to cope emotionally with what other often more senior occupational therapists outside the service expect them to do. Some of the issues are now further unpicked.

## Being non-judgemental

Being non-judgemental and remaining open minded is a significant challenge, not least because individuals can repeatedly make unwise lifestyle choices and live in a continual state of chaos. For example, illegal drug taking, alcohol misuse and gambling, resulting in a significant negative impact on money management, social functioning, physical and mental health are not uncommon. It is often essential to be non-judgemental and avoid being directive, in order to maintain engagement and client-centred practice, whilst being mindful of the duty of care to the individual.

## Box 2.6: Reflection 6

An individual repeatedly spends 90 per cent of their income on illicit substances leaving them very little to purchase food and other necessities until they receive their next benefit payment. How do you feel knowing they will be cold and hungry at several points in the week?

# A friendly approach versus friendship

Engagement requires many of the skills associated with forming a friendship. The approach is much more informal than in many settings, and as a result you may share more of your own experiences within assertive outreach than in other services. Often individuals at the point of referral have very little, if any, support from family or friends; hence the assertive outreach team can be perceived by the individual as a surrogate version of this. Indeed, this has great benefits for engagement, but in reality professional boundaries mean you are not a true friend/family member, and once discharged from assertive outreach, contact will cease. This raises the issue of how ethical it is to encourage the individual to believe you are a friend.

## Box 2.7: Reflection 7

Can you think of clients in the past for whom you have been tempted to blur the boundaries of professionalism? What was helpful in this situation?

It is vital to ensure that you maintain professional boundaries; it is useful to self-monitor, using reflection and/or supervision to ensure information you share about yourself is done to meet the individual's needs in terms of initiating or maintaining engagement, not to meet your own needs. You must ensure your own physical and emotional safety in terms of what you share, so a focus on the fact that the approach is friendly but that you are not a friend may seem obvious, but is sometimes helpful to keep in mind.

# Non-engagement

Being faced with an individual's non- or disengagement can lead you to question not only your own skills and abilities, but also your own personality and suitability for the area of work. At points of non-engagement individuals can demonstrate behaviours which can be interpreted as rude, offensive and at times aggressive. Support, reflection and supervision need to focus on the reality of the situation to enable you to make an accurate appraisal of the individual's response to you. Consideration of whether there are aspects of your own performance you could develop, or whether in fact this is the nature of the client group, which is often the case, is essential in order to build your own emotional resilience to such situations.

## Admission/readmission

At points in assertive outreach involvement when an individual has to be admitted to hospital, there is a tendency to experience a high level of emotion. Unhealthy feelings can range from concern about the treatment the individual will receive as an inpatient, through to guilt that you or the assertive outreach team have let the person down, or anger that other aspects of the wider services or family members and friends have let the individual down, resulting in readmission. Guilt and fear may also be associated with the situation if the assertive outreach team's success is measured according to reduction in numbers of hospital admissions. Due to the whole-team approach it is likely that other team members will be experiencing some of these emotions. In some instances this can be supportive, but if team members' feelings differ, this can in itself be challenging.

## Dependency versus discharge

Dependency versus discharge in assertive outreach initiates varied emotions. Often individuals remain on the caseload for some time, engagement that you worked hard to create has been successful, their mental health has stabilised. Potentially the boundary between friendly approach and friend can feel more blurred as on an emotional level you find the person easy to be with and you have spent a significant amount of time with them. Without conscious acknowledgement of these issues, you can unknowingly encourage dependency on the team. Once you do acknowledge this and the decision is made to discharge the individual, it can be an emotional time for both the individual and team members. Fear and anxiety about the individual and their future care without assertive outreach is often experienced, and, ultimately, the less emotionally challenging work that has recently been undertaken with that individual ends, and that client is replaced by a new individual with whom you are starting the challenging work of engagement for the first time.

# Maintaining personal safety

When working in assertive outreach, it is essential to maintain a focus on personal safety. It has already been noted that individuals often make unwise lifestyle choices; hence the environment can pose many risks. For example, if an individual is using illicit substances, it is likely their social networks are built around this. Assertive outreach services usually work extended hours and this also means there are environmental risks associated with certain times of day in some localities. This highlights risks with behaviours associated with drug taking, crime and weapons that require thorough, dynamic risk assessments. The term dynamic is important to take on board; the idea of making a risk assessment that is never updated or doesn't allow for changes in circumstance is a risk in itself.

Some best practice tips for maintaining safety follow. Whilst not exhaustive, they have been found both helpful and practical to achieve.

# Who knows where you are, who you are with and when to expect you back?

There will be local arrangements for storing this information and this should be one of the first things to find out when working in assertive outreach. Most teams will have a signing in and out system and it is usually the administrative staff who monitor this, but you need to be clear what happens prior to or after the hours they have finished. If you are visiting a number of properties, give an estimate of what time you will be at each property and the order in which you are visiting. This will ensure that if you need to be located at any time, the team will have a clear picture of where you should be. If this plan changes, telephone the team and make them aware. You will need to ensure your phone is fully charged and that the team have your mobile number so they can contact you if needed.

## Blending into the community

It is possible that the locality you serve may have many environmental risks, not necessarily related to the referred individual. For this reason, it is important that you blend into the community where possible. Each employer will have a dress code policy which ideally should be followed. However, there may be local agreements that assist in keeping you safe – for example, when working in an area with low socio-economic status, it would be sensible to avoid wearing valuable jewellery, expensive/designer/smarter clothes and carrying an expensive bag to avoid being a target for theft.

## Managing the environment

It is important to be aware of your surroundings and the key message would be to follow your 'gut' instinct. If it doesn't feel safe, then maybe it isn't, and it is certainly not worth taking the risk. There will always be the temptation to carry out a visit regardless of risk with the good intention of meeting an individual's need. However, if you are not safe, you cannot offer a service. It is important to monitor your surroundings and look out for any subtle differences. For example, there may be large groups of young people in some areas during the school holidays undertaking more risky behaviours, or there may be more drug dealers waiting for individuals on days people get paid or collect benefits. It is wise to learn when these events are to assist in completing your risk assessments. Local police are often a good source of information regarding areas of increased risk and most forces should be able to arrange joint visits if you feel your safety is compromised. Find out who your local community police contact is and liaise with them regularly to keep up to date.

## Build links with community members

Individuals such as landlords, the concierge in the block of flats, local shopkeepers, faith leaders, neighbours and in some instances the GP may be aware of both the mental health of the individual you are visiting, and of wider risk factors in the community. The issues mentioned earlier of confidentiality are important to consider, but these contacts can provide you with up to date information to inform your risk assessment, and may often be able to assist in visiting the individual, or at least in accompanying you to the person's front door and waiting for you to return to your car.

## Utilising social media and text updates

Social media can be useful, especially when working in a large city or rural areas. Sites such as Facebook, Twitter or city/county council text update services often have regular updates regarding major events within your area, and coverage of issues such as roadworks, traffic, security alerts and adverse weather conditions.

It is vital that you discuss any concerns you have with your team and that you feel comfortable doing so. It is likely that if you have concerns, someone else will share these, but may be apprehensive about voicing them. Your safety is paramount.

### Box 2.8: Case study – Gino

Gino was proud of his Italian heritage. He had a diagnosis of schizophrenia and had experienced four acute hospital admissions, primarily due to becoming very paranoid, a danger to himself and due to very low body weight. Prior to each admission he had stopped taking his medication and stopped attending appointments with the community mental health nurse. Gino was discharged from his last two admissions with a care package that included a support worker visiting every other day to help motivate him to prepare food. Gino let the support workers in, but refused the practical support for the first 3–4 weeks after discharge, reporting he was eating out. After this, Gino would not answer the door.

At his fifth admission Gino's body weight was dangerously low, and the length of time between admissions was becoming gradually shorter. Gino was referred to assertive outreach and the team agreed that immediate occupational therapy input would be valuable regarding how food shopping and preparation linked to Gino's low body weight. The assertive outreach occupational therapist and mental health nurse began working with Gino every other day, visiting both jointly and separately in an attempt to engage him. Initially Gino reported everything was fine and he was eating, but there was no evidence of food in his flat other than takeaway cartons. Engagement focused on going out for coffee, and it became clear that Gino had a passion for strong espresso, which his grandfather used to drink when he was a child. This led to general discussions around Gino's love of Italian food and the fact that preparing it was part of his previous identity.

Gino quickly started to decline opportunities to go out, occasionally not answering the door. There was no evidence of basic shopping or takeaway food. The occupational therapist or nurse started to call in every day, offering to order and collect pizza takeaway which Gino mainly accepted. The occupational therapist then started to take ingredients to prepare simple Italian meals for Gino ('doing for'). For several weeks he purely watched the food preparation, then gave verbal advice, and gradually started to become involved in some of the preparation ('doing with'). Gino gradually discussed paranoid ideas that any opened or unpackaged food was tampered with overnight.

The occupational therapist discussed progress with the wider team, especially that Gino's concern about food being tampered with was stopping him from moving to 'doing independently'. There was a dilemma around whether supporting Gino to shop just for one meal immediately before he prepared it would collude with Gino's fears that food was tampered with overnight. However, the team agreed this may enable him in the longer term to be 'doing independently'. Gradually, with encouragement, Gino would agree to store basic items like dried herbs and then pasta in the kitchen overnight. Although Gino developed a method of sealing food in several bags so he could be sure it hadn't been tampered with, he was able to move to cooking independently and remained engaged with the team.

# The future of assertive outreach services

Flexible assertive community treatment is currently advocated as the way forward for assertive outreach services within the UK. Despite its limited evidence base, many believe that as CMHTs have adopted more of a Recovery orientated approach, the need for assertive outreach services will over time continue to decline, as mainstream services improve their acceptability. The National Institute for Health and Care Excellence (NICE) guideline *Psychosis and Schizophrenia in Adults: Prevention and Management* (NICE 2014) continues to emphasise the need for engagement. It also identifies that whilst Early Intervention in Psychosis (EIP) services deliver evidence-based interventions with high levels of engagement, for people experiencing a first episode of psychosis, these gains are diminished once individuals are transferred to primary care or CMHTs. It could thus be interpreted that whilst CMHTs provide an appropriate service for some individuals with psychosis, others, upon leaving EIP teams, still require a more specialist service, with a focus on, amongst other things, engagement. This raises the question of whether historically these individuals would have been successfully transferred to an assertive outreach-specific team (showing many similarities in service delivery to EIP teams), rather than being transferred to CMHTs with a FACT component. The NICE guidelines advocate one potential answer could be to replicate successful elements of EIP services into mainstream services, not dissimilar to the concept of FACT. Another solution could be to consider a trial to re-establish dedicated assertive outreach teams. A strict set of referral criteria would be essential, for example being limited to (a) individuals leaving EIP who have not engaged with the FACT aspect of CMHTs or the CMHT as a whole, and (b) individuals who need the constant continual support of the FACT component of CMHTs, who never successfully transition between the FACT level of support and the less intensive CMHT support. A rigorous research project would be required to identify the subtle differences between each of these models of service delivery.

To conclude, it is evident that individuals will for the foreseeable future have needs that require assertive outreach type services, and that within these needs, occupational therapy has a significant contribution to make. It is imperative that, as part of all models of assertive outreach service delivery, occupational therapists begin to generate profession-specific evidence to determine the success or otherwise of occupational therapy-specific involvement, as well as generating whole-team evidence to either support or refute the model of assertive outreach delivery being used. If you have a passion for working with this group of individuals in the future, a passion for research into this area is a necessity that can't be ignored.

# Useful resources

- National Forum for Assertive Outreach, www.nfao.org
- Parkinson, S., Forsyth, K. & Kielhofner, G. (2006). *The Model of Human Occupation Screening Tool (MOHOST) version 4.0.* Chicago, IL: The Model of Human Occupation Clearing House.
- Taylor, R. & Melton, J. (2009). 'Therapeutic use of self: a model of intentional relationship' in *Skills for Practice in Occupational Therapy,* ed. E.A.S. Duncan. London: Churchill Livingstone.
- Taylor, R.R. (2008). 'Knowing ourselves as therapists: introducing the therapeutic modes' in *The Intentional Relationship: Occupational Therapy and Use of Self,* ed. R.R. Taylor. Philadelphia: F A Davis Company.

# References

Addis, J. & Gamble, C. (2004). Assertive outreach nurses' experience of engagement. J*ournal of Psychiatric and Mental Health Nursing* **11** (4), 452–460.

Bond, G.R. & Drake, R.E. (2007). Should we adopt the Dutch version of ACT? Commentary on 'FACT: a Dutch version of ACT'. *Community Mental Health Journal* **43** (4), 435–438.

Burns, T. (2004). *Community Mental Health Teams, a Guide to Current Practice.* Oxford: Oxford University Press.

Cameron, M., Edmans, T., Greatley, A. & Morris, D. (2003). Community renewal and mental health: strengthening the links. London: Kings Fund.

College of Occupational Therapists (2006). *Recovering Ordinary Lives: the Strategy for Occupational Therapy Services 2007–2017, a Vision for the Next Ten Years.* London: COT.

Creek, J. & Bullock, A. (2008). 'Planning and implementation' in *Occupational Therapy in Mental Health*, eds. J. Creek and L. Lougher, 4th edn. Edinburgh: Churchill Livingstone.

Fieldhouse, J. (2008). 'Community mental health' in *Occupational Therapy in Mental Health*, eds. J. Creek and L. Lougher, 4th edn. Edinburgh: Churchill Livingstone.

Fieldhouse, J. (2012). Community participation and recovery for mental health service users: an action research inquiry. *British Journal of Occupational Therapy* **75** (9), 419–428.

Firn, M., Hindhaugh, K., Hubbeling, D., Davies, G., Jones, B. & White, S.J. (2013). A dismantling study of assertive outreach services: comparing activity and outcomes following replacement with the FACT model. *Social Psychiatry and Psychiatric Epidemiology* **48** (6), 997–1003.

Hitch, D. (2009) Experiences of engagement in occupations and assertive outreach services. *British Journal of Occupational Therapy* **72** (11), 482–490.

Keilhofner, G. & Forsyth, K. (2009). 'Activity analysis' in *Skills for Practice in Occupational Therapy,* ed. E.A.S. Duncan. London: Churchill Livingstone.

Killaspy, H., Kingett, S., Bebbington, P., Blizard, R., Johnson, S., Nolan, F., Pilling, S. & King, M. (2006). The REACT study: randomised evaluation of assertive community treatment in north London. *British Medical Journal* 332, 815–820.

Killaspy, H., Kingett, S., Bebbington, P., Blizard, R., Johnson, S., Nolan, F., Pilling, S. & King, M. (2009). Randomised evaluation of assertive community treatment: 3-year outcomes. *British Journal of Psychiatry* 195, 81–82.

Killaspy, H.T., Boardman, J., King, M., Taylor, T., Shepherd, G. & White, S. (2012). The mental health recovery star: great for care planning but not as a routine outcome measure. *The Psychiatrist* **36** (5), 194.

Killaspy, H., Mas-Exposito, L., Marston, L., & King, M. (2014). Ten-year outcomes of participants in the REACT (Randomised Evaluation of Assertive Community Treatment) in north London study. *Biological Medical Central Psychiatry* 14, 296–302.

MacKeith, J. & Burns, S. (2008). *Mental health recovery star.* http://www.mhpf.org.uk (last accessed: 27.4.2015).

Marshall, M. & Lockwood, A. (1998). 'Assertive community treatment for people with severe mental disorders' (Cochrane Review). *The Cochrane Library,* 4.

National Institute for Health and Care Excellence (2014). *Psychosis and Schizophrenia in Adults: Prevention and Management Guideline.* http://www.nice.org.uk (last accessed: 22.10.2015).

Parkinson, S., Forsyth, K. & Kielhofner, G. (2006). *The Model of Human Occupation Screening Tool (MOHOST) version 4.0.* Chicago, IL: The Model of Human Occupation Clearing House.

Roberts-Jones, N. (2009). Development of the Concise Occupational Assessment. *OT News* **17** (9), 36–37.

Taylor, R. & Melton, J. (2009). 'Therapeutic use of self: a model of intentional relationship' in *Skills for Practice in Occupational Therapy*, ed. E.A.S. Duncan. London: Churchill Livingstone.

Van-Veldhuizen, J.R. (2007). FACT: a Dutch version of ACT. *Community Mental Health Journal* **43** (4), 421–433.

Vygotsky, L.S. (1978). *Mind in Society.* Cambridge, MA: Harvard University Press.

Wilcock, A. (1997). The occupational brain: a theory of human nature. *Journal of Occupational Science* **2** (2), 68–72.

# Chapter 3

# Occupational therapists working in a Crisis Home Treatment Team

## Anne-Marie Jerman

## Introduction

Working in Crisis Resolution and Home Treatment (CRHT) as an occupational therapist is fulfilling and rewarding. The CRHT is uniquely positioned between inpatient and outpatient adult mental health services and offers the opportunity to work with people with a wide variety of mental illness during times when they are often acutely unwell. The role is diverse, and an occupational therapist can often bring a much-needed alternative approach to the service. Working as an occupational therapist in a service which is invariably nurse led does, however, bring certain challenges.

## Key points

- The occupational therapy philosophy lends itself to the CRHT approach where being an alternative to inpatient care maintains and maximises independence in a home environment.
- Occupational therapy philosophy is different from other disciplines and therefore an occupational therapist working in the team brings a new perspective.
- A collaborative, multi-disciplinary approach to working allows the person who is unwell a greater resource of treatment.
- Working as an occupational therapist in CRHT poses challenges to usual working hours. Night, weekend and evening work are part of the job.
- CRHT imposes a greater emphasis on knowledge of medication than many other traditional occupational therapy roles.
- Assessment of risk is an integral part of the role. Occupational therapists have many skills which lend themselves to effective risk assessment.

- Occupational therapists' ability to assess function is beneficial when assessing risk in the home environment and can help with facilitating early discharge.
- It is easy to become a generic practitioner and it is important to maintain professional identity within the role and consider where occupational therapy specific skills can be used.

# What is crisis resolution and home treatment?

A CRHT service comprises a team of mental health clinicians who predominantly work with acutely and seriously ill people with the aim of expediting recovery and maximising quality of life. There are many aspects of the role. The four main responsibilities of CRHT are:

- To provide urgent assessments for people who are at risk of hospital admission
- To provide an alternative to inpatient care by providing treatment in the home
- To facilitate early discharge from hospital
- To act as 'gatekeeper' for acute hospital beds.

The CRHT service works with people who present with a vast range of mental illnesses, including psychotic illness, depression, bipolar affective disorder, personality disorder and anxiety. People often have comorbid alcohol and substance misuse. In addition to this the CRHT occasionally offers brief support for people who do not have psychological distress which is usually secondary to life stressors.

Risk assessment is a key part of CRHT work and team members need to be able to conduct sophisticated risk assessments in a range of clinical settings. The risk of deliberate self-harm, including suicide, is usually of paramount concern. However, the risk of harm to and from others, the risk of accidental self-harm and neglect, the risk of vulnerability, and the risk of significant deterioration of a person's health are also considered.

Invariably most team members are registered mental health nurses supported by healthcare support workers. Most CRHTs do not have an occupational therapist. Crisis resolution and home treatment teams usually have medical input from a psychiatrist and work closely with on-call junior doctors. The hours of work vary, with some CRHTs working 24 hours a day and others working from about 9am until midnight.

## Assessment

The CRHT team is responsible for assessing people who urgently present to mental health services. Referrals may come from a variety of different sources including emergency departments, general practitioners, community mental health teams and, in some areas, direct patient referrals. As part of an assessment a detailed history is taken, a mental state examination is conducted, and a person's previous history and collateral history from relatives is considered. A thorough assessment is essential in order to assess risk and safely plan any further intervention. The possible outcomes following assessment are: admission to hospital, home treatment by CRHT, referral for psychological intervention, referral to substance misuse services or discharge to primary care. There are also many other third sector agencies which CRHT can signpost onto.

## Home treatment

Home treatment is a way of providing intensive care for people in their own home. It provides an alternative to hospital admission and enables people to maintain independence in their own environment. Sometimes people are seen up to four times daily at home and the CRHT role includes monitoring the person's mental health, risk, compliance with medication and response to treatment.

## Facilitating early discharge

The role of CRHT does not end in the event that a person is admitted to hospital. Close liaison with the acute ward takes place to ensure that people do not remain in hospital for any longer than is necessary. Each person admitted to hospital is assessed the following day and quite often they can then be discharged with CRHT support in their home environment. The highest risk of suicide is in the first two weeks post discharge from hospital (Wise 2014). According to research by Manchester's national confidential inquiry into suicide and homicide by people with mental illness (Wise 2014), approximately 3,225 people died by suicide in the UK in the first three months of their discharge from hospital; this was 18 per cent of all suicides from 2002 to 2012; short admissions especially require careful and effective care planning. CRHT is part of this planning process and often involved in the admission of the person; therefore a good assessment of changes in risk can be carried out. Occupational therapy lends itself well to assessing function and risk within the home; often motivation and goal planning can give a better understanding of risk. Taking a holistic approach to the person and the risk is a key part of occupational therapy philosophy. Assessing a person when they are talking about something meaningful to them gives a good insight into protective factors in order to better assess risk.

## Gatekeeping to mental health acute beds

The CRHT team is responsible for coordinating all admissions to hospital. Often there is a high demand for hospital beds for people who cannot be home treated and this role demands excellent communication and organising skills. In some teams the CRHT chairs a twice daily telephone conference with all wards and relevant teams or services. This ensures that priority is given to the people who are at greater need of admission. There is a great strain on beds in mental health acute hospitals at present. A survey conducted by the Commission on Acute Adult Psychiatric Care (2015) reported that 91 per cent of the wards they surveyed were operating above the recommended level. Facilitating early discharge is an imperative in creating beds for those most in need. People needing an admission may be informal or detained formally under the Mental Health Act (UK Parliament 1983/2007).

# What an occupational therapist brings to CRHT

A considerable proportion of my CRHT role is not what would be considered core occupational therapy work and is often generic work, which would otherwise typically be carried out by a nurse. However, as an occupational therapist I bring a different skill set, a different philosophy and a different approach to the role. As an occupational therapist I am more likely to take both a holistic and person-centred approach, along with a core philosophy of doing 'with' a person, rather than doing 'to' a person. Occupational therapists are excellent at seeking out strengths, and this is highly useful at a time when people are very unwell. The philosophy of occupational therapy promotes enablement and independence in the person's own home and is ideally suited to CRHT. As an occupational therapist, I explore a person's core values and beliefs in order to motivate and engage. This can facilitate independence and promote wellbeing.

## Assessment

As an occupational therapist I assess holistically and evaluate each part of a person's life including the key domains of: self-care, productivity and leisure (Townsend & Polatajko 2007). Additionally, I need to explore the person's roles, relationships and home environment. No person or assessment is the same and the ability to be flexible and resourceful is imperative. Core occupational therapy domains which are commonly explored include: sequencing, hygiene, sleep, mobility, road safety, cooking, feeding and nutrition (Bryant et al. 2014).

Functional impairment is often present when a person's mental health deteriorates. Assessing the degree of this impairment provides invaluable information and is often relevant when considering whether someone is suitable for home treatment or requires admission. As an occupational therapist I am more inclined to investigate the person's functional impairment in detail, and a good assessment of a person's functional status can frequently highlight areas of risk including vulnerability, self-neglect and accidental self-harm.

Although most of my work is fast paced there is occasionally a need to use standardised occupational therapy assessments including the Occupational Circumstances Assessment Interview and Rating Scale (OCAIRS) (Forsyth et al. 2005), Canadian Occupational Performance Measure (COPM) (Townsend & Polatajko 2007), Client-centred Community Occupational Performance Initial Interview (CCOPII) (Orford 1995) and other Model of Human Occupation (MOHO) assessments – most commonly the Interest Checklist (Heaseman & Salhotra 2008). Significantly as an occupational therapist I can bring much more to CRHT than only assessing functional ability; my approach to an assessment is different to that of a nurse or a doctor. Some people are more inclined to engage with less 'medical' professionals; by using various strategies I can sometimes engage with a person who would not suit the more medical approach of my colleagues. This highlights how different professionals bring different strengths and skills, and a truly multi-disciplinary approach is much more likely to inform an accurate picture of a person, secure engagement, and thereby make an expedited recovery more likely.

# Intervention

Occupational therapy interventions within CRHT are as diverse as the person with whom we are working and are certainly not prescriptive. There are numerous interventions which an occupational therapist is particularly suited to, and we can often provide different and sometimes more specialist input than other multi-disciplinary colleagues. Occupational therapy promotes independence in all parts of intervention, putting the person at the centre of the treatment.

## Psychoeducation

This consists of providing information and educating a person about their condition. People often present to CRHT during their first episode of illness and this is particularly important in these circumstances. Providing information and knowledge empowers the individual, giving more independence and responsibility to the person.

## Goal setting

During an acute illness or a period of despair even simple tasks can seem unachievable, particularly given that motivation is often impaired. The setting and reaching of realistic and achievable goals provides a sense of accomplishment which in itself aids motivation. Goal setting often involves short-, medium- and long-term goals. Accomplishing small and achievable short-term goals can often be the first step towards achieving long-term goals. Whilst on the CRHT team's caseload, people often live on a day-by-day or hour-by-hour basis. Goal setting is a useful tool in this instance.

## Environmental adaptation

A person's home or personal environment is often a significant factor in their presentation or a barrier to their recovery. Addressing such issues is key and this is one area where more traditional occupational therapy intervention is particularly useful. For example, sometimes an occupational therapist in a CRHT team needs to consider providing aids and adaptations for the person's home. Additionally, if a person becomes aware of the impact that environment (either positive or negative) has on their illness, this provides an opportunity for making change. As occupational therapists are 'dual trained' it is evident that we can liaise well with and refer on to the right service. Often joint assessments can be carried out or correct short-term equipment can be assessed and distributed directly from CRHT.

## Roles and responsibility

Excess pressure and expectation can be both precipitating and perpetuating factors for someone's ill health. Occupational therapy is the ideal discipline to explore the person's roles and responsibilities, and, together with the person, consider what could be done to reduce the pressure they are under. Equally, there are people who lack meaningful roles or responsibilities; this can frequently contribute to a person's core negative beliefs, and an occupational therapist can help them explore what roles and responsibilities they would like to develop.

## Graded practice

This is particularly useful when a person has severe anxiety. Some people have social anxiety and others have specific phobias. Collaboratively devising a plan for gradual exposure and a gradual increase in activity can be invaluable, and offers a complementary approach to other intervention such as medication.

## Health promotion

This intervention is providing information, advice and signposting to encourage the person to make informed choices about health and lifestyle choices such as smoking, exercise, diet and stress management.

## Volitional support

Supporting a person in this area can aid recovery. If a person can develop meaningful interests and activities they are more likely to maintain remission of illness and less likely to engage in substance or alcohol misuse.

## Coping strategies

Supporting a person to identify and utilise coping strategies when they are in an acute crisis can be an invaluable intervention. Anything that a person can instigate themselves immediately, before services can assist them, can often make the difference between whether or not the person self-harms or attempts suicide. A practical coping strategy implemented with the assistance of the occupational therapist can be used daily to maintain wellness.

## Crisis and contingency

Collaboratively identifying a person's relapse indicators and early warning signs means that any future relapse can be identified and addressed promptly. In turn, early intervention means that the person is less likely to become seriously unwell and is more likely to be able to remain in the community as a functioning individual.

# Challenges faced

There are challenges whilst working as a lone occupational therapist in a predominantly nurse-led CRHT. There is a misconception that I'm a 'nurse who can't give meds'.

## Risk assessment

Many professions can carry out risk assessment effectively. It may not be a key part of the graduate occupational therapist's tool bag, and it was something that I saw as the biggest challenge when I started working in this area. However, I quickly learned that occupational therapy skills lend themselves to assessing risk: occupational therapists work 'with' not 'to' a person being assessed to ensure safety, working collaboratively, using a person's strengths as a way to promote personal responsibility. A holistic approach allows us to see a bigger picture and highlight safety measures such as distraction and other coping strategies. Specific people or places which are positive influences or triggers to the person can be easily identified if the correct questions are asked. The person's functionality with activities of daily living is a good indicator of whether they are currently coping and what risks are present.

## Medication

A good knowledge of medication such as antidepressants, neuroleptics and anxiolytics is important for CRHT clinicians. Occupational therapists generally don't graduate with a comprehensive working knowledge of these, but with a little reading and experience an understanding and appreciation is quickly acquired in order to allay fears about medications and be equipped to give information on how to take them and what side effects may be encountered. Crisis resolution and home treatment team clinicians monitor side effects of medications, especially during titration stages, which are often carried out in the community with CRHT.

Medication concordance is another area for CRHT – to maintain wellness and independence at home and to prevent hospital admission. Whilst never 'administering' medication I would collect it and provide information, advice and give reassurance about taking it. I feel this is an essential part of the role, but not an occupational therapy-specific skill. This leads to my colleagues' misconception of me as 'a nurse who can't give meds' – which is very frustrating.

Alcohol withdrawal is an aspect of the work which occupational therapists may well be required to know about; hospital staff may seek knowledge or reassurance about the use of the Clinical Institute Withdrawal Assessment for Alcohol (CIWA) (MDCalc 2016). It is important for occupational therapists to know about drug and alcohol services and to have strong working links with them.

There is misunderstanding from some about the role of a mental health occupational therapist: many colleagues assume that occupational therapists offer functional support only. Education of other clinicians is important. Volunteering to speak at any team days, one to one informal discussions about what the occupational therapist can offer, using a personal development review as an opportunity to focus on ways to promote full understanding of the occupational therapist's role are all ways of addressing this. As occupational therapists are dual trained in mental and physical health, we can offer assessments and interventions in both areas, as well as make ideal practitioners where there is a need to understand the interaction between physical and mental health.

## Time management

Limited time resources present another challenge. If one member of the team makes the initial assessment, it may not be them who then carries out the intervention in the care plan. This is due to shift work. It is difficult to pass on pieces of intervention to non-occupational therapists when the intervention requires specific occupational therapy knowledge and skills.

## Intensity of illness

People are typically acutely and seriously unwell when they are referred to CRHT at the crisis point of their illness and possibly also not ready to engage in long-term intervention. Time for rapport building is limited and so must be used skilfully to gain rapport. Concentration is difficult for people when affected by acute episodes of depression, psychosis, mania, and/or ruminating thoughts, which impact on the assessment process. Care plans are often basic and are written around self-care and maintenance.

## The allocation process

Once a care plan is written, it needs to be short-term as CRHT interventions are no longer than six weeks; often people are only just starting on their long journey of recovery. Parts can be passed on to a care coordinator, who could be an occupational therapist in a Community Mental Health Team (CMHT). However, it can be frustrating when when there are lengthy referral processes and allocation, often work started could not be continued in a timely fashion due to work restrictions and pressures of the CMHT.

## Occupational therapy networks and supervision

Keeping up to date with Trust-wide occupational therapy meetings and training is difficult with shift work – events are often scheduled on a day when you are not working, or when you are expected to carry out the obligations of the shift; being flexible and adaptable to change is a 'must'. Caseload management during team supervision and discussion is invaluable. However, with occupational therapy-specific supervision, this is difficult, as the supervising occupational therapist is often unfamiliar with the role in CRHT.

## Problem solving

- Be true to your professional identity: professional isolation is difficult, especially if you have never experienced working outside an occupational therapy team before.
- Be clear about the role from the beginning: be mindful that occupational therapy intervention is more likely to be short-term and goal-specific, time pressures make practice restricted, and people at their most unwell cannot concentrate for lengthy assessment.
- Consider your role in maintaining wellness to be important.
- Encourage people to identify their strengths, be patient-focused, stick to a holistic approach to care.
- Reflect on your practice: in order to grow and develop as a clinician, use supervision effectively.
- Be positive about the richness that your skills offer the team, and remind other clinicians of how they can be used regularly.
- Be adaptable and resourceful to fit your shifts around when your interventions may need to be carried out, or meetings which may be useful to attend.
- Offer occupational therapy ideas in handovers and other forums; use opportunities to ensure that occupational therapy is clinically very effective within CRHT.

I have worked in CRHT for six years in two very different teams with different models of working, and I would like to have done a lot more occupational therapy-specific work, where I had days for occupation-based assessments and interventions.

# Conclusion

Working as an occupational therapist in CRHT can be rewarding, although it is easy to work only as a generic practitioner. There are many interesting and diverse roles and responsibilities which are unique to CRHT; occupational therapists are very well suited to the work. However, there are challenges to face along the way. Through our work as occupational therapists we need to remain mindful of our professional identity, and remain true to it. It is a historical legacy that there is usually just the one 'token' occupational therapist in such a team; however, there is no reason why occupational therapists cannot be a larger proportion of the disciplines which make up CRHT teams.

## Box 3.1: Case study

A 50-year-old male presented with his first episode of anxiety which led to psychotic depression. He lived at home with his wife and one daughter. He had worked all his life, had an interest in football, and used to be outgoing and sociable. His brother killed himself several years ago.

For this gentleman building rapport was difficult as he initially did not want to engage, had almost constant ruminating thoughts and needed regular reassurance. Basic ADLs were discussed with him and his family (sleeping, eating and washing). Medication was also addressed and the importance of concordance.

I carried out an interest checklist with his wife present in order to ascertain what meaningful activity he might engage in, which could be used to distract him from the unhelpful intrusive thoughts which he was experiencing. I looked beyond the label of his illness and wanted to find the person who had become lost during illness. We completed a daily schedule in order to engage and motivate him. This included basic ADLs such as showering and changing his clothes, spending time doing both passive and active activities (such as skyping his friends in Australia, talking to his children on the phone, and watching football on the TV). I asked him about the football games which he had watched to assess memory, cognitive state and concentration. I encouraged him to think about going back to refereeing a football game or going to watch a local game. I also prompted him to think about the future and consider pursuing one of his goals to be a pet owner and subsequently he did get a kitten.

I considered his employment: he was a mechanic at a garage and there were issues around working relationships which contributed to ruminating thoughts. A return to that environment was not possible at the time. With his wife's support he had spoken with his previous employer. He was given the details of where to go for information and advice around benefits he may be able to claim whilst he is too unwell to be in employment. I also accompanied him to the local volunteering agency. I gave him a lift as he could not drive at this time. He was motivated to engage in activity and he spoke about his strengths. The remoteness of where he lived and not being able to drive posed problems. He decided that he would do more internet-based research before making a decision.

He continued to have a great relationship with his wife and children, who were very supportive. They used graded activity and set out small achievable tasks such as grating cheese as a part of meal preparation. This progressed to participating in the laundry, lighting the fire, doing the washing up, and hanging out the clothes. He went on to have an occupational therapist care coordinator with whom I liaised. The aim was to continue with the motivation generated and for this person to continue to improve functionally and volitionally as well as maintaining wellness and maximising independence. (See Figure 3.1.)

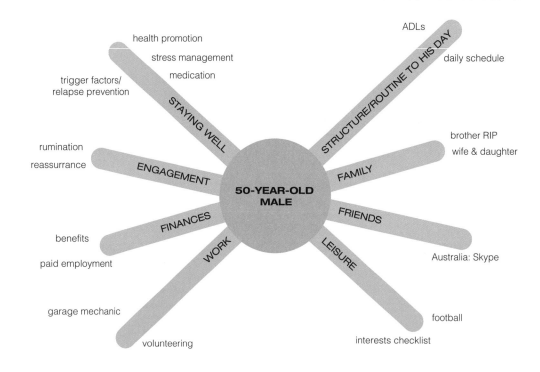

*Figure 3.1: Spider diagram illustrating case study.*

4

# Useful resources

- Barber, P., Brown, R. & Martin, D. (2012). *Mental Health Law in England and Wales: A Guide for Mental Health Professionals*, 2nd edn. London: Sage.
- Hart, C. (2014). *A Pocket Guide to Risk Assessment and Management in Mental Health*. Abingdon: Routledge.
- www.hafal.org
- www.mind.org.uk
- https://pathways.nice.org.uk/pathways/depression
- Wilson, M. (ed.) (1996). *Occupational Therapy in Short Term Psychiatry*, 3rd edn. London: Churchill Livingstone.

# References

Bryant, W., Fieldhouse, J. & Bannigan, K. (eds) (2014). *Creek's Occupational Therapy and Mental Health,* 5th edn. Oxford: Churchill Livingstone Elsevier.

Commission on Acute Adult Psychiatric Care (2015). *The Commission to Review the Provision of Acute Inpatient Care for Adults in England, Wales and Northern Ireland.* http://www.caapc.info (last accessed: 15.8.2016).

Forsyth, K., Deshpanade, S., Kielhofner, G., Henriksson, C., Haglund, L., Olson, L., Skinner, S. & Kulkarni, S. (2005). *The Occupational Circumstances Assessment Interview and Rating Scale (OCAIRS), Version 4.0.* Chicago: University of Illinois.

Heaseman, D. & Salhotra, G. (2008). *Interest Checklist.* http://www.cade.uic.edu (last accessed: 9.2.2016).

MDCalc (2016). CIWA-Ar for Alcohol Withdrawal. http://www.mdcalc.com (last accessed 9.2.2016).

Orford, J.E. (1995). Community mental health: the development of the CCOPII, a Client-Centred Occupational Performance Initial Interview. *British Journal of Occupational Therapy* 58 (5), 190–196.

Townsend, E.A. & Polatajko, H.J. (2007). *Enabling Occupation II: Advancing and Occupational Therapy Vision for Health, Well-being, and Justice through Occupation.* Ottawa Canada: CAOT Publications ACE.

United Kingdom Parliament (1983/2007). *Mental Health Act.* London: TSO.

Wise, J. (2014). Mental health patients pose high suicide risk in first two weeks after discharge, inquiry finds. *British Medical Journal* 349, http://www.bmj.com/content/349/bmj.g4659 (last accessed: 16.7.2016).

# Chapter 4

# Occupational therapy on a Psychiatric Intensive Care Unit

## Rachel Hickey and Rachel Nias

---

## Introduction

This chapter addresses the major gap in literature available for occupational therapists working within psychiatric intensive care units. It sets out some of the practical aspects of the role which provides a helpful guide to those interested in working in this rewarding field. This chapter also presents some of the challenges and contentious issues faced by occupational therapists working in this area, such as use of standard assessment tools, risk and restraint. The chapter provides practical suggestions for those embarking on a career as an occupational therapist within a Psychiatric Intensive Care Unit (PICU) through discussion about grading activities. Special attention is given to the future of the role and potential avenues.

---

## Key points

- The occupational therapist on PICU provides a valuable contribution by being a role model for others in promoting patient-centred approaches and positive risk taking.

- The occupational therapist has a unique role to play in risk assessment and works closely within a multi-disciplinary team.

- A ward-based occupational therapist has the challenge of role blurring and the positive element of timely patient engagement.

- The problem solving process within PICU is mostly focused on assessment which is a continuous process.

- There is a need for more research into this field to enable the occupational therapist to develop effective assessments and interventions appropriate for PICU patients.

# The Psychiatric Intensive Care Unit

A PICU is a locked unit which is located within an adult acute hospital (Sims 2014). It is common that PICUs will be gender-specific or have designated single sex areas. Most PICUs have multidisciplinary teams which may include art therapists, nursing staff, occupational therapists, pharmacists, psychiatrists, psychologists, and support staff. Patients on PICUs have similar diagnoses to patients on adult acute mental health wards, such as schizophrenia, bipolar and psychosis (Best 1996). The PICU has much higher staffing levels than traditional adult acute wards as part of a heightened focus on safety and risk assessment. To this end, there are often restrictions around access to toiletries, sharps and equipment (McNeill & Bannigan 2014). The PICU is often characterised by having a fast turnover of patients with high risks, working at a fast pace, with patients who may be in crisis or experiencing a particularly distressing time (Sims 2014). McNeill and Bannigan (2014) liken PICUs to low secure units.

> Psychiatric intensive care is for patients compulsorily detained usually in secure conditions, who are in an acutely disturbed phase of a serious mental disorder. There is an associated loss of capacity for self-control, with a corresponding increase in risk, which does not enable their safe, therapeutic management and treatment in a general open acute ward.
>
> (National Association of Psychiatric Intensive Care and Low Secure Units 2014, p. 5)

In addition, the PICU usually has a more rapid turnover of patients than inpatient acute wards (Sims 2014).

# The occupational therapy role on a PICU

The occupational therapist within a PICU has an important, varied, and multi-faceted contribution to make. The role is characterised by working with patients towards recovery and discharge from adult acute settings to the community. Patients on PICU are often detained under a section of the Mental Health Act (UK Parliament 1983/2007) which means that they may feel a reduced sense of control over their environment (Best 1996). The overall aim of the occupational therapist on a PICU is for the patient to increase his/her level of functioning and skills, and to promote recovery (Sims 2014). Occupational therapy engagement within a PICU is often ward-based, with engagement in other parts of the hospital or community where possible and appropriate (McNeill & Bannigan 2014).

The evidence base to support occupational therapy within PICU is very limited. This absence of a clear evidence base poses a difficulty for clinicians in defining their role and identifying training needs. In a rare inclusion in the literature, Sims (2014) likened occupational therapy in PICU to that of an adult acute unit but did not acknowledge the increased risk. The literature on PICU and occupational therapy is so sparse that it is commonplace for research from adult acute and general mental health settings to be (rightly or wrongly) generalised to all inpatient mental health settings to cover the work of occupational therapists.

# Too unwell to engage?

Due to the acute nature of the PICU patients' mental health, it can be said that they are 'too unwell to engage'. Sutton *et al.* (2012) suggested that 'disengagement' is part of the process of recovery for those with mental health problems; it may be a time when they disengage from the world and themselves, for example remaining in bed. This presents a challenge for the PICU occupational therapist.

Occupational therapy philosophy highlights activity as a basic human need which encompasses all aspects of a person, and wherein most can engage irrespective of other factors. The theorist Yerxa (2000, pp. 195–196) considered humans to be 'occupational beings', with occupation involved in every part of a person, their 'biological, psychological, socio-cultural and spiritual levels of being'. It could be suggested that for patients on a PICU engaging in occupations is vital to regain a sense of self in an unfamiliar environment. For example, Dewey (1933) suggested the human need for action is embedded in a person's sense of who they are, and Sutton *et al.* (2012) found that engaging in an activity assisted people to reconnect with themselves and their priorities.

# Grading

A key skill of the occupational therapist on a PICU is to modify and grade occupations to the individual and the environment to enable people to reengage with themselves and their world. Grading can be achieved through the 'just right challenge', when the activity is of suitable intensity to engage the person, but within the limits of his/her current potential. The challenge should balance the person's strengths and needs in occupations (Walters *et al.* 2014). An example is making a sandwich with someone who has difficulty in both choosing from a wide variety of ingredients and the functional skills involved. Grading is used to limit choices and the required elements of the task to let the person gain confidence and skill in this area before introducing more choices and sequences. These interventions, and the environment itself, require careful and detailed analysis on a daily basis to maintain safety and to limit adverse risks. For example, the behaviour of one patient may affect the planning of group interventions, or the timing of activities may require modification in relation to sleeping patterns and motivation levels. Engaging patients on a PICU is both challenging and rewarding; it entails exploring the possibilities of activities in a locked ward environment, negotiating the competing factors of risk, motivation and engagement.

# The problem solving process on a PICU

Assessment is the focal aspect of the problem solving process used on PICU and is continuous. The Accreditation for Inpatient Mental Health Services (AIMS) (2014, p. 14) suggested that patients on PICU: 'must have access to an occupational therapist for assessment within 72 hours of admission'; although this requires that assessment must take place it does not dictate its nature, either verbal or observation. Anecdotally, there is a general consensus that assessment in its traditional format is not always possible when working with patients on PICU. Sims (2014) acknowledges these patients may be frightened, confused and distressed. In this regard a formal assessment characterised by an occupational therapist asking questions may not be appropriate and may be an unwelcome stressor. Instead, Sims (2014) documents the importance of rapport building within any acute mental health unit. Within PICU, rapport building is particularly essential in building trust and familiarity while also observing the patient's level of function. Through this process, it may be that interests can be identified which may facilitate a more formal assessment (Sims 2014). Sims (2014) further suggested the use of observational assessments such as the Model of Human Occupational Screening Tool (MOHOST) (see Kielhofner et al. 2009). This assessment is invaluable within the PICU setting and can be used during an individual or group session through observation whilst gathering collateral information from notes and staff reports. The importance of applying a creative approach throughout the problem solving process was highlighted by Hickey (2016). Specific attention was paid to the importance of building rapport and carrying out assessments with patients in a non-traditional manner. Part of the recommendations suggested by Hickey (2016) have focused on the development of specific assessment and outcome measures to better meet the needs of this patient group. Traditional self-report or lengthy verbal assessments were identified as incongruent with the patients' needs and abilities whilst on PICU (Hickey 2016).

## Risk assessment

The occupational therapist has a special role in contributing to risk assessment due to the occupational focus of the interaction with the patient. Risk assessments are a focal point of all professions working on a PICU; they are used for PICU ward and community-based activities to ensure the safety of patients and staff engaging in activities. Throughout the patient's admission, risk assessment and grading activities are central to supporting the patient's level of functioning (Best 1996). McNeill and Bannigan (2014) acknowledge the importance of balancing risk assessment while working with core occupational therapy principles such as remaining patient-centred. Risk assessment is carried out on both a formal and informal basis, and communication with other professionals about risk is a pivotal aspect of multi-disciplinary working within a PICU. Positive risk taking is a key concept within mental health settings though it must be ensured that risk is minimised and patients are given the opportunity to achieve goals and to gain satisfaction through these achievements. An example of practical positive risk taking was use of a blender to make smoothies with the associated risks of accidental or intentional injury, balanced with an increase in engagement and interaction with patients. Introducing risk may seem counter-intuitive but is important in building a recovery-focused environment.

Occupational therapists have a unique role in risk assessment, due to the very nature of the discipline and its focus on occupation and patient-centredness. Risk management involves supporting a patient to function by reducing or limiting specific risks. Through engagement and observation the occupational therapist gathers information around the patient's current mental state, strengths and needs, and this provides a foundation on which to base risk decisions.

Risk management on a PICU may differ from other areas due to the risks of aggression to others and self which are frequently imminent. One of the issues with risk assessment is the variety of opinions about risk, as identified in a study of forensic occupational therapists (Cordingley & Ryan 2009). They suggested risk assessment can be affected by a professional's role, views and previous experience. Decisions which arise through risk assessment impact hugely on decisions around the patient's interventions and treatment. For example, following a thorough risk assessment, a patient may be required to remain on the ward, and be unable to engage in activities elsewhere within the hospital or in the community. This again highlights the fact that different professional viewpoints may shape risk decisions as occupational therapists see engagement as part of a recovery which must be balanced with current risk management plans.

# The use of restraint and the occupational therapist

One of the most contentious issues around the role of occupational therapy within the PICU is the role of restraint, such as using safe holds or 'positive management of violence'. The use of physical restraint remains controversial in mental health settings: some patients on a PICU are restrained due to the imminent risk of harm to themselves or others. Settings may also offer seclusion as an alternative to restraint, i.e. where the patient is put into a minimal hazard environment, and/or kept isolated from others, in order to reduce risk to others or self.

Often the occupational therapist is required to be trained in these methods for the safety of all people on the PICU. This decision tends to be based on the setting and whether the occupational therapist is included in the safe working numbers for the ward. It is, however, often suggested that the involvement of the occupational therapist in a restraint would have a negative effect on the therapeutic relationship with that individual. Duxbury and Wright (2011) suggested that some nurses have similar concerns about physical restraint, which can be seen by patients as distressing and at odds with a philosophy of care.

Occupational therapy has a lot to offer in de-escalating, or preventing situations before they occur, through offering occupations which fulfil a need for routine, pride in achievement, and meaningful engagement. It is interesting to note that some authors acknowledge the role of engagement in reducing violence and aggression (Bowers 2006, Stubbs & Sengupta 2008). This assertion advocates the use of purposeful activities particularly within a high risk environment such as a PICU. Bowers (2006) carried out a literature review based on PICU research and concluded that occupational therapy activities support routine and also reduce feelings of agitation. In particular, reference is made to the role of occupational therapy in promoting wellbeing and positive mental health which can avoid and reduce aggression on the PICU (Bowers 2006). This puts occupational therapy at the forefront of risk management and ties in with the earlier discussion that no one is ever too unwell to engage in occupational therapy.

# Environment

The inherent assumption that the environment is an essential component in health promotion is widely accepted within the field of occupational therapy. Occupational therapists are acutely aware of the role of the environment and how to adapt and shape it to increase function, e.g. reducing distraction around meal times to make it easier for the patient to focus on eating. The environment is all the more relevant within a locked environment, such as a PICU, in which individuals have restricted access, or are limited to the locked area; for a patient it can present as either a positive or a negative factor (COT 2012). A positive factor may be the security and safety the patient experiences; negatives include the various restrictions in place.

Despite numerous references within the national guidelines to maintaining a safe environment (AIMHS 2014, NAPICU 2014), little effort is made in terms of access to, or provision of, specific environments (art room, kitchen) within a PICU. Often PICUs have a sparse and limited space without access to a kitchen or creative area. The focus on safety also shapes the environment and makes it difficult to find a space that is quiet or without interruptions; patients often voice their dissatisfaction within a PICU because they feel restricted and they lack control and choice. The occupational therapist can be well placed to offer suggestions on the design of the environment and also how to adapt it to promote function and wellbeing. Simple adaptations seen in older adult mental health settings are now being seen in PICUs, such as sensory rooms and quiet rooms for relaxation. Occupational therapists should continue to work with other professionals to convey the impact of environment on function, and to offer their unique perspective on environmental design within a PICU.

# Occupational therapy identity

The role and identity of the occupational therapist in the PICU is the subject of frequent debate. The College of Occupational Therapists' (COT 2006) *Recovering Ordinary Lives* strategy for occupational therapy in mental health services found that in mental health settings, occupational therapy lacked a clear professional role and purpose. Role blurring, a lack of clear evidence base, and the impetus for generic working were considered as factors affecting the identity of occupational therapy in mental health services, and these factors correlate with the PICU occupational therapy identity. Role blurring can be a threat to occupational therapy identity but can also be considered an opportunity (Brown *et al.* 2000). On a PICU, the role of occupational therapy is often blurred with those of nursing staff and consultants in areas such as self-care and engaging in activity.

The scarcity of research as an evidence base about the role of the PICU occupational therapist threatens their identity. The polarisation of PICU settings and other mental health inpatient settings has been further increased by the establishment of the *Psychiatric Intensive Care Journal* which many occupational therapists working in PICUs have used as a platform rather than the profession-specific

*British Journal of Occupational Therapy.* In this regard it has highlighted PICU occupational therapy as a specialist area but has distanced itself from occupational therapy and chosen instead to align itself with PICUs. Lloyd *et al.* (2004) warn that within occupational therapy and mental health it is difficult to maintain occupational therapy identity and also be fluid and work to meet patient needs.

The identity of the PICU occupational therapist can be established through involvement with other occupational therapists, utilising occupational therapy philosophy and occupational therapy's unique contribution to the team. Liaison with other acute mental health occupational therapists assists with maintaining an identity, preventing isolation and creating a seamless step-down approach from the PICU. A further positive influence is for a higher grade occupational therapist to oversee acute mental health occupational therapists; this facilitates service improvement, a common approach and a unified service, and thus enables the PICU occupational therapists to develop their role.

Another way to maintain identity as an occupational therapist is through use of a model. Cook (2012) suggested the use of Model of Human Occupation (MOHO) to avoid some of the pitfalls of generic working; this model is effective for PICU assessments and to structure reports and records. Raising the profile of occupational therapy is essential in development of the PICU role; this can be achieved through input at multi-disciplinary discussions and professionals' meetings, and daily promotion of the contribution and perspective of the occupational therapist. In addition, collaborating with nursing staff on ward interventions such as the Safewards' 'mutual help meetings' (Safewards 2015), and healthy eating regimes, has developed understanding of the occupational therapy approach. The role of the PICU occupational therapist is indeed challenged by the aforementioned role blurring, generic working and isolation from other occupational therapists; however, it also provides valuable opportunities to promote occupational therapy and its philosophy to the benefit of the service and its patients.

# Safe staffing

The national minimum standards for PICU (NAPICU 2014) highlighted the need for safe staffing levels agreed at a local level. The NAPICU's recommendation is that therapy and management staff should not be included in the staffing levels. In practice, some services have an occupational therapist included in these numbers who is based on the ward and is responsible for generic duties alongside the occupational therapy role. In contrast some occupational therapists are based within an occupational therapy department and attend PICU as part of their working day. The AIMS scheme (Lemmey *et al.* 2011) reported 70 per cent of PICUs have a permanent occupational therapist but did not distinguish whether this role is ward-based or based in an occupational therapy department.

A ward-based occupational therapist has the difficulties of role blurring which is further tested by the lack of clear differentiation between the generic and occupational therapy-specific tasks required. The patients on PICU can require close supervision. Anecdotal evidence suggested that involving an occupational therapist in such close observations could restrict their ability to plan and organise interventions. Another challenge for a single occupational therapist on a nursing-led ward is the lack of understanding about occupational therapy, as reported by Duffy and Nolan (2005): the occupational therapists in this study were regularly explaining why they were carrying out interventions and that their role was not simply to 'entertain' patients. A reason for this situation was suggested to be the dominance of the medical model in that setting which was incongruent with the role and philosophy of occupational therapy. Ashby et al. (2015) highlighted the need for occupational therapists to develop strategies, such as reflection, to manage these incongruences to work effectively alongside the medical model whilst maintaining occupation-focused practice. This is vital for preventing burnout for the PICU occupational therapist.

There are many benefits for a ward-based occupational therapist. They can utilise their skills as a role model for managing such tasks as close observation. This could include demonstration of appropriate ways to engage individuals, using the time to investigate the interests of the person and to consider suitable occupations. Being ward-based and amongst the safe staffing levels, an occupational therapist can also embed the theory and practice of occupational therapy within the environment and practice of the ward. Brown et al. (2000) refers to the role of group normalisation and development of group norms which may develop if an occupational therapist is based on a PICU rather than part of an occupational therapy department. This may shift the occupational therapist identity through proximity and team decision making (Brown et al. 2000). Research by Bowers et al. (2005) suggested that if the occupational therapist was based in an occupational therapy department, the role would focus on the assessment of activities of daily living and running groups. This research also highlighted the role of nurses in building rapport and engaging patients in different activities through their 'presence' on the ward throughout the day and night. The occupational therapist's role on PICU incorporates some aspects of both of these roles, building rapport, assessment and interventions. This enables a more comprehensive assessment of each patient through a proactive approach to engaging patients at a time when they are ready and motivated to engage, without the concern of missing an appointment time.

## The future of occupational therapy and the PICU

This field seems to be under researched and there is little or no literature on the role of occupational therapy on a PICU. In a rare inclusion in the *British Journal of Occupational Therapy,* Best (1996) highlights the need for more dissemination of PICU occupational therapy practice guidelines. Despite this publication in 1996, no further developments have been documented in the literature. More individual and tailored research and theory related to PICU and occupational therapy would be helpful to support those working in this area. The research should also explore specialised assessments which are relevant to the PICU setting and useful in practice, which would lead to a more efficient identification of the patient's strengths and needs, and in doing so, a more appropriate intervention while the patient is on the PICU. The lack of established outcome measures, surely, is in tandem with the absence of available research within PICUs. Development or identification of an appropriate outcome measure would be useful in building the sought after evidence base for occupational therapy within the PICU.

There is considerable opportunity to develop the role of the occupational therapist within the PICU, and this could lead to the future inclusion of a greater variety of activities. For example, sessional specialists could be a useful addition to the therapeutic activities. Art therapists have been used on PICUs for some time; drama therapists could introduce another therapeutic activity to the ward. The difficulty for sessional workers is the conflict between their designated and fixed time on the ward, and the changeable nature of motivation and behaviour within their patient group. However, a sessional worker can bring a fresh outlook and different perspective to the ward and the patients, leading to a more rounded view of each individual's abilities. The occupational therapist's role with sessional workers can be to act as a liaison, co-facilitator and/or supporter, helping to ensure that their time on the ward is both safe and effective; this can include promotion of a role within the PICU and identification and encouragement for those who may be interested.

A further role as mentor could also be developed through engagement with someone with personal experience of mental health. They would require supervision and debriefing to ensure their safety and ongoing wellbeing; this could be facilitated by the occupational therapist. The involvement of people providing vocational activities of interest to patients may be another useful addition, providing role models and positive experiences from people outside the health professions. The use of external sources of support may have a positive influence on rapport building and care on the ward.

## Conclusion

This chapter has highlighted the unique and often challenging role of occupational therapy within PICUs. The role may often feel like a juggling act which has to balance both function and risk, but professionals have a lot to offer through their occupational therapy skills in grading activities appropriately so that the patient can achieve success and experience feelings of satisfaction, and also through shaping the environment to meet the needs of the patient at a period of crisis. Special attention has been paid to the positive and negative aspects of the role of occupational therapy in safety, encompassing risk assessment, restraint and environmental factors. It is clear that more research is needed to determine whether professionals are more effective when ward-based or operating within occupational therapy departments, and how best the role may be supported within any professional environment.

# Useful resources

- College of Occupational Therapists – Specialist Section, Mental Health: https://www.cot.co.uk/
- Creativity and PICU – Hickey, R. (2016). An exploration into occupational therapists' use of creativity within psychiatric intensive care units. *Journal of Psychiatric Intensive Care*, published online March 2016. doi:10.20299/jpi.2016.011
- National Association of Psychiatric Intensive Care Units: NAPICU: http://napicu.org.uk
- Psychiatric Intensive Care Journal: http://journals.cambridge.org/action/displayJournal?jid=JPI
- Safewards (Intervention for PICU): http://safewards.net

# References

Accreditation for Inpatient Mental Health Services (AIMHS) (2014). *National Minimum Standards*, 3rd edn. London: Royal College of Psychiatrists.

Ashby, S., Gray, M., Ryan, S. & James, C. (2015). Maintaining occupation-based practice in Australian mental health practice: a critical stance. *British Journal of Occupational Therapy* **78** (7), 431–439.

Best, D. (1996). The developing role of occupational therapy in psychiatric intensive care. *British Journal of Occupational Therapy* **59** (4), 161–164.

Bowers, L. (2006). *Psychiatric Intensive Care Units: A Literature Review.* London: Department of Mental Health and Learning Disability.

Bowers, L., Simpson, A., Alexander, J., Hackney, D., Nijman, H., Grance, A. & Warren, J. (2005). The nature and purpose of acute psychiatric wards: The Tompkins Acute Ward Study. *Journal of Mental Health* **14** (6), 625–635.

Brown, B., Crawford, P. & Darongkamas, J. (2000). Blurred roles and permeable boundaries: the experience of multidisciplinary working in community mental health. *Health and Social Care in the Community* **8** (6), 425–435.

College of Occupational Therapists (2006). *Recovering Ordinary Lives: The Strategy for Occupational Therapy in Mental Health Services 2007–2017.* London: COT.

College of Occupational Therapists (2012). *Occupational Therapists' Use of Occupation Focused Practice in Secure Hospitals, practice guideline.* London: COT.

Cook, S. (2012). 'Personal reflections on understanding and using the Model of Human Occupation in Practice' in *Using Occupational Therapy Theory in Practice*, eds. G. Boniface and A. Seymour. Chichester: Blackwell Publishing.

Cordingley, K. & Ryan, S. (2009). Occupational therapy risk assessment in forensic mental health practice: an exploration. *British Journal of Occupational Therapy* **72** (12), 531–538.

Dewey, J. (1933). *How We Think*. Boston: D. C. Heath & Co.

Duffy, R. & Nolan, P. (2005). A survey of the work of occupational therapists in inpatient mental health services. *Mental Health Practice* **8** (6), 36–41.

Duxbury, J. & Wright, K. (2011). Should nurses restrain violent and aggressive patients? *Nursing Times* **107** (9), 22–25.

Hickey, R. (2016). An exploration into occupational therapists' use of creativity within psychiatric intensive care units. *Journal of Psychiatric Intensive Care*, doi:10.20299/jpi.2016.011.

Kielhofner, G., Fogg, L., Braveman, B., Forsyth, K., Kramer, J. & Duncan, E. (2009). A factor analytic study of the Model of Human Occupation Screening Tool of Hypothesised Variables. *Occupational Therapy in Mental Health* **25** (2), 127–137.

Lemmey, S., Bleksley, S., Cresswell, J. & Lelliott, P. (2011). *Accreditation for Inpatient Mental Health Services – Psychiatric Intensive Care Units (AIMS-PICU).* London: Royal College of Psychiatrists/National Association of Psychiatric Intensive Care & Low Secure Units.

Lloyd, C., King, R. & McKenna, K. (2004). Generic versus specialist clinical work roles of occupational therapists and social workers in mental health. *Australian and New Zealand Journal of Psychiatry* **38** (3), 119–124.

McNeill, S. & Bannigan, K. (2014). 'Forensic and prison services' in *Creeks Occupational Therapy and Mental Health*, eds. W. Bryant, J. Fieldhouse and K. Bannigan, 5th edn. London: Churchill Livingstone.

National Association of Psychiatric Intensive Care and Low Secure Units (NAPICU) (2014). *National Minimum Standards for Psychiatric Intensive Care in General Adult Services.* Glasgow: National Association of Psychiatric Intensive Care and Low Secure Units.

Safewards (2015) *Mutual help meetings*. http://www.safewards.net/interventions/mutual-help-meeting (last accessed: 2.8.2015).

Sims, K.L. (2014). 'The acute setting' in *Creeks Occupational Therapy and Mental Health,* eds. W. Bryant, J. Fieldhouse and K. Bannigan, 5th edn. London: Churchill Livingstone.

Stubbs, B. & Sengupta, S. (2008). Aggression: is it a problem for occupational therapists? *British Journal of Occupational Therapy* **71** (8), 313.

Sutton, D.J., Hocking, C.S., & Smythe, L.A. (2012). A phenomenological study of occupational engagement in recovery from mental illness. *Canadian Journal of Occupational Therapy* **79** (3), 142–150.

United Kingdom Parliament (1983/2007). Mental Health Act. London: TSO.

Walters, J.H., Sherwood, W. & Mason, H. (2014). 'Creative activities' in *Creeks Occupational Therapy and Mental Health*, eds. W. Bryant, J. Fieldhouse and K. Bannigan, 5th edn. London: Churchill Livingstone.

Yerxa, E.J. (2000). Confessions of an occupational therapist who became a detective. *British Journal of Occupational Therapy* **63** (5), 192–199

# Chapter 5

# Prison inreach: the occupational therapist role

Carmen Lewis

## Introduction

This chapter sets out to outline the opportunities for occupational therapists working in the prison environment. It introduces the history and legislation behind the development of mental health inreach teams and occupational therapists working in this setting. It explores the occupational therapy role, including generic duties and multi-agency working, occupational-based groups, psycho-educational groups, one-to-one work, follow-on community work, and the use of the Model of Human Occupation. The chapter goes on to identify the challenges and barriers to working in this environment, as well as highlighting the skills required to work in a prison and similarities to other fields.

## Key points

- The ever-changing landscape of the prison and frequent changes to policies and legislation make it a challenging environment. However, occupational therapists have a valuable and unique role in supporting clients to add meaning and purpose to their lives which ultimately helps prevent them from returning to substances, crime and prison.

- Multi-disciplinary working and generic duties are a vital part of the occupational therapy role in the prison setting. However, it is important to remain true to your occupational therapy values and promote the unique role of occupational therapy with an occupational-focused service.

- The use of the Model of Human Occupation (MOHO) helps provide a common core of occupationally focused language to support profiling and occupational identity. This is vitally important working in an environment where you are a minority profession.

- It is essential when working in this environment with limited resources and staffing to 'think outside the box' and explore other ways of securing resources.

# Mental ill-health in prisoners

The belief still held by many is that a person is sent to prison for punishment, that merely being confined is inadequate and that life in prison should be harsh and as difficult as possible. However, more recently there has been a growing belief that prisons should be places where prisoners should be given the opportunity to improve themselves and prepare for successful reintegration into the community (Molineux & Whiteford 1999). This would include having appropriate mental healthcare to support the mental health needs of the prison population. The recent *Prison Mental Health Needs Assessment* undertaken by Public Health Wales (2013) estimates that only 8 per cent of the 3,300 prisoners held in Wales, at any given time, *do not* suffer from any type of diagnosable mental health problem; the majority have one or more presenting difficulties with a range of severity.

# The development of mental health inreach teams

The *Changing the Outlook* (DoH 2001) document brought about the birth of the prison inreach teams. Although there were a small number of occupational therapists working within prisons before this point, they were few and far between and working in isolation. *Changing the Outlook* (DoH 2001) uses the terminology applying to mental health services in England but there was also very close cooperation with the National Assembly for Wales in taking forward a similar programme of improvement in Wales: this was the plan entitled *Improving Health in Wales – A Plan for the NHS with its Partners* also published in 2001 (National Assembly for Wales 2001). These documents were informed by the principle that improvements in prison mental health services need to be based on the *National Service Framework (NSF) for Mental Health*, published in September 1999 (DoH 1999). The NSF sets out seven standards for the provision of effective mental healthcare for all those who need it, including prisoners.

The *Changing the Outlook* (DoH 2001) document states that 'services should be provided as far as possible in the same way as they are in the wider community' (p. 26). This saw the development of the mental health inreach teams and the NHS funding multi-disciplinary teams, similar to Community Mental Health Teams (CMHTs), within the prison. The first phase of inreach schemes started in 2001–2002 in 12 prisons in England and the four Welsh prisons, including HMP Cardiff. The inreach team was to provide a whole range of services which included occupational therapy and other therapeutic interventions.

There are large differences between inreach teams across England and Wales. This is partly due to different levels of funding and staffing, different mixes of disciplines, constraints of levels of security in different prison environments and different prison populations, i.e. longer-term prisoners are more stable as a population than remand prisoners. The original remit of inreach teams was to provide secondary care. However, the volume of mental health need within prisons and difficulties in creating or sustaining primary mental healthcare services has resulted in a gradual broadening of inreach criteria in some prisons.

# Cardiff inreach team

Cardiff prison mental health inreach team has been in existence since 2002. The inreach team is the equivalent of a CMHT but working within the confines of a prison environment. The team therefore works to the standards and procedures of CMHTs provided by the Cardiff and Vale University Health Board in the wider community. The team accepts referrals for prisoners who are thought to be suffering from serious mental illnesses/mental disorders.

The multi-disciplinary team consists of two full-time community psychiatric nurses (CPNs) (one also being the team leader), a full-time occupational therapist, full-time administrative assistant, part-time consultant psychiatrist, part-time psychotherapist and part-time occupational therapy technical instructor. The psychotherapist also set up a student counselling service within the prison.

Although the team works primarily with severe and enduring mental illness, there is overlap with primary care clients. The CPNs work solely with the secondary care clients as there are registered mental health nurses (RMNs) who work within primary care. However, the occupational therapist, psychotherapist and psychiatrist bridge the gap and also offer services to complex primary care clients with specific needs.

The team automatically accepts clients who are already open to secondary care services such as CMHTs and have been transferred in from secure hospitals or under other inreach teams. The team holds a weekly multi-disciplinary team referral meeting jointly with primary care where all mental health referrals are discussed. Referrals to inreach are primarily received from nurses who have completed the reception screen and identified someone as being open to services, or by the primary care team nurses following their initial assessments. Any staff member can make a referral, including prison officers, offender supervisors and the substance misuse team.

# Current legislation

As well as following the Care Programme Approach (CPA), the team adheres to the *Mental Health (Wales) Measure* (National Assembly for Wales 2010). This is a law that places legal duties on local health boards and local authorities about the assessment and treatment of mental health problems. For secondary care this includes allocating a named care coordinator and formulating care and treatment plans. It also enables clients who have previously been discharged from secondary services to be able to refer themselves back. Many clients who come into the prison under the care of a CMHT will continue to have a named care coordinator through this team and the inreach team would be co-workers. However, if they are sentenced to a long length of time, the CMHT may close them and the inreach team would take over those care responsibilities and refer them back on release.

In 2006 a Prison Mental Health Collaboration in Wales produced the *Prison Mental Health Pathway* (Welsh Government 2006), a step-by-step guide for the commissioners and planners of mental health services in prisons, and for practitioners. In 2012 the Welsh Government published *Together for Mental Health: A Strategy for Mental Health Wellbeing in Wales* (Welsh Government 2012b) and a corresponding *Delivery Plan for 2012–16* (Welsh Government 2012c). This was the first mental health strategy in Wales that covered all ages and it reinforced the need to promote better health and wellbeing among the whole population. This document outlines efforts to improve mental health services which can support offenders, and includes statutory provision under the mental health measure. The document highlighted a need to further help prisoners in Wales with the difficulties they face in relation to their mental health problems. This has led to the development of a consultation document for a *Policy Implementation Guide: Mental Health Services for Prisoners in Wales* (Welsh Government 2014) which sets out the minimum levels of service required in all local health boards to address this matter.

The Care Act (UK Parliament 2014) was implemented in England in April 2015, followed by *The Social Services and Wellbeing (Wales) Act* (Welsh Government 2014) which was due to come into force on 6 April 2016. These acts outline the way in which local authorities should carry out carers' assessments and needs assessments, which includes outlining practices for the care of prisoners. This new legislation will affect not only the prison service but local authorities. Prisoners who meet set criteria and are deemed to require extra support will have services provided by their local authority rather than individuals employed directly by the prison service. For the first time, the prison service and local authorities will work in conjunction to share a legal duty of care. The introduction of these acts, which places a legal obligation on local authorities to address the social care needs of the prison population, provides further opportunity to profile the role of occupational therapy in being able to meet these needs.

# Introduction to Cardiff prison

Her Majesty's Prison (HMP) Cardiff is a category B local/training prison with a current capacity of 820 prisoners. Category B is the second highest of four categories of prison and is for those who do not require maximum security, but for whom escape still needs to be difficult. Men on remand are usually held in category B conditions. Category A is for those whose escape would be highly dangerous to the public or national security; there are no category A prisons in Wales. Category C is also a closed prison and is for those who cannot be trusted in open conditions but who are unlikely to try and escape. There are also no category C prisons in Wales; Stoke Heath prison in Shropshire is the most local category C prison which accepts prisoners from Cardiff. Category D prisons are for those who can be reasonably trusted not to escape, and are given the privilege of an open prison. There is one category D prison in Wales which is HMP Prescoed. A high number of category C prisoners will remain in HMP Cardiff as it is their local prison.

Cardiff prison holds adult (over 21 years) male remand and short/medium-term convicted prisoners. Any prisoner sentenced to two years or over would be transferred to Parc prison in

Bridgend. There are a small number of prisoners serving life sentences who remain in Cardiff prison. The prison also holds young adult offenders (prisoners aged between 18 and 21) while they are on remand; however, once sentenced, they would also be transferred to Parc prison regardless of length of sentence.

Cardiff prison has six main wings which have different functions, including an induction wing where all new receptions are located, a remand wing, and enhanced wing and working wings. In addition to this there is a care and separation unit (previously known as segregation), a detox landing and a therapeutic landing. The therapeutic landing houses vulnerable prisoners who would struggle to cope in the main location. In addition to this there is a healthcare unit which houses prisoners with either physical or mental health needs. Cardiff prison is the only prison in Wales which still has an inpatient healthcare unit. The inreach team will support clients in all the different areas of the prison.

The prison regime is continually changing. Currently prisoners are expected to work or attend education from Monday to Friday. Prisoners also have opportunities to attend gym, chapel and visits. If they are sentenced and refuse to work they will be placed on basic regime which consists of: restricted visits, restricted money to spend, no television, and very little association time (time out of cell), and inability to attend activities such as the gym. Many prisoners with mental health difficulties can struggle to conform or cope with the prison environments. The prison regime is very rigid and the concept of occupational deprivation is one that has been applied to understanding the phenomenon of inmates' restricted occupational engagement in traditional penal settings (Molineux & Whiteford 1999). Whiteford (2000) describes occupational deprivation as 'a state of preclusion from engagement in occupations of necessity and/or meaning due to factors that stand outside the immediate control of the individual'. Simple opportunities to engage in routine activities of daily living such as preparing food or doing the laundry are often unavailable in prison. It is a very rigid and structured routine with lack of choice or decision making, e.g. meals are always at a set time.

## Generic duties and multi-agency working

The CPNs carry out the majority of initial mental health assessments. However, if there is a specific need identified that is more appropriately met by another team member, such as an occupational therapist, then that person will carry out the initial assessment and care coordination duties if applicable. Occupational therapists are detailed as core members of CMHTs and are legislated to fulfil the role of care coordinator within both the mental health (Wales) measure (part 2) and the *Delivering the Care Programme Approach in Wales Interim Policy Implementation Guidance* (Welsh Government 2010). This will include duties such as completing care and treatment plans with clients and arranging care and treatment planning meetings. This involves close liaison with CMHTs that clients are under and transferring of care.

Multi-disciplinary working is a vital part of the role for any discipline. This will include risk management, liaising with probation officers and offender supervisors, attending sentence planning meetings, joint working with the substance misuse team, attending Multi-Agency Public Protection Arrangements (MAPPA) meetings, etc. The MAPPAs are in place to ensure the successful management of violent and sexual offenders who pose a risk to the public. It is not a legal framework, but a set of arrangements for supervising offenders in the community. They are principally a structure by which the various agencies an offender comes into contact with can share information and thereby monitor risk factors after the person is released. The occupational therapist will also work closely with other members of the prison community (such as gym staff, education and workshop staff) to support clients in engaging in these activities.

The occupational therapist is the inreach lead for Safer Custody and Violence Reduction (SCVR) and inputs into monthly meetings for this. The occupational therapist is appointed as the lead due to having a special interest in this area and also as it fits in well with occupational therapy philosophy. Research has indicated that for those with complex needs, time out of the cell and higher rates of purposeful activity are associated with lower levels of self-inflicted death (Prisoner Ombudsman for Northern Ireland (PONI) 2011). As a result, occupational therapy can play a vital role in the improved response for offenders to reduce suicide, self-harm and challenging behaviour (COT 2012). The occupational therapist will also attend Assessment, Care in Custody and Teamwork (ACCT) reviews for clients on caseload. The ACCT process allows the prison to monitor the prisoner closely, engaging them in planning ways of reducing their difficulties and helping them to build up their own sources of support. It is acknowledged that whilst some prisons are not therapeutic environments, some prisoners require a therapeutic approach during periods of vulnerability (Curran & Wilkinson 2010) which is a role for occupational therapists.

# The role of occupational therapy

The key role of the occupational therapist within the inreach team involves enabling service users with mental health difficulties to learn, regain and maintain skills in order to carry out everyday activities such as self-care, leisure or work activities, and live as independently as possible. Occupational therapists are able to assess and identify the mental health issues which are affecting clients' abilities to cope effectively in the community and work with the individual to improve their skills and enable them to live a more fulfilling life. This will include improving and maintaining independent living skills as much as is possible within the restraints of the prison environment. Many clients will not be able to gain employment or engage in vocational opportunities immediately on release. Therefore, it is important to explore other ways in which they can structure their time, work towards their goals and have meaning in their lives, which will ultimately prevent them from returning to substances, crime and prison. A vital part of this will include them engaging in leisure activities which they value, are meaningful to them and give them a sense of purpose.

A healthy balance of occupations includes a variety of physical, mental and social occupations, so that the individual is able to develop and exercise their capacities in all these areas (Creek &

Lougher 2008). In reality the intent of the prison environment is to prevent individuals engaging in some activities and from having choices, which can result in depression, anxiety and apathy. Occupational therapists are able to use therapeutic occupation not only to improve mood but also to reduce challenging behaviours which is also a means of addressing offending behaviour by improving everyday life skills (Curran & Wilkinson 2010).

When the prison inreach teams were first implemented in order to reflect the services being offered in the community, the idea was for prisons to move away from prisoners with mental health difficulties being automatically located in healthcare facilities. The provision of day care services with greater opportunities for prisoners to engage in a purposeful regime and join in other prison activities was seen as important to mirror what was happening in the community. Day care services would provide a timetable of different activities and therapies. The *Changing the Outlook* (DoH 2001) document supports occupational therapists as having an effective role to play within the provision of day care: '[d]ay care provides the opportunity for work with occupational therapists, who can assess individual capabilities and identify a therapeutic approach to enhance the patient's skills both in prison and after release' (p. 19).

However, since 2001 there has been a move away from providing dedicated day care services in the community for individuals with mental health problems. The drive has been more towards integrating these individuals into mainstream activities. This shift has also been seen in some of the prisons, including Cardiff, with the ending of funding for a number of day care facilities that were being offered such as art, yoga and music therapy. This has meant that occupational therapists have needed to rethink their role, not having such easy access to resources and facilities.

# The occupational therapy process

The mental health occupational therapy service within the Trust set up a service model working group that pooled resources regarding the various occupational therapy models. The Model of Human Occupation (MOHO) (Kielhofner 2008) which addresses motivation, performance and organisation of occupational participation in everyday life was chosen as the preferred model because it:

- supports person-centred practice
- provides a common core of occupationally focused language to support profiling and defining professional identity
- offers a comprehensive range of assessment tools that can be applied across a range of clinical settings
- has elements of validity and reliability with future-proof eligibility of data for research.

Occupational therapists use this model to gather information on a client's occupational identity and occupational competence in order to work in a person-centred way to identify key occupational issues, set measurable goals and occupational therapy interventions.

Where possible within the prison setting, the occupational therapist will use the forensic Occupational Circumstances Assessment and Interview Rating Scale (OCAIRS) (Forsyth et al. 2005) as an initial interview. It is not always appropriate to complete a MOHO assessment on initial contact due to a client's mental state or circumstances. For individuals who are more acutely unwell and without the attention span for a structured interview, the Model of Human Occupations Screening Tool (MOHOST) (Parkinson et al. 2006) is a more appropriate tool. The occupational therapist also uses the Occupational Self-Assessment (OSA) (Baron et al. 2006) on occasions and will find this particularly helpful to use prior to release planning.

From completion of the initial assessment the occupational therapist would identify the client's strengths and needs and use these to formulate an occupational therapy intervention plan in collaboration with the service user. This may include a combination of one-to-one and/or group interventions. These intervention plans will regularly be reviewed and adapted with the client. If the occupational therapist is the care coordinator for an individual then in line with the mental health (Wales) measure they will also need to complete a care and treatment plan with the client. Where possible the MOHO assessments will be repeated to gather outcomes on any improvement in the clients' level of functioning.

## Barriers

There are difficulties with completing a MOHO assessment as an initial interview when the occupational therapist has been allocated as either care coordinator or first assessor for this person. With these individuals, as part of the CPA process, the occupational therapist would need to complete the CPA assessment form on initial interview. This is an overview assessment which gathers background information on an individual such as: past contact with mental health services, substance misuse history, personal history, current concerns and mental state. This generally takes an hour to complete and it would not be appropriate to also complete an occupational therapy-specific assessment at this time. However, the occupational therapist would be able to derive a number of personal strengths and needs from this assessment and formulate an intervention plan. An additional MOHO assessment could be completed at a later date.

Due to the prison being remand and having a high turnover of prisoners, it is often not possible to repeat the assessment and gain outcomes. This is because clients can be released from Court or transferred to other establishments without prior warning. However, if a client is sentenced to over two years and consequently transferred to Parc prison, the client will be referred on to the occupational therapist in Parc who will have access to the original assessment and will therefore be able to review and evaluate this.

## Box 5.1: Case study – non-standardised assessment

Client A was on remand for murder and facing a life sentence. He was very low in mood and continually thinking that his life as he knew it was over. It was not appropriate at this time to complete a structured interview asking him about his roles, interests, etc. which would cause him great distress. Therefore, it was more appropriate to gather this information in a gradual and less formal way, i.e. through discussions when attending the art group. Following a number of weeks of observing skill levels and having informal discussions with client A, the occupational therapist was then able to complete the MOHOST as an assessment.

# Occupation-based groups

Many prisoners with mental health difficulties can struggle to access mainstream courses both in prison and on release. A fundamental part of the occupational therapist's role is to use activity to improve social and communication skills, improve mood, self-esteem and confidence, create structure and routine, and encourage participation in hobbies and interests. Groups can also be used as a stepping stone to improve skills and confidence in order for service users to be able to participate in mainstream prison and education activities. The occupational therapist grades activities to ensure successful rehabilitation and recovery.

There is a demand for a variety of different activity groups to be run. However, due to staffing levels there is a limit to how many can be timetabled. Therefore, groups are continually changing depending on the needs and interests of the clients at the time. Different groups that have been run include art, games, creative writing, drama, music and gardening.

It is important when working within this environment with limited resources to 'think outside the box' and explore other ways of securing resources. When working within HMP Swansea, links were developed with the volunteer coordinator, who coordinates volunteers within mental health settings across the Trust. A pilot project of volunteers was recruited to assist with facilitating occupational therapy groups. The volunteers recruited had a skill mix and aided with the running of art and creative writing groups.

Within HMP Cardiff, prisoners residing on the therapeutic landing have access to participate in gardening as part of their work programme. The individuals who accessed this resource valued the therapeutic activity highly. Fieldhouse (2003) found a gardening group has two key benefits: the first involves cognitive benefits of enhanced mood, reduced arousal and improved concentration; the second is the social nature of the group – the need to cooperate with each other to achieve the end goal. However, it could only be accessed by this small number of the prison population. The occupational therapist therefore set about liaising with the appropriate governor and workshop staff to set up a gardening group that could be accessed particularly by the inpatients but also by other occupational therapy clients with an identified need from the main wings. One session a week was agreed when the workshop would not be using it and it was also agreed that workshop staff would be available to support the running of this group.

# The Koestler Awards

The occupational therapy service supports and actively encourages prisoners to participate in and enter the Koestler Awards. The Koestler Trust is the UK's best known prison arts charity and has been awarding, exhibiting and selling artworks by offenders for over 50 years. The aim and purpose of this is to help offenders lead more positive lives by motivating them to participate and achieve in the arts. Participation in the arts can lead to employable skills, high self-esteem, collaboration with others and a feeling of purpose in life. Every prisoner who enters the awards receives a certificate and they can win cash prizes which gives a sense of achievement. The awards can also be used by occupational therapists to develop ideas for group projects that clients can engage in, for example within the art group.

Box 5.2: Case study – 'An award-winning prison drama – Occupational Therapists Support Prisoners' Mental Health Recovery', won runner-up in 2014 NHS Wales awards

A client questionnaire was distributed to ascertain what activities prisoners would be interested in. Drama was highlighted as something which people were keen to try. Although the occupational therapy technician had experience of facilitating drama groups in a specialist behaviour unit, the occupational therapists had never run a prison-based drama group and were keen to support clients' interests and explore how this could be achieved.

The Arts Alliance reports that arts used with ex-offenders can awaken an interest in learning and help build new positive identities. Engaging in the arts can lead not only to employment, but the skills and desire to actively engage in community and culture.

Establishing the group did not present insurmountable barriers; however, participants wanted to film their performance and enter the Koestler Awards. Initially there was uncertainty around the possibility of filming within a prison and collaboration with prison staff was required. Permission was needed to film and additional barriers had to be overcome such as who would film, provide the equipment and other resources and funding that were needed. The tight timeframe also posed a challenge as there was less than two months until the application deadline for the award. The project proposal secured the approval of the prison governor who allocated the security governor as a contact to support the project. In support of the rationale for the project he put the team in contact with an existing National Offender Management Service (NOMS) employee who already had filming equipment approved. She enthusiastically agreed to do the filming and advised about the associated restrictions. This highlights the benefits of working with other agencies as they have access to additional knowledge and resources.

Scheduling sufficient rehearsal time, while adhering to the prison regime, was a challenge. Participants were keen to use their initiative to overcome lack of resources by making props and adapting things from available resources.

A non-standardised evaluation form, completed pre- and post-project, measured the benefits and improvements clients experienced from participating in the project. This combined qualitative and quantitative methods using open-ended questions and Likert scales.

At the end of the finished DVD the clients gave feedback on their reasons for participation and what they perceived as the benefits. Attendance was measured as very high; clients only missed sessions if they clashed with another appointment.

Using Likert scales, clients rated their confidence between 0 and 4 prior to the course and between 7 and 10 afterwards. One of the participants said 'I lost a lot of confidence in my life with issues in the past, but this has made me come out of my shell a bit'. All participants reported an increase in confidence by the end of the course and this was reflected in the development of the story. As rehearsals progressed, the clients offered an insightful portrayal of prison life by incorporating their feelings and experiences, creating a powerful and emotive performance.

Wellbeing was impacted positively for clients with low self-esteem. Through drama they found a voice and shared personal experiences in a safe and creative environment. Due to the practical nature of drama, one group member built self-esteem and confidence, noting 'this could be a big thing as I can't read or write but played a good part in the drama and I'm very happy with this'. At the end of the DVD participants recommended that drama be offered to all prisoners as many have stories to tell but may not be able to write or even talk about them, but could maybe express themselves through drama.

The DVD won the Koestler Awards Renee Cressey Highly Commended Award. The success of the project created a 'buzz' on the healthcare wing with a number of prisoners showing interest in participating. As the groundwork has been done, this will enable future projects to be facilitated more quickly which is vitally important in a remand prison where there is a fast turnover of prisoners.

Although participants were given certificates in recognition of their contribution, it was felt these did not accurately reflect the progress made and skills learnt and developed. Therefore the occupational therapy technician is developing an 'Agored Cymru accreditation'. Although this cannot be awarded retrospectively, it will be in place for future groups.

# Psychoeducational groups

Within the scope of the *Psychological Therapies in Wales Implementation Guidance* (Welsh Government 2012a) occupational therapy is included as a psychologically focused intervention. Part one of the *Mental Health (Wales) Measure* (National Assembly for Wales 2010) is to improve and expand primary care mental health services. As well as assessment, this includes offering a person short-term treatment or support where appropriate. Examples of this include counselling and psychological interventions such as stress management, anxiety management and cognitive behavioural therapy, etc. This could be offered individually or through groupwork. The prison environment is a good opportunity to offer this to a client group who are generally difficult to engage in the community as they are a captive audience. These are interventions which occupational therapists can effectively offer as a part of their core role within the prison environment.

Within HMP Cardiff the occupational therapist uses psychosocial approaches to improve coping skills and life skills and groupwork is an effective way of doing this. Current groups that are being run are anxiety management, anger management and 'living life to the full'. These interventions are currently offered to both primary and secondary care clients, depending on level of need and suitability to attend groups following a risk assessment.

## Barriers

It can be a challenge to facilitate psychoeducational groups within HMP Cardiff due to it being a remand prison and consequently having a high turnover of prisoners. Nevertheless, there is still a core number of clients who do fit the criteria for these interventions and do reside in prison long enough to engage and complete these. It may be that the way groups are run and the interventions offered need to be adapted to meet the needs of the remand prison but this is possible, e.g. rolling groups and providing self-help materials.

Due to lack of staffing, there is only one member of staff available to run groups, and this limits how frequently groups can be run. It also means that, due to the complex client group, group numbers need to be kept low and group size tends to be a maximum of six clients. This limits the number of clients who can complete these interventions.

# One-to-one work

A number of individuals may not be suitable to attend groups and may need interventions on a one-to-one basis, i.e. if they are too high risk or not mentally well enough. Some clients may need one-to-one work to build up their confidence prior to being able to attend groups. Nearing release, the occupational therapist will focus on goal setting and planning for managing in the community and transferring the skills learnt in prison. It has been difficult to facilitate a pre-release group to address this, due to prisoners being from a large catchment area where they would have access to different resources. A high proportion of prisoners are also homeless and do not know their address prior to release.

After three years of fighting for this, the occupational therapist now has access to a kitchen facility which is an invaluable development. Activities of Daily Living (ADLs) and developing cooking skills are a fundamental part of the occupational therapist's role. As well as being vital for the occupational therapist to assess a client's level of ability and amount of support required in the community, a high proportion of clients on the occupational therapists' caseloads have identified having very poor cooking skills and the lack of a kitchen facility has been consistently highlighted as an unmet need. Unfortunately, the occupational therapist is currently limited on how often the kitchen facility can be used as there is not always a second staff member available as is required due to safety policy.

# A role in the community

It is the first couple of weeks following release that is the most difficult period for this client group. They have numerous appointments to attend and issues to sort out, e.g. housing, job centre, probation, etc. Individuals with mental health problems can struggle to cope with the stress and expectations of this initial period which can result in them missing appointments, using substances and being homeless. Intensive support is needed in this initial period to help reduce anxiety, to solve problems and cope with these situations. Occupational therapists are able to assess and identify the mental health issues which are affecting their ability to cope effectively in the community and work with the individual to improve these skills. Following this initial period, occupational therapists can help the clients to structure their time, pursue vocational aspirations, hobbies and interests, work towards their goals and have meaning in their lives, which will ultimately prevent them from returning to substances, crime and prison.

The Centre for Mental Health (2011) has shown that there is poor continuity of care both into and out of prison. There are reports that CMHTs are reluctant to accept responsibility for released prisoners. While clients are in prison there is a real opportunity to be able to engage with them and build a rapport while they are not using substances or involved in a chaotic lifestyle. However, CMHTs have little contact with their clients while they are in prison. This is a missed opportunity to be able to start working with these individuals. One difficulty with this though is that the prison covers a large catchment area and some CMHTs may be based a couple of hours away.

At HMP Cardiff, it was agreed that the occupational therapist could continue to work with a select number of clients for a set period of time following release. Occupational therapists can access community resources and use a 'hands on' approach to reintegrate clients back into the community. This would be for a handover period to the CMHT or to continue with some of the occupational therapy goals for those who do not have a community occupational therapist. This role is vital to continue the work started in prison and to support clients to transfer these skills into practice in the community. The Prolific and Priority Offender

(PPO) scheme (Box 5.3) highlights the benefits of occupational therapists working with this client group in the community.

## Box 5.3: Case study – secondment with Prolific and Priority Offender scheme

In 2010 I had the opportunity to work as part of a unique and dynamic project between Abertawe Bro Morgannwg University Health Board and South Wales Probation Trust. This was a time limited pilot scheme offering occupational therapy to individuals who are known to the Prolific and Priority Offender service (PPO) and the Integrated Offender Management cases (IOM).

Research carried out in 2001 concluded that of a total offending population of around one million, only approximately 100,000 offenders (10 per cent of all active offenders) were responsible for half of all the crime committed in England and Wales (Home Office 2001). In other words, it appears that a relatively small number of offenders were far more criminally active than others and contributed disproportionately to the overall crime levels. The most active 5,000 of this group were estimated to be responsible for one in ten offences (Home Office 2002). The National PPO programme aims to tackle this small number of offenders who commit a disproportionately large amount of crime. The PPO scheme is a government initiative that brings a multi-agency approach to the PPO in order to reduce offending.

Funding was sourced through Swansea Bay Partnership Deprived Areas Fund (DAF). Initially the project was funded for 12 months; however due to delays in this being set up, it only ran for approximately seven months. The occupational therapy team consisted of a band 7 and a band 6 occupational therapist and a band 4 technical instructor, all on secondment.

The majority of PPOs have substance misuse problems, chaotic lifestyles, no fixed abode, mental health problems, poor education, poor occupational histories and deprived backgrounds. Offending is seen as a culturally acceptable occupation within this client group in order for them to support their substance misuse or lifestyle choices.

A key effective strategy was being able to offer support prior to and following release from prison, enabling a seamless service. This was beneficial in enabling occupational therapists to engage with clients and build rapport and therapeutic relationships whilst they were relatively clean from illicit substances, and stated they were motivated to change/ engage. It gave us the opportunity to develop coping skills in preparation for release, increase and maintain motivation for community work, and support in planning and setting goals. Some assessments were completed in prison allowing for forward planning and goal setting. From evaluation it was noted that there was a greater/longer engagement with clients who had been seen in prison prior to release rather than those first seen in the community.

Evaluation of the project was difficult due to the short length of time the project had been running. Nevertheless, the evaluation highlighted the key areas that the occupational therapy team effectively assisted clients with, including: assisting clients to engage with other services such as health services and substance misuse services; coping skills work such as anxiety and anger management; attending courses, voluntary work or gaining employment (some for the first time); being supported with maintaining or gaining housing; reducing offending; assistance with benefits claims; and independent living and work skills. It should be noted that this was in collaboration with other agencies within the PPO scheme.

Although other agencies such as probation also look at a lot of these areas, the occupational therapy approach differs and has been found to complement the work of these other agencies. A key difference in the occupational therapy role from others has been the more 'hands on' approach and flexibility to see clients in many different environments. Unique to occupational therapy has been the assessment of the underlying areas of dysfunction that is often hidden and the assessment of the client's level of ability. It has also been the ability to use graded approaches and to offer intensive support when required that has proved positive.

Another key reason highlighted for differences in how clients engage with occupational therapists, in contrast to the police and probation, is because they are not forced to engage with an occupational therapist. It is voluntary and is not a condition or part of any licence or contract. A lot of clients with antisocial attitudes can find it hard to accept this sort of support from the police or probation. Some clients commented that they felt they could trust occupational therapists more and be more honest with us because of this.

Evaluation questionnaires for both other professionals working within the PPO scheme and the clients themselves were disseminated. Several clients stated that this is the longest period they have managed to stay out of prison and they would not have been able to do that without occupational therapy. It would have been useful for this to have been part of a research project and would definitely be an area where the impacts and the benefits of occupational therapy in this area would prove a useful area to be researched.

# Challenges for occupational therapists working in HMP Cardiff

## Low levels of staffing

Currently the qualified occupational therapist spends clinical time engaging in activities that could be completed by the technical instructor. However, there is not enough technical instructor time to be able to delegate these tasks as she is only part-time. This includes some one-to-one sessions for clients unsuitable for groups as well as administrative duties such as group preparation, photocopying and ordering resources. There is also a high demand for groupwork but the occupational therapy team is limited in how many can be run due to time constraints. Having additional support staff time would free the occupational therapist up to do more occupational therapy-specific assessments and interventions, reports and community follow-up work.

## Lone working

Working in the prison is a challenging environment with a complex client group; this can be hard in such an isolated role. Although the inreach team is supportive, it is important to maintain support and contact with the occupational therapy profession. This is achieved through having regular monthly supervision with the head occupational therapist and additional peer supervision. There is also the opportunity to attend Professional Development Groups (PDGs). In addition the occupational therapist attends senior occupational therapists' meetings to keep up to date with other service developments and have team support. There are also in-house training sessions and journal clubs regularly held. It is also important to network with occupational therapists working in other prisons to build a support network and share ideas and practice.

## Continual changes to prison regime/wing functions

For example, Cardiff prison did have a lifer wing with prisoners serving life or Indeterminate for Public Protection (IPP) sentences. However, in 2014 HMP Cardiff changed this function and no longer holds a high number of lifer or IPP population. Consequently, this has resulted in a higher number of remand and shorter stay prisoners who form a less stable population, increasing the demand for occupational therapy input. This shows how occupational therapists need to continually adapt to meet the changing needs and functions of the prison.

As well as the changes to the overall prison population, there have been a number of changes to prison regime in recent years. Last year the regime was changed so that prisoners could only work or attend education for half a day on Monday to Friday, as opposed to full days. This consequently had an impact on clients' mental health and an increased demand for occupational therapy and additional groups (particularly activity-based). Inreach clients became increasingly anxious as they were struggling to cope with the additional isolation time, as well as a lowering of mood due to having less distraction and time to engage in purposeful and meaningful activity.

The prison regime changed again with *New Ways of Working*. This is a benchmarking programme under which the budgets of public sector prisons are to be driven down to match selected private sector jails. The purpose is to contribute to the further efficiencies of public prisons and to optimise the effective delivery of services (Ministry of Justice 2013). The implementation of this saw the introduction of a new 'core' day to standardise the time spent by prisoners out of their cells with increased time in work. This was seen as beneficial as it meant our clients had more opportunity to engage in occupations for longer in the day. However, this change meant that team members needed to revise working hours in order to fit in with the new regime.

## Environmental factors

When the occupational therapist came into post there was a holding cell, consultation room and group room in healthcare solely available for the inreach team to use. However, the prison decided they needed these rooms to serve another purpose and this was knocked through and changed into a staff dojo training room. As this room was only going to be used once a month it was agreed that occupational therapy staff could still use it for some sessions such as relaxation and drama. However, once completed this was no longer agreed due to risk issues. This meant the only group room available was now a shared resource and occupational therapy was not allowed to put anything on the walls such as clients' work to enhance the therapeutic milieu.

## Lack of suitable rooms on the wing

There are no suitable rooms to see clients on the wings. Some wings have no rooms at all; one has a room which is like a cupboard and overheated; others allow you to use the office where you get interrupted; on others there are rooms referred to as 'goldfish bowls' as they have windows all the way around with people walking past and looking in. If there are no rooms available you can sit with prisoners on the wing landing. None of these options are therapeutic or confidential environments and it would also not be possible to carry out any interventions in these rooms.

## Lack of a movements officer

There has been an ongoing drive with inreach for many years to have a movements officer and/or clinic slots. This would be an officer who collects prisoners from the wing to bring them over to healthcare for either one-to-one or group sessions. There are already movement officers in place who collect prisoners for other health appointments such as the GP, dentist, optician, etc. However, there was no agreement with the partnership board for mental health services to have access to this facility. Eventually, after the occupational therapist had been in post for two years, it was agreed for inreach to have two slots in a week, which was later increased to three. This meant that occupational therapy could run groups or have one-to-one sessions at this time in healthcare and clients would be escorted over.

Outside these slots, in order for the occupational therapist to see patients in healthcare, the occupational therapist has to collect a prison radio prior to escorting the patients over. This process can take half an hour pre- and post-session for individual sessions and longer when collecting a group. Also having a prison radio can affect the therapeutic relationship which occupational therapists strive to build. The technical instructor is not allowed to escort at all due to prison policy and in order for the technical instructor to carry out any interventions in healthcare, the occupational therapist would have to use clinical time to escort the clients.

Due to there being no prison officer present, groups have to be limited to very small numbers in order to manage risks. As a consequence some clients would also be excluded from attending occupational therapy sessions due to their risk levels being too high with no officer in the vicinity.

## Punishment versus rehabilitation

Working in the prison environment is difficult. Engaging with officers and improving their understanding of mental health difficulties is vitally important. For example, one client with Attention Deficit Hyperactivity Disorder (ADHD) was continually receiving written warnings and being on basic regime for not following staff instructions. Consequently, being in this confined environment and bored for this length of time made his mental health worse and his behaviour was more problematic when out of cell. Occupational therapy worked with staff to understand his difficulties and they became more understanding and lenient. The occupational therapist provided him with in-cell activities to keep him occupied when locked in the cell – he loved card making and matching. This helped him to get off basic regime and progress through the prison system.

## Development of an occupational therapy materials budget

When an occupational therapist was first in post there was no budget allocated. This meant that there was very limited choice in the groups that could be run due to the limited resources available. This did not enable individualised client-centred practice. A key part of the occupational therapy role is to encourage clients to engage in in-cell activities to distract from anxiety, depression and self-harming thoughts. Resources were needed in order to be able to purchase items to loan out, e.g. art materials, wordsearch books. A valuable skill of the occupational therapist is to be resourceful where possible. It was possible to run an art group due to the occupational therapist finding resources such as paint that were no longer being used since the ending of day care facilities. The occupational therapist also liaised with the education department and was given some old guitars that were no longer being used over there to start a music group. A guitar loaning service was also developed so that prisoners could borrow guitars to use in cell. The occupational therapist also printed off wordsearches and pictures from the internet for in-cell activities. After writing a case and lots of negotiations an occupational therapy materials budget was agreed which has improved the occupational therapist service greatly.

## Box 5.4: Case study – life choices changes

### Background

A 25-year-old man was serving an IPP sentence in Swansea prison which meant he had a minimum tariff to serve before being eligible to apply to the parole board for release. He had an 18 month tariff and had already been in prison for three and half years (two years over his tariff). His current offence was committing actual bodily harm and he had had numerous convictions and been in and out of prison since the age of 15.

He had a diagnosis of Borderline Personality Disorder (BPD) with associated anxiety and depression. He had also previously had a diagnosis of Attention Deficit Hyperactivity Disorder (ADHD) and was a prolific self-harmer with additional substance misuse issues.

Funding had been applied for transfer to a medium secure personality disorder service but this was declined as it was felt that the prison service should be able to meet his needs. However due to his current level of self-harming and unstable mental health he was not suitable to be transferred to another prison establishment with more specialist services to meet his needs, such as a prison with a therapeutic community.

## Occupational identity

He had numerous interests such as: sports, football (watching and playing), poetry, art, painting, gardening, woodwork, computer games. He highly valued his family, animals and helping others.

## Occupational competence

He had difficulty dealing with relationships and struggled to trust people. He had fluctuating moods from low to elated, became easily frustrated and had difficulty controlling his anger. He had fluctuating concentration/attention span and difficulty dealing with stress/anxiety. He used self-harm as a coping mechanism. He had poor ADL abilities due to lack of opportunities. He had low self-esteem and did not recognise his positive qualities such as being very talented at sports and quick to learn, and being creative and skilled in poetry and art. He had a good sense of humour and was well liked; he also enjoyed helping others.

## Environmental impact

He was unable to hold down a job or education in the prison and excluded from safer custody groups due to his behaviour. Consequently he was locked up for long periods, had poor structure and routine, limited opportunities to engage in interests and struggled with boredom. He was unable to get away from people he did not like and was increasingly self-harming to release frustrations. This self-harming also restricted him from being allowed to participate in activities he enjoyed such as football.

## Role of occupational therapy

To increase his structure and routine through starting to attend occupational therapy groups – art and creative writing. He was supported with having a decorating job in healthcare and given trust and respect as well as being provided with in-cell activities for distraction. The occupational therapist liaised with gym staff who gave him a helping role when he was unable to engage in sports. He also had a regular one-to-one slot to engage in anxiety/anger/relaxation/DBT skills, as well as working on ADL skills by attending cooking sessions.

## Benefits

Reduced self-harming. Previously the hospital were refusing to operate as he was repeatedly continuing to replace objects after their removal. After six months of no self-harming the hospital agreed they would operate to remove items from his arm. He had improved behaviour and no adjudications or written warnings for a year. Outcomes included increased confidence, self-esteem, and positive results for work and leisure. He received a Koestler award for poetry he had written and gained an Open College Network (OCN) qualification for his decorating work.

# Key similarities with other fields of work

A lot of students and staff can be put off from working in the prison as they picture the client group as being high risk. However, the majority of clients would not meet the criteria for specialist forensic community teams and would be under standard CMHTs prior to and on release from prison. In a lot of ways the prison is similar to working with clients in a CMHT. This is because the prison has its mainstream activities such as work, education and gym, and the role of occupational therapy would be to support and enable clients to be able to engage in their community.

Certain areas of the prison may be more similar to inpatient ways of working. For example, some individuals located in healthcare may be acutely unwell and awaiting transfer to hospital. Therefore, the occupational therapist may start work with them which would be similar to what occupational therapists would continue within the receiving hospital. Working with individuals on the therapeutic landing is also similar to working on a rehabilitation ward environment. Individuals are not acutely unwell but are vulnerable and have poor independent living skills. They need rehabilitation from occupational therapy staff, wing staff and workshop staff to help learn and develop skills similar to a rehabilitation setting.

# Challenges for students

The occupational therapist does take students in the prison. This, though, is more difficult than in other settings as students require extra prison vetting before being able to start a prison placement. This means that the placement needs a lot of coordination in advance. There are many environmental issues which need to be overcome due to it being a locked environment. Students are not able to have keys and consequently have to permanently rely on other staff to get anywhere or do things. This can make it hard for them to plan their own time and manage a caseload. There is a dearth of literature in this field and this makes it hard for students to research into prison occupational therapy practice. There are a lot of prison policies and procedures to contend with, as well as the usual NHS protocols.

# Opportunities for students

Despite these challenges it is a unique and invaluable experience for students. There are very limited opportunities to gain any forensic jobs at band 5 level, and there are currently no band 5 occupational therapists in prisons in Wales. Being able to gain this experience as a student will help anyone with an interest in this field. The student experience will always be very varied with the whole range of mental health conditions, from primary to secondary care, and clients being supported at all stages along their recovery journey. With limited access to community resources the occupational therapists are also very holistic and need to address physical occupational needs on a regular basis.

## Key skills required to work in this setting

Adaptability and patience are essential. For example, you could have a session planned and then be informed that the prison is on stand still roll check. This means that the prison has been unable to account for all its prisoners. If this happens no one is allowed to go anywhere that involves passing through a locked gate or door until the missing prisoners have been found. This means that you would not be able to take prisoners to a group and your group would come to an end.

It is also important to have strong occupational therapy values, promote the unique role of occupational therapy in this setting, and not get drawn into too much generic work, particularly keeping the focus on occupations and groupwork. In order to achieve this you need to be proactive, such as in procuring suitable group rooms and facilities you can use around the prison. As previously mentioned, it is important to 'think outside the box' in how you can access equipment and resources with a limited budget. It is important to be resilient and not give up as things take a long time to get sorted in this environment. If you have the skills to overcome the barriers, it is a rewarding environment to work in with positive outcomes.

## Conclusion

The role of the inreach teams has continued to develop and change over the 13 years they have been in existence. The ever changing landscape of the prisons and changes to policies and legislation have made it a challenge for occupational therapists to establish their role. This chapter has outlined the valuable and unique role that occupational therapy has to offer working with this client group and the positive impact this can have. Occupational therapists working in prison settings need to continue to offer student placements in order to develop enthusiasm and drive to work in this area. Prison occupational therapy would benefit from further research to evidence the effectiveness of their role and follow-on community work is a particular area where research could be conducted.

# Useful resources

- OT News **19** (1), (2011) has a feature practice section on prisons entitled *Prison inreach: focus on occupational therapists delivering mental health services in prisons.*

- *OT News* **24** (6), (2016) has a feature section on occupational therapy in prison services.

- There is a Forensic Forum which is a sub-group of the College of Occupational Therapists' Specialist Section Mental Health. In 2012 this group published and launched COT Practice Guidelines for occupational therapists working in secure hospitals. This publication is an evidence-based resource to support occupational therapists working with adults in secure settings. It provides a practice guideline with recommendations for those occupational therapists currently working in this speciality, as well as offering a useful reference document for students. Although this does not include prison, it is a useful and relevant resource. The College of Occupational Therapists (2012) *Occupational Therapists' use of Occupation-Focused Practice in Secure Hospitals. Practice Guidelines.* London: COT.

- There is a Forensic Occupational Therapy Group on Yahoo which enables occupational therapists working in forensic care to network with each other and share ideas on research, clinical practice, CPD and other professional issues. There have been National Forensic Occupational Therapists conferences held yearly and other additional events held sporadically. In 2013 Staffordshire held a Regional and National Occupational Therapists Prison Inreach Service Conference, 'Few and far between'.

# References

Baron, K., Kielhofner, G., Iyenger, A., Goldhammer, V. & Wolenski, J. (2006). *Occupational Self Assessment (OSA), Version 2.2.* Chicago: University of Illinois.

Centre for Mental Health (2011). *Mental Health Care and the Criminal Justice System.* London: Centre for Mental Health.

College of Occupational Therapists (2012). *Scottish Prison Service: Women in Custody – a Consultation Response from the College of Occupational Therapists.* London: COT.

Creek, J. & Lougher, L. (2008). *Occupational Therapy in Mental Health.* 4th edn. Edinburgh: Churchill Livingstone Elsevier.

Curran, A. & Wilkinson, C. (2010). *Development of Regional Forensic Mental Health Occupational Therapy Services.* Belfast: Northern Ireland Occupational Therapy Managers Forum.

Department of Health (1999). *National Service Framework for Mental Health.* London: TSO.

Department of Health (2001). *Changing the Outlook: A Strategy for Developing and Modernising Mental Health Services in Prisons.* London: TSO.

Fieldhouse, J. (2003). The impact of an allotment group on mental health clients' health, wellbeing and social networking. *British Journal of Occupational Therapy* **66** (7), 286–296.

Forsyth, K., Deshpanade, S., Kielhofner, G., Henriksson, C., Haglund, L., Olson, L., Skinner, S. & Kulkarni, S. (2005). *The Occupational Circumstances Assessment Interview and Rating Scale (OCAIRS), Version 4.0.* Chicago: University of Illinois.

Home Office (2001). *Criminal Justice: The Way Ahead.* London: TSO.

Home Office (2002). *Justice for All. Government White Paper.* London: TSO.

Kielhofner, G. (2008). *Model of Human Occupation: Theory and Application*, 4th edn. Philadelphia: Lippincott, Wilkins and Williams.

Ministry of Justice (2013). *Freedom of Information Request.* http:www.gov.uk (last accessed 13.2.2016).

Molineux, M. & Whiteford, G. (1999). Prisons: from occupational deprivation to occupational enrichment. *Journal of Occupational Science* **6** (3), 124–130.

National Assembly for Wales (2001). *Improving Health for Wales: a Plan for the NHS with its Partners.*

http://www.wales.nhs.uk/Publications/NHSStrategydoc.pdf (last accessed: 14.10.2016).

National Assembly for Wales (2010). *Mental Health (Wales) Measure 2010.* http://www.assemblywales.org (last accessed: 2.1.2016).

Parkinson, S., Forsyth, K. & Kielhofner, G. (2006). *The Model of Occupation Screening Tool (MOHOST), Version 2.0.* Chicago: University of Illinois.

Prisoner Ombudsman for Northern Ireland (2011). *Summary and Issues of Concern Raised in the Report into the Circumstances Surrounding the Death of Allyn James Baxter.* Belfast: PONI.

Public Health Wales (2013). *Prison Health Needs Assessment: Thematic Review 2013: Mental Health Needs and Provision across the Welsh Prison Estate.* Public Health Wales NHS Trust.

United Kingdom Parliament (2014). *The Care Act.* London: TSO.

Welsh Government (2006). *Prison Mental Health Pathway.* http://www.wales.gov.uk (last accessed: 14.2.2016).

Welsh Government (2010). *Delivering the Care Programme Approach in Wales Interim Policy Implementation Guidance.* http://www.wales.gov.uk (last accessed: 14.2.2016).

Welsh Government (2012a). *Psychological Therapies in Wales Implementation Guide.* http://www.wales.gov.uk (last accessed: 14.2.2016).

Welsh Government (2012b). *Together for Mental Health and Wellbeing in Wales.* http://www.wales.gov.uk (last accessed: 14.2.2016).

Welsh Government (2012c). *Together for Mental Health: Delivery Plan 2012–16.* http://www.wales.gov.uk (last accessed: 14.2.2016).

Welsh Government (2014). *Consultation Document, Policy Implementation Guidance: Mental Health Services for Prisoners in Wales Consultation Document.* http://www.wales.gov.uk (last accessed: 14.2.2016).

Welsh Government (2014). *The Social Services and Wellbeing (Wales) Act.* http://www.legislation.gov.uk (last accessed: 10.7.2016).

Whiteford, G. (2000). Occupational deprivation: global challenge in the new millennium. *British Journal of Occupational Therapy* **63** (5), 200–204.

# Chapter 6

# Social groups within an intensive mental health team, and creative methods for evaluating the service

## Hazel Bryce

## Introduction

This chapter discusses the usefulness of social groups for people with severe and enduring mental health problems, taking as example certain groups facilitated by Sheffield outreach team (SORT) in collaboration with other partners.

The chapter explores:

- the key value base, including Recovery principles and strengths-based practice
- the continuously changing and developing roles of the group facilitator
- a member's view of how his role has changed through becoming a volunteer
- the consumption of alcohol during groups
- the relationships between these groups and social enterprises, together with perceived challenges
- the creative evaluation of interventions.

It is hoped that readers will feel encouraged to devise novel solutions to the challenges discussed, and to revise their perceptions of what data may be recorded as 'knowledge'.

# Key points

● As occupational therapists we have the challenge of how not just to work towards risk management and maintenance but to instil hope and optimism.

● As a facilitator in a social group you will have many roles to potentially adopt and draw upon at any time. It is essential to recognise the pull from your many roles and the effect that this is having on group dynamics.

● Use of volunteers can help to redefine the relationship between service users and staff, and help to shift ways of working from 'us and them' to more of a collaborative approach.

● It is increasingly necessary to work with other services and share resources and form partnerships with other organisations which can provide services through social care budgets rather than seeing the NHS as sole providers.

● Art exhibitions and other visual displays can be seen as a form of knowledge production. They can generate knowledge that can be used alongside other information gained from more traditional forms of research and evaluations, such as questionnaires and interviews.

# Introduction to Sheffield outreach team

Sheffield outreach team is an intensive community mental health team which has developed over time from an assertive outreach model. The team aims to provide a high level of support, working with service users according to Recovery principles. It offers an intensive service to people who have complex mental health needs and a primary diagnosis of psychosis, usually with chaotic lifestyles and a history of numerous admissions to hospital. Sheffield outreach team has been in operation for over ten years and has roughly 160 service users. Staffing consists of the team's own consultant psychiatrist and five support workers, plus 16 care coordinators from a variety of professional backgrounds including social work, psychiatric nursing, and occupational therapy (the occupational therapists have a reduced caseload to allow for the facilitation of the groups).

Working in a service for those with severe and enduring mental health needs provides the challenge of focusing not just on risk management and maintenance of individuals, but how to instil hope and optimism in users of the service. This means working with users towards their own goals and aspirations, a fundamental principle of occupational therapy (e.g. Sumsion 1999). This aligns itself to the Recovery approach, which is about hope and finding a way to live a meaningful and productive life alongside having severe mental health difficulties. It is about making sure that people, no matter what their diagnosis, have the opportunity to do things that they enjoy and enhance their lives.

# Strengths Approach

The groups in SORT are facilitated according to the Strengths Approach as defined by Ryan and Morgan (2004). The Strengths Approach focuses on and prioritises working with users' strengths and values, and what they want to work on, rather than focusing on managing medication and risk.

The seven principles of the Strengths-Based Approach are:

1. The focus of the helping process is upon the service user's strengths, interests, abilities and capabilities, not upon their deficits, weaknesses or problems.

2. All service users have the capacity to learn, grow and change.

3. The 'service users–assertive outreach' relationship becomes a primary and essential partnership.

4. The service user is viewed as the director of the helping process.

5. Continuity and acceptance are essential foundations for promoting Recovery.

6. The helping process takes on an outreach perspective.

7. The local neighbourhood is viewed as a source of potential resources rather than as an obstacle; natural neighbourhood resources should be considered before segregated mental health services.

(Ryan & Morgan 2004, p. 52).

From the principles above it can be seen how this approach aligns itself with occupational therapy and Recovery philosophy. It is full of hope and optimism and about working with service users' strengths and aspirations to produce meaningful lives. The seven principles can be used to map and guide the development of the groups, and as a checklist to see if they are still being run according to strengths approach principles.

# Applying the principles

The Monday group can be used as an example of application of the above principles. The group has developed over time; it started with a social group which was meeting every Monday with the aim of visiting areas of interest in the locality. The same community location and time is used every week to provide consistency, and this is midday at the local leisure centre café. This venue allows people to come and go as they please in a fluid, natural manner, and it is easily accessible by public transport. We always aim to have a drink together and gather before we carry out our activity, and this allows people to join us for the drink but not for the activity if they so prefer. We recognise that not everyone will want to do all the activities, so anyone can stay for all or part of a session (as long as they have sufficient leave if subject to the Mental Health Act 1983/2007). The group uses community resources and public transport wherever possible. A list of the activities that we are going to do is produced in advance and posted to people's homes, enabling people to plan their attendance. Examples include: a walk in the peak district, a walk in the park, a picnic, a pub meal, cinema visit, a trip to a local town centre. The activities incorporate suggestions from group members, taking into account their aspirations. This means that the range of activities is constantly changing depending on who is attending the group at any given time.

# Mental capital and wellbeing

The Government Office for Science's review *Mental Capital and Wellbeing: Making the most of ourselves in the 21st century* (2008) was produced after critiquing a wealth of research. It concludes that five things can help lead to increased wellbeing in the population. These are illustrated in Box 6.1, together with their application to the Monday group. All five can be used as tools to reflect and measure the activities in which people participate, leading to ideas of how to increase wellbeing both for individuals and for communities.

## Box 6.1: Five ways to wellbeing

**Connect...**

With the people around you. The Monday group allows each person the opportunity to connect with other group members and members of the public whom we encounter during the activities (for example, during a bus ride or when bowling).

**Be active...**

The Monday group always involves some form of activity even if this is just walking to the bus stop. It also gives people a chance to try new activities, such as walking, and gives suggestions regarding places to go.

**Take notice...**

Be curious. Catch sight of the beautiful. Remark on the unusual. Savour the moment. Be aware of the world around you and what you are feeling. This happens through talking about the activities and encouraging people to take notice when out and about. Reflecting on experiences helps people to appreciate what matters to them, and, in consequence, more key activities can be scheduled in.

**Keep learning...**

Try something new, or rediscover an old interest. The Monday group is all about this; we promote trying other people's passions as they just might become your own.

**Give...**

This is about doing things for others. We have found that, as the people in the group become more familiar with each other, they start helping each other out. This could be lending a book, or sharing a recommendation, or talking about how they have overcome a difficulty in their lives.

# The development of groups

The Monday group was the first group that was established. From this, other groups emerged, as members wanted to explore activities and interests that could not be accommodated in the Monday group. The development of new groups comes from shared passions and interests, as all members (including staff) get to know each other. There needs to be a fit between the passions of the worker and those of the service users. (For example, I think gardening is a good activity but I do not get inspired by it; as this is an activity that my colleague really enjoys, it makes sense for him rather than me to facilitate a gardening group.) The groups can be considered as a dynamic ever changing programme, with the focus and content shifting to keep pace as people's lives change and they develop different aspirations.

Here is a brief outline of the current groups, to give an idea of what SORT is facilitating at the time of writing.

- Weekly Monday group: this is a social out-and-about group, meeting at midday at the leisure centre café and then going to visit a local attraction using public transport.
- Weekly Tuesday allotment group: we have an allotment where people can help to grow produce or just enjoy the good view, social company and cup of tea. Our allotment volunteer maintains the allotment throughout the year for us.
- Weekly spirituality session: a couple of service users attend a church in town for a 'pause for thought' lunchtime reflection.
- Weekly Thursday exercise group: we meet at the leisure centre café for the afternoon. Some people chat and socialise whilst others play badminton, go to the gym or swim.
- Weekly Friday jam session: service users throughout the Trust meet and jam together at a local studio.
- Fortnightly women's group: planned social activities.
- Monthly evening meal for women: in a local pub or restaurant.
- Monthly evening meal: a different group of people, this time mixed, meet in a pub or restaurant.
- Monthly 'Sunray': this happens as part of the exercise group. A service user is paid to come and tell the group what is happening about service user involvement throughout the wider NHS Trust.
- Yearly respite stay: we facilitate three week-long respite stays in a caravan park. The amount of support provided in each of these varies as members progress towards Recovery. The first is heavily staffed, progressing to the last one having very minimal staff input.

Sheffield outreach team and the mental health recovery ward in Sheffield have been combining resources and sharing some of their groups. Many of the service users who are on the recovery ward will at some time have contact with SORT, and for service users on the recovery ward, having increased opportunities in the community is good. This model of shared resources is a model that we are looking to expand.

Over time a shift has been noticed, as group members have been taking more ownership of the groups. The culture has been developed that these are shared groups and not owned by the occupational therapists who facilitate, and the development has been aided by joining with other partners such as the recovery ward. This is part of a journey, with all taking time to adjust to the shift in power dynamics. The groups have moved from being solely occupational therapist-led to adopting a model of co-production, recognising each person's expertise and knowledge.

The journey is a continuous one, with values and norms being redefined and adapted as new members join the groups, and others leave. Group members are increasingly having a greater say in the day to day running, but as yet are not as involved in wider decision making affecting the groups.

With time it is hoped to involve group members in any development discussions, and an ideal opportunity to do this would be for people to have an opportunity to be involved in annual reviews.

# My experience of the role of facilitator

Personal experience as the group facilitator and occupational therapist in the SORT groups sometimes led to my feeling pulled in many directions. Was I a participant taking part in bowling, a facilitator being aware of what everyone was doing, or a care coordinator listening to individuals' concerns and triumphs? In reality I fulfil all these roles to varying degrees within the group. To consider this and understand the dynamic, insider/outsider positions can be used (Coghlan & Casey 2001, Corbin-Dwyer & Buckle 2009, Humphrey 2007, McCulloch 2008). Insider/outsider positions are sometimes presented as a dichotomy where a researcher is either an insider or an outsider in relation to their research (McCulloch 2008), or in this case to the group that they facilitate. This did not make sense for the group facilitator role in the group, as I occupied multiple identities that simultaneously made me an insider and an outsider. I was an insider as I took part in the group activity and had become part of the fabric of the group, but at the same time an outsider as I am employed as a mental health professional and not a service user.

Corbin-Dwyer & Buckle (2009) argue that we can perhaps only ever occupy the space in between the insider/outsider role. This means that, due to our position as both facilitators and participants in the group, we are neither an outsider nor an insider. We may be closer to the insider or closer to the outsider position.

Our perspective is shaped by our position, which as occupational therapists includes having completed a university degree, being paid, and having statutory responsibilities. I was aware of this gap in knowledge and roles between the group members and myself; I could never be a full group member. Initially I chose to position myself closer to the outside, but then journeyed towards an insider position. This happened as I got to know the strengths and aspirations of the group members and they got to know mine; it consequently allowed me to feel more a part of the group and move towards more shared decision making.

I would suggest that the position of the group facilitator is not static, but changes and develops throughout the group.

Humphrey (2007) refers to being both an insider and outsider in her research on self-organised groups among black people, disabled people, and lesbians and gay men within trade unions in Britain. She talks about journeying between the different life worlds, which she terms as 'activating the hyphen between insider-outsider'. By taking control of this 'hyphen', I am defining my own identity within the group. An example of one way in which I negotiated my own identity is by going to the gym and completing a workout alongside other group members. This identified me as the same as the other group members exercising in the gym. Initially I situated myself as group facilitator talking to members in the café area and encouraging them to participate in activity. Then I went to the gym but exercised alongside the group members before finally exercising on separate machines. At other times group members pushed me towards the outsider position as a mental health professional by asking questions about meetings, or about their medication.

Coffey (1999), describing fieldwork, suggests that identities are managed, crafted and shaped by the dialectic between the researcher and the researched. This applies to groups, where the identities of all group members including the facilitators are influenced by each other.

Thus as a facilitator in a social group you will have many roles to potentially adopt and draw upon at any time. It is essential to recognise the pull on you from your many roles and the effect that this is having on group dynamics. Once you have recognised this, you can choose to take control of this unique ever changing in-between space that you occupy.

# Communication

The acronym 'CUE' can be used as a guide to encouraging good communication:

## C: Connecting

- through eye contact, touch, conversation, and action
- relatives and friends with the life of the individual
- with the community and outside world

## U: Understanding the person's life

- past and present

## E: Encouraging

- conversation
- getting out and about and physical activity
- normal everyday activities.

Adapted from the *Living Well in Care Homes Tool Kit* (College of Occupational Therapists 2013, p. 10).

## Example of communication

The recovery ward has support workers who attend the groups when needed. These workers are often only used to working in a restrictive environment. They may be slowly moving towards adopting Recovery principles in their everyday practice, but this change takes time and needs to be modelled to workers and reinforced through supervision and training. Sometimes this is obvious, as illustrated in the example (see Box 6.2).

### Box 6.2: Supervision case study

> John, a staff member, has been asked to come with service user Jenny to the exercise group. The group usually get the bus down to the leisure centre, but John thinks this is a waste of time when he could order a taxi. On arrival at the leisure centre, John sits with Jenny at a different table from the rest of the group. He wears his NHS name badge so all can identify that he is a worker. John does not know what to talk to Jenny about and so both look bored and awkward. He buys Jenny a drink, rather than encouraging her to buy her own. He does not let Jenny out of his sight and stands with her whilst she has a cigarette.

Thankfully this experience is rare now, with all workers understanding the ethos and values of the groups. We have found that some workers, who are not familiar with operating in a relaxed Recovery-focused way with service users, may require more direction. Often, getting the worker engaged in an activity such as playing badminton is much more successful than asking the worker simply to be with the group. If any staff member seems to be uncomfortable in the group situation, using a prop can help – for example, having a newspaper with articles to discuss.

# Types of volunteers

To support the running of the groups we have used volunteers in a variety of capacities. This section highlights some of the potential roles that volunteers can play: the volunteers may adopt several of these roles or move between these roles at different times, as part of their Recovery journey if they have previously been service users.

People apply to the NHS Trust to become a volunteer; this can be a lengthy process, as volunteers have to attend NHS Trust induction and have vetting and a Disclosure and Barring Service (DBS) check done. On the positive side, once checks are completed, volunteers gain access to a wealth of training and resources, and opportunities to apply for paid jobs within the Trust. These volunteers may have been service users themselves, past students who want to continue working with SORT, or members of the public who want to gain experience of working in mental health. Volunteers mainly take part in the group activities and liaise between service users and staff. They are unpaid but have their expenses reimbursed. (Our allotment volunteer is essential to the running of the group as she maintains the allotment between the scheduled group sessions.)

In addition, there is a facility to provide financial remuneration to service users who carry out specific forms of identified NHS work. This is through the 'service user appreciation scheme'. Service users who are registered with this scheme can be paid to attend formal meetings, and one person is also paid to produce a monthly flier. To register on this scheme people are first interviewed at the Citizens Advice Bureau (CAB) to ensure that they understand the financial restrictions attached to the work; individuals can usually earn a small amount a week without affecting their benefits.

Use of volunteers can help to redefine the relationship between service users and staff, and help to shift our ways of working from 'us and them' to more of a collaborative approach. This can be further developed by the creation of opportunities for more permanent paid work, through the creation of peer support worker jobs.

The social enterprises with which we work in partnership have more flexible opportunities for volunteering. Their opportunities include management (via some form of governing committee) or practical help with the work of the particular organisation. Volunteering through social enterprises can be more flexible than it is within the NHS, as their volunteering systems and procedures are easier to access.

## Box 6.3: Interview with volunteer

Mark, who is both a service user with SORT and a volunteer on the recovery ward, shares his experiences.

Mark started off as a group member and now acts as a volunteer.

Q: What made you want to volunteer with SORT?

A: *I wanted to expand my horizons, to be useful, and help people.*

Q: What are the challenges about volunteering with SORT? What was your initial voluntary position?

A: *Initially I tried to volunteer at the exercise group that I already attended. This did not work because people did not have membership at the gym and did not want to go swimming with me. Then I started volunteering at the recovery ward. I knew some of the service users from the exercise group and through the occupational therapist.*

Q: What works about volunteering with the recovery ward? What do you do?

A: *My role is generally around socialising. I play pool a lot. I come on to the ward and go to the communal areas and chat to people and get involved. I get people involved in what is going on. I also try to support new and existing groups.*

Q: What is good about volunteering on the recovery ward?

A: *People get involved, I know the people from the joint groups. They have welcomed me. I feel confident now. The volunteering has worked around my routine. I am not a morning person so I tend to volunteer in the evening. The role is flexible and when I am not so good I can stay off. The activities fit with who I am and what I like doing.*

Q: What does volunteering mean to you?

A: *Being active.*

Q: How has it changed you?

A: *It has made me more confident and more sociable.*

Q: Where do you see yourself going with it?

A: *Hopefully into a paid job.*

# Alcohol consumption

One of the ongoing and recurring discussions is around the appropriateness of alcohol, and members drinking whilst attending the group. It is important to facilitate the groups using the principles of Recovery, and members' own aspirations. We found that some members wanted to drink alcohol, and it can be an expected cultural norm to drink when out, especially in the evenings. As workers, if we go out for a meal outside working hours and use public transport, we have the option of consuming alcohol, and this should ideally be the same for group members. We wanted our groups to be as natural and normal as possible, but it was not felt appropriate to adopt a 'blanket' approach. For some people, drinking alcohol would not be advisable, as it could lead to a worsening of their mental health conditions or be disruptive to the group dynamic. After much consideration an alcohol agreement was formulated, and this is discussed with, and agreed to, by each service user (see Box 6.4).

## Box 6.4: The alcohol policy

**The policy states:**

It is not the intention to:

- limit the enjoyment of our users
- place demands that are not consistent with social norms.

But the excessive use of alcohol can be detrimental to the health and wellbeing of the users and those in the vicinity.

We ask users to monitor and know their own limits and to stop drinking alcohol especially if:

- It is having an adverse effect on their mental health, such that the user is becoming depressed, suicidal, paranoid, over-anxious.

- It is causing the user to display socially unacceptable behaviours, e.g. being over loud, physically or verbally aggressive, which are affecting other people's enjoyment of the social event.

- The user's drinking is causing him/her not to have adequate control over their actions and judgements, so placing self or others at risk of injury.

- A member of staff, or of the establishment supplying the drinks, requests that a user stops drinking alcohol, and/or leaves the area. We ask that the user please respects this decision and complies.

If excessive drinking continues, the user may be asked to leave the event/service permanently, which may have consequences for attending future SORT activities.

If it is considered that a user has not met the above guidelines, the case will be discussed with the wider team. It may be decided that the user will not be able to return to the event, or attend future SORT events. In extreme cases users will be asked to leave the event and/or abstain from drinking alcohol whilst on SORT events.

Users sign to agree to the guidelines and the consequences of breaking them, as well as receiving information about the NHS guidelines around safe alcohol use.

For those members who require leave to attend the groups as they are under a Mental Health Act (1983/2007) section, whether or not they can consume alcohol is written as part of it.

# Partnership working

Sheffield outreach team has been increasingly forming partnerships with other service areas and third sector organisations. Each sector used to run its own programme, and SORT would refer into other programmes but have no direct input into their running. Working together means that we have been able to pool resources and make better use of community facilities. These groups or activities also act as a bridge between services, which provides extra stability for our groups. The pooled groups are not reliant on a couple of staff, so can continue if, for instance, a staff member is on leave. They also provide more consistency for service users, who benefit from having a service or activity that they can continue to access when they are discharged or are referred from one team to another.

There are challenges to this type of working including: funding, data sharing and recording, letting go of ultimate control and thinking that the paid workers inevitably 'know best'. These new ways of working take time and commitment and can be meeting-heavy initially. As with any new relationship, it takes time to get to know and understand the cultures from which others work and the value bases of their organisations. The process can be helped by recognising and openly acknowledging some of these different values and aims. Creative Arts Steering Team (CAST) is an example and is discussed in Box 6.5. The music project is another example (see Box 6.6).

**Box 6.5: First example – interview with creative arts steering team staff member**

Q: How would you describe CAST?

A: *The creative arts steering team is a group of service users, staff and governors who are interested in promoting the use of arts throughout Sheffield.*

Q: How has it developed?

A: *It started after an art exhibition that was held in the centre of Sheffield. A focus group met to evaluate this. There was a lot of enthusiasm to continue to meet and plan events together and CAST emerged from this.*

Q: What does CAST look like now?

A: *We have a different organisational structure; we come under a social enterprise and charity with a core group of regular organising members. We have our own volunteer system and bank account. We run art and writing workshops which are service user led, we support the artist gatherings (an open mic music and poetry gathering), organise exhibitions and run stalls.*

Q: What has been your journey with CAST?

A: *It grew out of my passion with arts and helping promote service user artists; initially I did this alongside my work as an occupational therapist in SORT. Then I left my work in SORT in order to focus on CAST.*

Q: Since leaving your job as an occupational therapist, how have things changed?

A: *I have more time for CAST, and am more relaxed. When I had to meet more objectives and outcome measures through demands placed on me, it became less organic. There was more conflict and people were more disillusioned. Now I am not working as an occupational therapist I no longer have these pressures. There are objectives to be met to attract funding bids but people see these as more useful. If a SORT service user came to a CAST meeting I felt that I had to document it, and monitor and assess their mental health. Now I do not have clinical responsibility for people which makes things easier. It is a clearer co-production relationship which is better.*

## Box 6.6: Second example – the music project

The music project started out as a SORT activity group; several SORT service users who played musical instruments formed a band which rehearsed and played several gigs. The rehearsals grew into a regular weekly jam session which was financed by the SORT activity budget. Several service users who were not direct SORT service users became involved and the idea grew of forming some sort of project that would provide opportunities for service user musicians to meet, play instruments, network and socialise around music.

The idea of becoming a social enterprise with outside funding was conceived and several service users formed a committee with a constitution. Increased NHS funds were provided to obtain more musical rehearsal time. We began advertising internally for musicians and secured the support of workers from the day service. By this time there were two functioning bands of musicians, the jam session and a committee. Funding was applied for and links were made with the Trust's 'Recovery Enterprises' initiative to help support funding bids. We began supporting the 'Artists Gathering' and facilitated service users producing a show with local gigging bands called the 'Jamboree'.

These bids for funding failed and the local NHS withdrew day services support. As a consequence of service reorganisation/cuts in funding, the committee suffered difficulties and fractured. Currently we retain the jam session once a week, attracting musicians from across the Trust and supporting the artists' gathering and Jamboree.

# Difficulties

Service user involvement on the committee was difficult. There was a requirement by the Trust to register them as volunteers. Service users could be paid expenses through the Trust scheme but many could not see the point of all the paperwork and training. They did not want to travel to the unfamiliar Trust headquarters.

The bidding process was long, and demanded business plans, etc. Some assistance was available but it demanded service user involvement that they did not have the skills to take on.

The gap between big ideas and small starting steps proved too difficult to bridge.

Personality clashes – different ideas about how to develop more sophisticated social skills led to schism.

Lack of Trust support – occupational therapy services did not have time to provide enough support. Initially the Trust were wary of service user-led philosophy.

# What does the future hold?

The development of the groupwork programme as previously described is influenced by the unique mix of the service users and staff, but it is also influenced by the political climate. Occupational therapists and mental health workers need to be aware of the political climate and how this may influence and affect service design and funding. Current considerations include the move towards personalisation, where service users are increasingly able to buy individual care, especially social care services, from within a personal budget. It is increasingly necessary to form partnerships with other organisations which can provide services through social care budgets (such as CAST) rather than seeing the NHS as sole providers.

# Creative evaluation

Over the years SORT have tried numerous ways of gaining and evaluating feedback about our groups. Some methods are shown here, and how successful they have been. Each provides a glimpse into some aspects, functions and experiences of the groups but together they paint a bigger, fuller picture.

## Surveys

We have completed surveys, including both open and closed questions, periodically asking group members about their experiences. We did gain some useful information but found that people were often 'surveyed out' and preferred general conversation. The advantage of a survey meant that all were offered the chance to provide feedback, but it was felt that this method came from the occupational therapist's need for evaluation, rather than group members' desire to give feedback.

## Focus groups

We have completed several focus groups and identified themes that occurred from them. Focus groups can take the form of a discussion in a pub rather than sitting in a room with a tape recorder.

## Six hats

Edward de Bono's 'six thinking hats' (1985) method was used, as this allows a group to explore a topic from a variety of different perspectives in turn (for a description of hats and an example of responses see Box 6.7). This method allows a topic to be explored thoroughly within a short time, and encourages individuals to put their points across. It provides a structure for discussion and encourages a spirit of play which again can encourage participation.

The short timeframe does, however, limit the group in terms of the depth of discussion, and the method necessitates a level of abstract thinking that some service users may find difficult.

**Box 6.7: Evaluation example using the six hats method: evaluating the SORT service user respite stays (holidays)**

**Black hat**: negative judgement/devil's advocate: why will it not work?

- Holidays should be longer.
- The weather was not that good on the last holiday.
- There was only one pub nearby.
- There was nowhere for a pub meal.

**White hat**: information known or needed

- The group have been going away on holidays for four years.
- They have stayed in caravans and youth hostels.
- It was self-catering this year.
- Some service users preferred their own bedroom.

**Green hat**: possibilities, alternatives and new ideas

- Some service users would prefer to go to Butlins next year.
- They would all like to go when the weather is good!
- Two different styles of holidays may be preferred.
- Having a guide like a holiday rep would be a good idea.

**Blue hat**: managing the thinking process

- A choice of different styles of holidays is a possibility.
- This would make it easier for staff (if there were 2–3 separate holiday groups).
- Different rules on each of the holidays need to be observed.
- It depends on the weather.
- The quality of accommodation was a factor, e.g. the cottage was nice last time.

**Yellow hat**: optimism: values and benefits; why will it work?

- The weather is a key factor; it's good when it is sunny!
- More group holidays with variation would be good: holidays in the countryside, near facilities, e.g. shops, country pubs, holidays tailored for particular needs.

- There are still benefits with big groups.
- It is good for holiday groups to be made up of people who get on with each other.
- It was good that there was a wheelchair available for one service user.

Following the groupwork the service users said they had enjoyed previous and recent holidays. They gave the following suggestions as to what would make a successful holiday in the future:

- having a choice and variation of where to go (a choice of different styles of holidays if possible)
- the weather was a key factor (it had to be warm and sunny)
- the accommodation had to be near amenities (such as pubs that provided food, and shops)
- there were still benefits to going away in this group because everyone got on
- the accommodation had to be nice.

The 'six thinking hats' method offered a productive and thorough means of exploring people's views about the SORT holidays, and could be used to evaluate one or a variety of the groups.

## Photovoice

Photovoice is a participatory action research methodology based on health promotion principles, critical consciousness from education, feminist theory, and a community-based approach to documentary photography, which emerged from the work of Wang in the USA (Wang & Burris 1997). It values and shares people's expertise and intimate knowledge of their own communities through the use of photographs, written descriptions and stories which are produced by the participants (Andonian & MacRae 2011).

Photovoice has three broad aims:

1. To record and reflect the community's assets and concerns
2. To discuss issues of importance to the community in large and small groups, promote critical dialogue and produce shared knowledge
3. To reach policy makers.

(Wang & Burris 1997, p. 369)

Photovoice involves a group of individuals meeting together and deciding on a topic or theme that they want to explore and about which they wish to raise awareness. Participants take photographs which are shared and discussed in a group format. Captions are produced by the individuals and the

**100**

group to illustrate and tell the story of the images. The group then decides which photographs and captions are used to form an exhibition. People are invited to see the Photovoice exhibition which, it is hoped, may then influence change. Photovoice has been used in numerous contexts including vulnerable populations (Catalani & Minkler 2009) and mental health communities (Andonian 2010, Fleming *et al.* 2009, Thompson *et al.* 2008).

The theme for the SORT group project was: the experience of participating in social activity groups that were facilitated by the outreach team. People had an interest in taking photos; it was part of their aspirations and so it seemed a natural way to consider the groups. People generally were very positive about this method which is detailed below.

The possibility of doing a Photovoice project together was discussed with other people who had been involved in similar projects. After an initial meeting, a group of five people then met each week for a total of ten sessions. In the first session the nature of Photovoice was discussed, images from the project 'mental wealth' (Brandling & Wall 2009) were viewed, and ground rules were established. A regular meeting venue, time and duration was agreed: using the leisure centre café which was familiar to the participants and conveniently timed to follow on from an exercise group.

The second session covered the ethical use of the camera, and the importance of consent. Following a group discussion, the theme was agreed to be 'our experience of groups'. In context, 'groups' meant the activities that were organised for the community by this specific mental health team. After this second session it was agreed that photograph taking should start. At the third, fourth and fifth sessions, discussion covered consent issues and how to get others involved; photographs that had been taken were reviewed and consideration given as to their display. At the end of the fifth session, each participant (including myself as a participant) selected photographs that they felt best represented their experiences of 'groups'; they were asked to select about five photographs each. The sixth, seventh and eighth sessions consisted of reviewing, and composing captions for each participant's photographs in turn, some of which was done initially by individual work and some through group discussion. Eventually the work done was reviewed again, with all photographs and captions now being considered as a whole series. This enabled the group to identify multiple photographs on the same theme, so some could be removed or combined. Displaying photographs and captions led to representing individuals and the work of the outreach team (Wang & Burris 1997). It was important to display both the individuals and the service in a 'true light'. Participants needed to be mindful of what was in their best interests both as individuals and for the service: for example, one photograph that was taken was of a hand holding a cigarette. This led to an interesting discussion as to whether the participants wanted to be represented by smoking, and in the end this photograph did not form a part of the exhibition. During the ninth session, the exhibition was assembled. The boards were then exhibited as part of one of the activity groups, and plans were made for a wider exhibition in the future. The group then met for one last time as a celebration of what had been achieved and to review the project.

Initially the sessions were planned, adapting structures found in Photovoice manuals (Palibroda *et al.* 2009, Photovoice Hamilton 2007). However, it soon became apparent that following a rigid structure was not going to allow the desired flexibility, shared ownership, or the ability to work at an appropriate pace.

## Autoethnography

It is important not just to evaluate the effect an intervention has on the group but also the role that the researcher has in providing this. Autoethnography provides a framework for doing this. Autoethnography can be seen as an extension of reflective practice. 'Ethnography' is a method which aims to make the familiar strange, 'auto' is where you focus on yourself. By developing an autoethnographical lens, exploration of my position within the group was enabled. This was achieved by making comments in a reflective practice diary, noting reflections regarding the role within the group. Foster *et al.* (2006) argue that autoethnography is of particular relevance to mental health nursing research and practice because of its reliance on the exploration of self, which is a fundamental component of mental health practice.

## Conversations with purpose

In everyday conversation people discuss the activities and their experiences of them. This information is often not recorded and yet provides a wealth of information. I started trying to make written records of these conversations to add to the other methods of evaluation.

## Evaluation through the arts

The creative arts steering team facilitates a Trust-wide art exhibition with a different theme each year, such as 'strength and softness and hope'. The exhibition, as well as displaying local talent, is also a forum for creating knowledge and understanding about how people experience and perceive the topics explored.

The art exhibition can be seen as a form of knowledge production. It can generate knowledge that can be used alongside other information gained from more traditional forms of research, such as questionnaires and interviews, or by itself to inform our understanding of how people experience the world. Beebeejaun *et al.* 2013 write about 'beyond text' forms of knowledge, of which this is one. In everyday life people utilise all our senses to interpret what they are experiencing and so it is logical to employ methodologies that draw upon all of the senses. Art exhibits can utilise many of the senses at once, with tactile, visual and auditory components.

As facilitators, before dismantling displays once an exhibition is over, we need to consider how we can capture, record and share this unique knowledge.

Interacting with art work can be very powerful. The CAST displays increasingly contain interactive elements where members of the public are themselves invited to contribute. Equally, group members can interact with, or produce displays on, themes that relate to their lives.

The activities that are facilitated by occupational therapists are only a part of any person's life, and the art exhibition may provide information that reveals how the said activities interact with other aspects of their lives.

## Conclusion

This chapter provides a description of the development, running and facilitation of the groupwork programme within SORT, an intensive community mental health team. It includes examples of considerations for the facilitator, such as aspects of the facilitator's role, partnership working, challenges which commonly arise, and effective evaluation. The principles described in this chapter are broad enough to be applied to groupwork within a variety of unique mental health settings.

# Useful resources

- PhotoVoice, https://photovoice.org
- de Bono, E. (1985). *Six Thinking Hats*. Little Brown and Company: London.
- College of Occupational Therapists (2013). *Living Well Through Activity in Care Homes: the Tool Kit*. London: COT.
- Government Office for Science (2008). *Mental Capital and Wellbeing: Making the Most of Ourselves in the 21st Century*. London: TSO.
- PhotoVoice, https://photovoice.org
- Photovoice Hamilton. (2007). *Manual and Resource Kit*. Hamilton Community Foundation. http://photovoice.ca (last accessed: 16.10.2016)
- Ryan, P. & Morgan, S. (2004). *Assertive Outreach: a Strengths Approach to Policy and Practice*. London: Churchill Livingstone.

# References

Andonian, L. (2010). Community participation of people with mental health issues within an urban environment. *Occupational Therapy in Mental Health* **26** (4), 401–417.

Andonian, L. & MacRae, A. (2011). Well older adults within an urban context: strategies to create and maintain social participation. *British Journal of Occupational Therapy* **74** (1), 2–11.

Beebeejaun, Y., Dunrose, C., Rees, J., Richardson, J. & Richardson, L. (2013). 'Beyond text': exploring ethos and method in co-producing research with communities. *Community Development Journal* **49** (1), 37–53.

de Bono, E. (1985). *Six Thinking Hats*. Little Brown and Company: London.

Brandling, J. & Wall, S. (2009). *United Response – UR in the Picture, Final Report. Bath: Mental Health Research and Development Unit*. http://www.Photovoice.org (last accessed: 12.12.2015).

Catalani, C. & Minkler, M. (2009). Photovoice: A review of the literature in health and public health. *Health Education and Behavior* **37** (3), 424–451.

Coffey, A. (1999). *The Ethnographic Self: Fieldwork and the Representation of Identity*. London: Sage.

Coghlan, D. & Casey, M. (2001). Action research from the inside: issues and challenges in doing action research in your own hospital. *Journal of Advanced Nursing* **35** (5), 674–682.

College of Occupational Therapists (2013). *Living Well Through Activity in Care Homes: the Tool Kit*. London: COT.

Corbin-Dwyer, S. & Buckle, J. (2009). The space between: on being an insider-outsider in qualitative research. *International Journal of Qualitative Methods* **8** (1), 54–63.

Fleming, J., Mahoney, J., Carlson, E. & Engebretson, J. (2009). An ethnographic approach to interpreting a mental illness: Photovoice exhibit. *Archives of Psychiatric Nursing* **23** (1), 16–24.

Foster, K., McAllister, M. & O'Brien, L. (2006). Extending the boundaries: autoethnography as an emergent method in mental health nursing research. *International Journal of Mental Health Nursing* **15** (1), 44–53.

Government Office for Science (2008). *Mental Capital and Wellbeing: Making the Most of Ourselves in the 21st Century*. London: TSO.

Humphrey, C. (2007). Insider-outsider: activating the hyphen. *Action Research* **5** (1), 11–26.

McCulloch, G. (2008). 'Historical insider research in education' in *Researching Education from the Inside,* eds. P. Sikes and A. Potts. London: Routledge.

Palibroda, B., Krieg, B., Murdock, C. & Havelock, J. (2009). *A Practical Guide to Photovoice: Sharing Pictures, Telling Stories and Changing Communities*. Prairie Women's Health Centre of Excellence. http://www.pwhce.ca (last accessed: 12.12.2015).

Photovoice Hamilton. (2007). *Manual and Resource Kit.* Hamilton Community Foundation. http://photovoice.ca (last accessed: 16.10.2016) .

Ryan, P. & Morgan, S. (2004). *Assertive Outreach: a Strengths Approach to Policy and Practice.* London: Churchill Livingstone.

Sumsion, T. (1999). *Client-centred Practice in Occupational Therapy.* Churchill Livingstone: London.

Thompson, N., Hunter, E., Murray, L., Ninci, L., Rolfs, E. & Pallinkkathayil, L. (2008). The experience of living with chronic mental illness: a photovoice study. *Perspectives in Psychiatric Care* **44** (1), 14–24.

United Kingdom Parliament (1983/2007). *Mental Health Act.* London: TSO.

Wang, C. & Burris, M. (1997). Photovoice: concept, methodology, and use for participatory needs assessment. *Health Education and Behavior* **24** (3), 369–387.

# Chapter 7

# Occupational therapists delivering Recovery

## Carol Savage

## Introduction

As a process that can take time, recovery can mean different things to different people. This chapter will provide a basic introduction to the concept of Recovery from mental illness that explores what appear to be key areas in the lives of many people working towards their goals and having hope for the future. It will consider the role occupational therapists have within Recovery services and the differences between types of mental health recovery, and recovery challenges around acceptance, gaining control and interdependence.

## Key points

- The occupational therapy profession emphasises a holistic approach to function, participation and partnership that is used to help support people with mental illness to develop skills, engage in activities of interest, and meet individual recovery goals.

- The practice of occupational therapy, like Recovery principles, is based on the philosophy and evidence that individuals diagnosed with mental health conditions can and do recover and lead meaningful, satisfying and productive lives.

- Fundamental Recovery principles are in full alignment with the philosophy of occupational therapy practice, which is inherently client-centred, collaborative and focused on supporting resiliency, full participation, health promotion and a wellness lifestyle (American Occupational Therapy Association 2016).

- Recovery clearly shares its philosophy of supporting people to stay in control of their lives despite experiencing mental health issues. Occupational therapists have long acknowledged the influence of the Recovery approach in mental health practice and the resulting opportunities for improved client and service outcomes (COT 2008).

# What is Recovery?

The concept of Recovery was essentially conceived by and for people with mental health issues to describe the significance of their own experiences and journeys, and to affirm that they are able to live a satisfying, hopeful and meaningful life, beyond the constraints of diagnoses. Interest in Recovery by mental health service providers has grown considerably during recent years. It has been suggested that Recovery ideas have their roots in apparently diverse threads of mental health service development: person-centred planning approaches, service user and carer involvement, social role valorisation, social inclusion, narrative research, radical political pressure groups, and self-management approaches (Davidson 2005). Roberts and Wolfson (2004) have even speculated that the origins of Recovery-oriented practice is to some extent a rediscovery of psychiatric care and practices initiated at the turn of the 18th century by the Tuke family in York where clinical philosophy and therapeutic practice was based on kindness, compassion, respect and hope of recovery.

# Defining Recovery

Recovery ideas are not easy; the word itself causes confusion because of its link to 'cure', and therefore what is meant by Recovery has proved somewhat difficult to define with any degree of specificity (Smith-Merry et al. 2011). The diverse ways the concept has been used have not helped, being explained as 'an approach, model, philosophy, paradigm, movement, vision and illusion' (Roberts & Wolfson 2004, p. 38); and having no particular set of therapeutic or preventive practices or services is suggestive of representing a more general if rather vague philosophy of mental healthcare (Smith-Merry et al. 2011). At the heart of Recovery, however, there appears to be a general consensus of a set of values about a person's right to build a meaningful life for themselves, with or without the continuing presence of mental health symptoms (Shepherd et al. 2008). A central tenet of the Recovery approach is that it does not necessarily mean cure ('clinical recovery'). Instead, it emphasises the unique journey of an individual living with mental health problems to build a life for themselves beyond illness ('social Recovery'). Thus, a person can recover their life, without necessarily 'recovering from' their illness.

Because Recovery is different for everyone and there is no single description or definition of Recovery it has been, and continues to be, something of a contested term. However, central to all Recovery paradigms are hope, self-determination, self-management, empowerment and advocacy. Also key is a person's right to full inclusion in a meaningful life of their own choosing, free of stigma and discrimination. Although much has been written on this subject, and there are many definitions, a widely agreed succinct definition by Bill Anthony, one of the intellectual founders of the Recovery movement, defines Recovery as: '[a] deeply personal, unique process of changing one's attitudes, values, feelings, goals, skills and roles. It is a way of living a satisfying, hopeful and contributing life, even with the limitations caused by illness. Recovery involves the development of new meaning and purpose in one's life as one grows beyond the catastrophic effects of mental illness ...' (Anthony 1993, pp. 11–23).

Based on ideas of self-determination and self-management, this definition highlights the fact that Recovery is about having a satisfying and fulfilling life, as defined by each person (Slade 2009). It represents a shift in who has authority to define and recognise Recovery away from the professional and towards the individual, and emphasises the importance of hope in sustaining motivation and supporting expectations of an individually fulfilled life (Shepherd *et al.* 2008). Therefore, putting Recovery into action means focusing care on supporting Recovery and building the resilience of people with mental health problems, not just on treating or managing their symptoms.

# Implementing Recovery: key organisational challenges

Strong interest in incorporating the Recovery philosophy into mental healthcare and in developing Recovery-oriented services has been particularly evident in countries such as the USA, New Zealand and somewhat more recently in England. The Recovery approach has emerged from the writings of people who used services in the 1980s in the USA, and in the 1990s in the UK (Chamberlin 1988, Coleman 1999, Deegan 1988, Leete 1989, Lovejoy 1984, Reeves 1999, Unzicker 1989). Many wrote about coping with symptoms, getting better, and regaining a satisfactory sense of personal identity that was not defined by illness experience. Personal accounts, alongside more systematic analysis, have been important contributions to the literature on Recovery. They highlight putting values into practice, being strongly influenced by what is personally meaningful, and being oriented around outcomes rather than inputs (Woodbridge & Fulford 2004).

In April 2002, in *Discovering Hope for Recovery from a British Perspective*, the concept of Recovery was described as only just beginning to be recognised (Allott & Loganathan 2002). Since then, Recovery ideas and concepts have been advancing rapidly throughout the mental health community (Davidson 2005), and although Recovery is not a new concept within mental health, it has come to the forefront of the policy agenda in recent times (Bonney & Stickley 2008).

# Implementing Recovery through Organisational Change (ImROC)

Recovery provides a new rationale for mental health services and has become the key organising principle underlying mental health services in New Zealand (Mental Health Commission 1998), the USA (Department of Health and Human Services 2003), and Australia (Australian Institute of Health and Welfare 2005). The ImROC programme (Implementing Recovery through Organisational Change 2012) was established by the Department of Health in England in 2008 to help local services become more supportive of Recovery for those using them and their carers (Shepherd et al. 2008). In April 2010 the Department of Health commissioned the NHS Confederation's Mental Health Network and the Centre for Mental Health to pilot a major national project involving 29 mental health provider sites. In 2012 the ImROC project set about establishing a new approach to helping people with mental health problems. The project also aimed to change how the NHS and its partners operated so that they could focus more on helping those people with their Recovery (Mental Health Network 2012).

In March 2014 the longstanding myth that mental health service providers, users and commissioners 'can't agree on what Recovery is, nor offer any evidence for it' (ImROC 2015) was finally laid to rest in a new briefing document published by the ImROC programme. The ImROC briefing paper 8 *Supporting Recovery in Mental Health Services: Quality and Outcomes* (Shepherd et al. 2014) set out three key frameworks for discussion at local level between commissioners, providers and service users:

● Quality indicators for services aiming to support Recovery at an individual level

● Quality indicators for supporting Recovery at an organisational level

● A set of individual level Recovery Outcome Domains.

(Shepherd et al. 2014, p. 1)

The frameworks aimed to help organisations in the mental health sector develop clear, empirically informed statements about what constitutes high quality services, and how these will lead to key Recovery outcomes for service users. It also included a series of recommendations for health and social care providers and commissioners, and for NHS England and the government that aimed to support development of an evidence-based approach to commissioning mental health services. Deliberately avoiding an overly prescriptive approach, the frameworks encourage discussion at a local level to agree the most appropriate quality indicators – at both individual and organisational level – and outcome measures for Recovery-focused mental health services.

The idea of Recovery has therefore not only evolved, but arrived, and has radical implications for the design and operation of mental health services and partnerships between health, social services and third sector organisations.

As Recovery-focused services appear to be a central component in making mental health services fit for the twenty-first century, occupational therapists need to think about how well placed they are to work alongside and in partnership with people who use their services. The closure of the large institutions, the development of community-based services and policy initiatives which emphasise Recovery all provide opportunities to make Recovery-oriented practices and services integral to the organisation and delivery of mental health services. As clinicians we need not abandon our traditional occupational therapy skills of assessment, treatment and evaluation. However, the challenge is for us to look beyond clinical recovery and to measure effectiveness of treatments and interventions in terms of the impact these have on the goals and outcomes that matter to the individual service user and their family. We therefore need to continually remind ourselves of the skills and competencies we are able to use and share so that we may evidence how effective we are at helping a person reach their Recovery goals. After all, occupational therapists have been working with this philosophy for years and are therefore well placed to be the discipline of choice when considering and developing services.

# Is Recovery possible?

The evidence about the prospects for people diagnosed with a severe mental illness is reasonably encouraging (Warner 2009). Research suggests that clinical recovery is possible, even if we may undervalue clinical recovery or the evidence for this is more favourable than we often believe. People with diagnoses get well and stay well. Even for 'major' diagnoses like schizophrenia, scientific studies demonstrate that a majority of individuals recover over time. While some individuals become free of psychiatric concerns altogether, others learn new ways of living in and adjusting to the world. Such evidence also points to the fact that people can also enter a process of personal Recovery beyond that and in the presence of ongoing symptoms and difficulties (Warner 2010).

To make Recovery possible for people, mental health services need to be designed and operated differently. Recovery ideas and approaches require a different relationship between service users and professionals, while the objectives of Recovery-oriented mental health services also need to be different from those of traditional, 'treat-and-cure' health services (Centre for Mental Health 2014). Clinical commissioning groups (CCGs) are a core part of the government's reforms to the health and social care system. In April 2013, they replaced primary care Trusts as the commissioners of most services funded by the NHS in England. They now control around two-thirds of the NHS budget and have a legal duty to support quality improvement in general practice (Kings Fund 2015).

# Recovery principles – what supports Recovery?

The principles of Recovery-oriented mental health practice ensure that mental health services are delivered in a way that supports the Recovery of mental health consumers. Some suggested principles of Recovery are shown in Box 7.1.

## Box 7.1: The principles of Recovery

- Recovery is about building a meaningful and satisfying life, as defined by the person themselves, whether or not there are ongoing or recurring symptoms or problems.
- Recovery represents a movement away from pathology, illness and symptoms to health, strength and wellness.

- -Hope is central to Recovery and can be enhanced by each person seeing how they can have more active control over their lives ('agency') and by seeing how others have found a way forward.

- Self-management is encouraged and facilitated. The processes of self-management are similar, but what works may be very different for each individual. There is no 'one size fits all'.

- The helping relationship between clinicians and service users moves away from being expert–patient to being 'coaches' or 'partners' on a journey of discovery. Clinicians are there to be 'on tap, not on top'.

- People do not recover in isolation. Recovery is closely associated with social inclusion and being able to take on meaningful and satisfying social roles within local communities, rather than in segregated services.

- Recovery is about discovering – or rediscovering – a sense of personal identity, separate from illness or disability.

- The language used, and the stories and meanings that are constructed, have great significance as mediators of the Recovery process. These shared meanings either support a sense of hope and possibility, or invite pessimism and chronicity.

- The development of Recovery-based services emphasises the personal qualities of staff as much as their formal qualifications. It seeks to cultivate their capacity for hope, creativity, care, compassion, realism and resilience.

- Family and other supporters are often crucial to Recovery and they should be included as partners wherever possible. However, peer support is central for many people in their recovery.

Source: Shepherd, G., Boardman, J. & Slade, M. (2008). *Making Recovery a Reality.* London: Sainsbury Centre for Mental Health.

These fundamental Recovery principles are in full alignment with the philosophy of occupational therapy practice, which is inherently client-centred, collaborative, and focused on supporting resiliency, full participation, health promotion, and a wellness lifestyle.

# Why should occupational therapists be interested in Recovery?

Historically mental health nurses (and other mental health workers) have been perceived as 'doing to' people who use services; more recently this has shifted to a desire to 'do with' people who use services. Within Recovery-focused practice the challenge is to 'be alongside' as service users take the lead in creating their own Recovery journey. The role of mental health workers therefore becomes that of 'facilitator', a resource person able to provide information and support to enable service users to identify their own goals and to take the steps to achieve them, recognising that at some times this may be more difficult than at others. This is a familiar position for occupational therapists, one where they are adept and comfortable, and therefore should be concerned with how they can facilitate Recovery.

If Recovery ideas are to have an impact then occupational therapists and other mental health professionals working in mental health services need to understand what Recovery means, and in partnership with service users and others, actively support its implementation across services. This will require occupational therapists and the profession to think about the way we work; about promoting the structure and organisation of our services; and about highlighting the diversity and fundamental contribution occupational therapy is able to offer when considering the culture of our profession in order to make our services more 'Recovery-oriented'. Recovery ideas and Recovery-oriented practice are not new but have the potential to radically transform mental health services for the better. Altering and challenging traditional profession-led services also provides a means of promoting occupational therapy as a key profession in Recovery services.

Recovery ideas are now a core part of Department of Health Policy and are supported by other mental health professional bodies in the UK. The development in English national policy, *New Horizons* (DoH 2009), offered the opportunity to make Recovery-oriented practice the core of our mental health services. For the white paper, *Liberating the NHS: No Decision About Me Without Me* (DoH 2012), with its clear focus on service user experience (quality) and shared decision making, there remains a central place in policy for Recovery-oriented practice.

In addition, the occupational therapy profession has been able to promote its philosophy and embrace changes. Alongside self-management approaches, there has also been increasing interest in shared decision making, self-care and patient choice, and greater recognition of the contribution of service users as experts in their own conditions. This brings together two sources of expertise – the knowledge, skills and experience of health and social care professionals and the individual's own knowledge and expertise about their own condition. Both forms of expertise are key to making good decisions. Used together, they enable individuals to make choices regarding treatment and management options that are most consistent with research evidence and with their own preferences and priorities.

Possessing and employing specialist skills, core competencies and expertise in particular areas, occupational therapists are able to meet the diverse needs of their clients for treatment and other interventions. The challenge to mental health professionals is, therefore, to look beyond clinical recovery and to measure the effectiveness of treatments and interventions in terms of the impact of these on the goals and outcomes that matter to the individual service user and their family, i.e. personal Recovery (Craig 2008).

# Opportunities and benefits of Recovery

Serious mental illness (SMI) affects 1–2 per cent of the population (Mind 2011), and people with SMI have an average lifespan that is 12.5 years shorter than the general population (Jones 2013). These people need to access services that are not only effective in treating their mental health but also increase their awareness of lifestyle choices and promote autonomy and independence, thereby reducing their need for inpatient services. Recovery has been described as a voyage of self-discovery and personal growth. Experiences of mental illness can provide opportunities for change, reflection and discovery of new values, skills and interests (Mental Health Foundation 2014).

# Obstacles to Recovery-oriented practice

One of the biggest obstacles to the implementation of Recovery-oriented practice has been the lack of clarity regarding what it really means. How can we recognise a 'Recovery-oriented' service? How will we know when we have made progress in achieving it? If we can succeed in creating Recovery-oriented services, what kinds of benefits would there be for service users? Mental health professionals need to see the productivity challenge as being their responsibility. As part of this, they should be encouraged to: develop quality dashboards to support improvement, make use of comparative performance information to reduce unwarranted variations in practice, and take advantage of opportunities to become more involved in redesigning processes of care and developing new service models (South London and Maudsley NHS Foundation Trust and South West London and St George's Mental Health NHS Trust 2010)

# Challenges to occupational therapy practice

It has been suggested that mental health services are best planned by bringing together the whole range of stakeholders who have an active interest in improving mental healthcare including: service users, family members, carers, professionals (mental health and primary care), other service provider groups (e.g. non-governmental organisations), policy makers, advocacy groups, planners (Thornicroft et al. 2008). Innovative service delivery is extremely important for mental health services, and designing a mental health infrastructure or system that accommodates all types of providers may prove challenging. However, in order to meet the needs of the people who use them, in the best possible way, an environment should be fostered in which people working in the mental health sector are encouraged to continually look at new and better ways of delivering services. This means ensuring that groups which are not powerful advocates for their own interests are also given equitable consideration in planning services (Mental Health Commission 1998).

During the development of community mental health services, staff have faced challenges. These include: anxiety and uncertainty, lack of structure in community services, how to initiate new developments, how to manage opposition within the mental health system, opposition from neighbours, financial obstacles, system rigidity, maintaining morale, and trying to identify what is the right answer.

The overall lessons learned to date appear first to suggest that robust service changes, improvements that will last, take time. Part of the reason for this is that staff will need to be persuaded that change is likely to bring improvements for patients, and indeed their scepticism is a positive asset, to act as a buffer against changes that are too rapid or too frequent. The second overall lesson is that it is essential to listen to users' and families' experiences and perspectives. Everyone involved needs to keep a clear focus on the fact that the purpose of mental health services is to improve outcomes for people with mental illness. The intended beneficiaries of care therefore need to be, in some sense, in the driving seat when planning and delivering treatment and care. The third lesson that emerges is that the team managing such a process needs clear expertise to manage the whole budget. When financial boundaries for mental health funds are not established and fiercely maintained, then money can easily be diverted to other areas of healthcare. In other words, financial mechanisms need to be created which ensure that money follows service users into the community (Thornicroft et al. 2008).

# Putting Recovery into practice

## What are the core elements of the Recovery paradigm?

The mental health literature attests to a paradigm shift from an emphasis on treatment towards a focus on fostering Recovery. This paradigm emphasises many constructs familiar to occupational therapists, including quality of life, empowerment, hope, meaningful activities and work (Jones 2013). The objectives of occupational therapy can focus on improving the Recovery of people with mental illness to reduce social and economic marginalisation, by increasing participation in society, increasing social integration and social inclusion. By helping individuals to identify personally meaningful goals to obtain optimal treatment and care, while learning how to best manage their illness in the process of achieving those goals, occupational therapists can develop an understanding of how to offer assistance (Lloyd et al. 2008).

## Relationship to 'Recovering Ordinary Lives' (COT 2006) and occupational therapy

Recovery describes the struggles of people with mental health problems to live meaningful and satisfying lives. The principles of Recovery now underpin developments in mental health services in a number of countries. In England, they figure prominently in *New Horizons* (DoH 2009) and have received widespread support from the major professional bodies.

*Recovering Ordinary Lives – the Strategy for Occupational Therapy in Mental Health Services 2007–2017* describes how:

> Occupational therapists will value Recovery and will work within a socially inclusive framework to achieve goals that make a real difference to people's lives. They will encourage people with mental health problems to make decisions and responsibilities for their lives by providing the necessary support.

(COT 2006, p. 4).

Historically, the aim of mental health services has been to achieve clinical recovery through the treatment of symptoms and the prevention of relapse. Personal Recovery, however, demands a different sort of support from mental health services. Mental health professionals still need to prescribe medication and offer therapy – but only if an individual wants this sort of treatment. To support personal Recovery, professionals need to work in partnership with people with mental health problems, making joint decisions about what treatment is appropriate, rather than 'knowing what is best'. Paradigm shifts are a necessary part of life. Things do change and we need to adjust to change. Recovery research is mirroring the process of life and our understanding of self. It may appear to be fragmented and uncoordinated, but shares many commonalities with individuation.

## Defining a Recovery-oriented approach

Whilst some people refer to a 'Recovery model', it is probably better to speak about Recovery ideas, approaches or concepts. A model would suggest that there is a Recovery manual somewhere that should be applied to all people to fix them, when the opposite is in fact true. Recovery is about individualised approaches. Recovery is a struggle for many people. The struggle might stem from severity of symptoms, side effects of medication, current or past trauma and pain, difficult socio-economic circumstances, or the experience of using mental health services. Practitioners can also struggle as a result of the constraints of their work environment or when they sense a person's despair (Davidson & Roe 2007).

Recovery approaches may also differ depending upon where a person is on their Recovery journey. During an acute phase of illness, the person's capacity may be impaired to the extent that alleviation of distress and the burden of symptoms, as well as safety, is the primary focus of treatment and care. Regaining capacity for self-determination or deeper engagement should be a focus in the next stage of treatment and support. At later stages, when capacity is improved, there are opportunities for the person to consider broader Recovery strategies.

Recovery-oriented mental health practice refers to the application of sets of capabilities that support people to recognise and take responsibility for their own Recovery and wellbeing and to define their goals, wishes and aspirations. Capabilities for Recovery-oriented practice and service delivery encompass underlying core principles, values, knowledge, attitudes and behaviours, skills and abilities. Individuals, teams and organisations need these capabilities in order to support people with mental health issues to live a meaningful and contributing life in their community of choice (Australian Health Ministers Advisory Council 2013).

A Recovery approach requires a shared decision making process that is person-centred and client driven. The client–provider partnership supports shared decision making from the time the individual first engages in services, through developing intervention plans, and in all other aspects of the therapeutic process. A primary goal of a Recovery approach is to facilitate resiliency, health and wellness in the community of the individual's choice, rather than to manage symptoms. The practice of occupational therapy, like the Recovery approaches, is based on the philosophy and evidence that individuals diagnosed with mental health conditions can and do recover and lead meaningful, satisfying, and productive lives. It is the profession's emphasis on holism, function, participation, and partnership that is used to help support people with mental illness to develop skills, engage in activities of interest, and meet individual Recovery goals (The American Occupational Therapy Association 2011).

## The importance of Recovery principles for occupational therapy practice

The purpose and principles of Recovery-oriented mental health practice are to ensure that mental health services are being delivered in a way that supports the Recovery of individuals (Australian Government 2010). Putting Recovery into action therefore means focusing care on supporting Recovery from the perspective of the individual with mental illness. For many people, the concept of Recovery is about staying in control of their life despite experiencing a mental health problem (Mental Health Foundation 2014). Building the resilience of people with mental health problems and not just treating or managing their symptoms is therefore imperative to Recovery if they are able to gain and retain hope, understand their abilities and disabilities, engage in an active life, attain personal autonomy, social identity, meaning and purpose in life, and a positive sense of self. Although Recovery is now widely accepted as a concept by people in the mental health sector, it would appear that there is still a long way to go to ensure that Recovery, as we have defined it, becomes embedded in mental health services (O'Hagan 2004).

## How are occupational therapy skills incorporated into Recovery services?

Contemporary understanding of Recovery continues to recognise the complexity of suffering associated with severe mental health problems. Such understanding suggests that it is therefore possible to live well despite any limitations caused by the disability or illness, and that it may be possible to reconceptualise otherwise wasteful and destructive experiences as a challenge with a potential for positive outcomes. Mental health services recognise the need to change radically to focus on Recovery. They also need to demonstrate success in helping service users to get their lives back and giving service users the chance to make their own decisions about how they live their lives. Recovery turns mental health services' priorities on their heads. Whereas traditional services wait until a person's illness is cured before helping them to get their life back, Recovery-focused services aim from day one to help people to build a life for themselves, and the medical care they give is in support of that bigger purpose (Rose 2001).

Occupational therapists develop a range of therapeutic skills, and for Recovery-oriented approaches, these may be formulated in terms of the ability to work with the service user and significant others to formulate a shared understanding of the problem and a positive, forward-looking plan, which is implemented with clear, structured feedback regarding progress. However, as occupational therapy is concerned with the normality of everyday activity and this is common to everyone, it is taken for granted and therefore not highly valued (Kielhofner 2002).

Occupational therapists work collaboratively with people in a manner that helps to foster hope, motivation and empowerment, as well as system change. Educated in the scientific understanding of neurophysiology, psychosocial development, activity and environmental analysis, and group dynamics, occupational therapy practitioners work to empower each individual to fully participate and be successful and satisfied in his or her self-selected occupations.

Occupational therapists assume a variety of roles such as direct care therapists, consultants, academic educators, managers, and administrators. They may also work in public, private and third sector organisations to help assist in local, regional, and national transformation efforts. For occupational therapists, the forces of change are creating opportunities for new practice areas. Occupational therapists could move into unique, individualised interventions and service developments or, indeed, develop innovation within teams and interdisciplinary groups that work together in order to provide services in any settings.

Box 7.2 provides examples of how the knowledge and skill base of occupational therapy may be used in the process of assisting individuals in all phases of mental health recovery.

## Box 7.2: Knowledge and skill base of occupational therapy used in the process of assisting individuals in all phases of mental health recovery

- Teach and support the active use of coping strategies to help manage the effect of symptoms of illness on one's life, including being more organised and able to engage in activities of choice.
- Help to identify and implement healthy habits, rituals and routines to support a wellness lifestyle.
- Support the identification of personal values, needs and goals to enable informed decision making, such as when considering housing and employment options.
- Support the creation and use of a Wellness Recovery Action Plan (WRAP) in group or individual sessions.
- Provide information to increase awareness of community-based resources, such as peer-facilitated groups and other support options.
- Provide information on how to monitor physical health concerns (e.g. diabetes management, smoking cessation), develop strategies to control chronic symptoms, and recognise and respond to acute changes.
- Support the ability to engage in long-term planning (e.g. budget for major purchases, prepare advance medical and mental health directives) that leads to meeting personal Recovery goals.

(Source: American Occupational Therapy Association (2011) *Occupational therapy's role in mental health recovery*)

Recognised as one of the five key professions in health services assisting in Recovery of those with mental health problems, occupational therapy is acknowledged as an approach that uses activity to promote good mental health, assist Recovery and help people achieve personally meaningful outcomes such as employment, self-care and leisure (COT 2006).

## Recovery colleges

Recovery colleges are developed and specifically designed to enable people to rebuild their lives, to develop the skills they need for living and working, and to enable people to ultimately become experts in their own self-care while developing skills and confidence to manage their own Recovery journey (Perkins 2012).

While Recovery colleges/education centres have been key to the development of Recovery-focused services in the USA (Ashcraft & Anthony 2005), they did not begin to emerge in England until 2011. Officially opened in April 2012, the Central North West London (CNWL) NHS Foundation Trust Recovery College was just the third in the country, and along with its partners played a central role in pioneering the UK development of such colleges (Perkins 2012).

## Defining features of a Recovery college

In a Recovery college individuals with mental health problems have the opportunity to access education and training programmes, workshops and courses. Designed to run like other colleges, individuals select courses they would like to attend from a prospectus, do their own research in a library, and attend courses that enable them to take control and pursue what is important to them. Seeking to break down destructive barriers between 'them and us' that perpetuate stigma and exclusion, Recovery colleges explicitly recognise the expertise of mental health professionals and the expertise of lived experience in a process of 'co-production'. Therefore, courses may be co-devised and co-delivered by people with lived experience of mental illness, and/or by mental health practitioners who share their expertise. Delivery of such courses enables students to see what people facing challenges due to mental ill health can achieve, whilst peer support offered by peer trainers and fellow students enables people to feel less alone, offers images of hope and possibility and allows people to learn from others who have faced similar challenges and use their lived experience to help others (Perkins 2012).

Recovery college courses are offered to service users, professionals and families alike, with the aim of providing education as a route to Recovery, not as a form of therapy. The ranges of courses available within colleges aim to help students take control and become experts in their own wellbeing and Recovery, despite challenges brought about through mental ill health, and give them the skills and confidence they need for work, and to get on with their lives as 'students' rather than 'patients' (ImROC 2012). Exploring what they can be, and recognising the unique contribution they can make, may then go some way towards helping them gain improved confidence and self-belief in their abilities and potential (Ashcraft & Anthony 2005). Accessing such courses also aims to promote inclusion and participation, break down the prejudice and discrimination that divide people facing challenges due to mental ill health from their friends, families and communities, and increase the understanding and confidence of those friends, families and communities in accommodating those trying to manage mental health difficulties.

A Recovery college may have a central role to play in the development of Recovery-focused services, but it cannot, and should not, replace all other services; it cannot, for example, offer specialist assessment and treatment; nor can it provide the outreach support that some people need to navigate their lives. Nor can the Recovery college stand apart from these other facets of services.

A Recovery college will be of little value if it is seen as 'the place where Recovery is done' while all other parts of the service carry on as they have always done. Promoting Recovery is everyone's business. If a Recovery college is to have a positive impact on the Recovery journey of individuals, the messages of hope and possibility, self-management and self-determination, must be reinforced and extended in other parts of the service that people use. If it is to have a positive impact on the development of Recovery-focused services, it must be a fully integrated part of the organisation and its work. A wide range of staff and people with lived experience must contribute to its courses and workshops, not simply the 'core staff' of a college, but a wide range of practitioners and people with lived experience across organisations and beyond. Although some organisations have started establishing Recovery colleges, it should not be considered the end of the road, but the start of a journey.

A Recovery college needs to think about how it can accommodate the diverse range of people using all aspects of its services, like older people, younger people, people who use forensic services, addictions services, eating disorder services. It might also think about the role it has in the pre-qualification training of mental health practitioners. Perhaps local training programmes might purchase places on college courses? Perhaps a Recovery college might constitute a placement for trainees? Depending on the resources available, there are many possibilities to be explored as a college grows and matures.

A college could also play a far greater role in bridging the divide between mental health services and the wider community, making the resources of those communities available to people receiving mental health services and increasing the capacity of our communities to accommodate and address mental distress. This might be achieved by greater involvement of people from outside the mental health diaspora in providing courses (such as from colleges, community safety partnerships, job centres, housing associations, community groups). This would both increase the range of expertise available to students and also give people from external agencies some contact with people who have mental health challenges, which is so important in breaking down prejudice. Recovery colleges could also become an important resource for the community. If one in four people face mental health challenges then there are many who might benefit from courses like coping with stress, living with depression, personal Recovery planning, mindfulness and returning to work. If courses were available to a greater range of people (and those close to them) outside secondary mental health services then understanding of mental health conditions within our communities could increase substantially.

An educational approach lies at the heart of Recovery-focused services (Ashcraft & Anthony 2005). An educational paradigm focuses on reinforcing and developing people's strengths, enabling people to understand their own challenges, and how they can best manage these in order to do the things they value and pursue their aspirations. A Recovery college lies at the heart of an educational approach and provides much of what has traditionally been provided within a traditional therapeutic paradigm in the form of individual work and groups. However, the relationship between mental health practitioners and those whom they serve is quite different.

# Recovery challenges

Building a successful life in Recovery requires plenty of effort. In order to keep Recovery on track, individuals will need to overcome many challenges. Once individuals become more skilled at dealing with obstacles in their path and learn to cope with different challenges, they become more skilled at facing them in the future. Although this has created a positive shift in focus in the clinical care provided to individuals, Recovery remains an ambiguous concept that is difficult to apply to policies and behaviours. It remains imperative therefore that services work to create cultures within their service that support the values underlying the Recovery concept, and that service users and service providers increase their understanding of the multiple dimensions of Recovery in order to apply values more effectively in clinical care.

# Conclusion

It would appear that Recovery is a highly individual and personal journey that, when led by people with experiences of mental ill health and their family members, can make a very positive contribution to the effectiveness of the services being delivered. However, the innate tensions that have existed within the concept of Recovery from mental ill health are not easily resolved. Research suggests that, as a process and an outcome that may be both measurable and immeasurable, it will take time and patience, amidst the confusion, to persevere and learn from the personal uniqueness of people's own struggles with their experiences and discoveries of effective coping mechanisms and strategies for wellness (Allott & Loganathan 2002).

To make progress means doing things differently, and this will require significant change across the whole system, including Recovery frameworks, models of care, workforce, data collection, culture, consumers, and families' expectations (O'Hagan 2004). Therefore helping people to find the right combination of services, treatments and supports, and eliminating discrimination by removing barriers to full participation in work, education and community life is the key to the promotion and adoption of a Recovery-oriented culture within mental health services. Application of such a framework is likely to contribute to improved mental health and wellbeing as people are supported in new ways to lead fulfilling and contributing lives. Adapting such a framework therefore has the potential to foster new and innovative service designs, and in particular services designed and operated by people with lived experience of mental health issues.

Occupational therapists are not only familiar with these terms, but have addressed Recovery-related constructs in both research and practice. Core occupational therapy beliefs and assumptions are strikingly similar to those that are thought to be important to fostering Recovery. Occupational therapists should consider taking a keen interest in the construct of Recovery. By virtue of professional beliefs and assumptions, occupational therapists are uniquely positioned to assume a leadership role in the area of Recovery-related research and practice, and take comfort in knowing that emergent paradigms are always like this and our service systems must recognise that.

# Useful resources

- Centre for Mental Health (2016). *What is Recovery?* https://www.centreformentalhealth.org.uk/recovery
- College of Occupational Therapists (2006). *Recovering Ordinary Lives: the Strategy for Occupational Therapy in Mental Health Services 2007–2017.* London: COT.
- Live it Well (2016). *Recovery.* http://www.liveitwell.org.uk/ways-to-wellbeing/recovery
- Mental Health Foundation (2016). *Recovery.* https://www.mentalhealth.org.uk/a-to-z/r/recovery
- Mind. (2013). Mental health problems – an introduction. http://www.mind.org.uk/information-support/types-of-mental-health-problems/mental-health-problems-introduction/recovery
- NHS England. (2016). Mental health. https://www.england.nhs.uk/mentalhealth
- National Institute for Mental Health in England (2005). NIMHE Guiding statement on recovery. http://studymore.org.uk/nimherec.pdf
- Shepherd, G., Boardman, J. & Slade, M. (2008). *Making Recovery a Reality.* London: Sainsbury Centre for Mental Health.
- Time to Change (2016). *Mental Health and Stigma.* https://www.time-to-change.org.uk/mental-health-and-stigma

# References

Allott, P. & Loganathan, L. (2002). *Discovering Hope for Recovery from a British Perspective: a Review of Literature.* UCE, Birmingham: Centre for Community Mental Health.

American Occupational Therapy Association (2016). *Factsheet: Occupational Therapy's Role in Mental Health Recovery.* https://www.aota.org (last accessed: 15.8.2016).

Anthony, W.A. (1993). Recovery from mental illness; the guiding vision of the mental health service system in the 1900s. *Psychosocial Rehabilitation Journal* **16** (4), 11–23.

Ashcraft, L. & Anthony, W. (2005). A story of transformation: an agency fully embraces recovery. *Behavioural Healthcare Tomorrow* **14** (2), 12–22.

Australian Government (2010). *National Standards for Mental Health Services: Principles of Recovery Oriented Mental Health Practice.* https://www.health.gov.au (last accessed: 10.7.2014).

Australian Health Ministers Advisory Council (2013). *A National Framework for Recovery-oriented Mental Health Services.* http://www.health.gov.au/internet/main/publishing.nsf/Content/mental-pubs-n-recovfra (last accessed: 18.10.2016).

Australian Institute of Health & Welfare (AIHW) (2005). *Mental Health Services in Australia 2003–04. AIHW cat no. HSE 40. Canberra: AIHW (Mental Health Series no. 8).* http://www.aihw.gov.au (last accessed: 17.6.2015).

Bonney, S. & Stickley, T. (2008). Recovery and mental health: a review of British literature. *Journal of Psychiatric and Mental Health Nursing* **15** (2), 140–153.

Centre for Mental Health (2014). *What is Recovery?* London: Centre for Mental Health.

Chamberlin, J. (1988). *On our Own.* London: Mind Publications.

Coleman, R. (1999). *Recovery: An Alien Concept.* http://www.workingtorecovery.co.uk (last accessed: 12.4.2015).

College of Occupational Therapists (2006). *Recovering Ordinary Lives: The strategy for Occupational Therapy in Mental Health Services: a Strategy for the Next Ten Years.* London: COT.

College of Occupational Therapists (2008) *Position Statement – The Value of Occupational Therapy and its Contribution to Adult Social Service Users and their Carers.* http://www.cot.co.uk (last accessed: 23.6.2016).

Craig, T.J.K. (2008). Recovery: say what you mean and mean what you say. *Journal of Mental Health* **17** (2), 125–128.

Davidson, L. (2005). Recovery, self-management and the expert patient – changing the culture of mental health from a UK perspective. *Journal of Mental Health* **14** (1), 25–35.

Davidson, L. & Roe, D. (2007). Recovery from versus recovery in serious mental illness: one strategy for lessening confusion plaguing recovery. *Journal of Mental Health* **16** (4), 459–470.

Deegan, E. (1988). Recovery: the lived experience of rehabilitation. *Psychosocial Rehabilitation Journal* **11** (4), 11–19.

Department of Health (2009). *New Horizons: a Shared Vision for Mental Health.* London: TSO.

Department of Health (2012). *Liberating the NHS: No Decision About Me, Without Me – Further Consultation on Proposals to Secure Shared Decision-making.* London: TSO.

Department of Health & Human Services (2003). *Major Management Challenges and Program Risks. United States General Government Accounting Office.* http://www.gao.gov/ (last accessed: 12.5.2015).

Implementing Recovery through Organisational Change (ImROC) (2012). *Recovery Colleges.* http://www.imroc.org (last accessed: 22.5.2015).

Implementing Recovery through Organisational Change (ImROC) (2015). *ImROC Conference: Next steps for Recovery-focused support.* http://www.imroc.org (last accessed: 15.2.2016).

Jones, M. (2013). *Are Rehabilitation Services in Mental Health Effective?* http://www.nursingtimes.net (last accessed: 20.5.2015).

Kielhofner, G. (2002). *Model of Human Occupation,* 3rd edn. Baltimore: Lippincott.

Kings Fund (2015). *Clinical Commissioning Groups.* http://www.kingsfund.org.uk (last accessed: 22.5.2015).

Leete, E. (1989). How I perceive and manage my illness. *Schizophrenia Bulletin* **15** (2), 197–200.

Lloyd, C., Waghorn, G., & Williams, L. (2008). Conceptualising Recovery in mental health rehabilitation. *British Journal of Occupational Therapy* **71** (8), 321–328.

Lovejoy, M. (1984). Recovery from schizophrenia – a personal odyssey. *Hospital and Community Psychiatry* **35** (8), 809–812.

Mental Health Commission (1998). *Blueprint for Mental Health Services in New Zealand.* Wellington NZ: Mental Health Commission. http://www.hdc.org.nz (last accessed: 15.8.2015).

Mental Health Foundation (2014). *Recovery.* http://www.mentalhealth.org.uk (last accessed: 4.7. 2014).

Mental Health Network (2012). *Supporting Recovery in Mental Health.* http://www.nhsconfed.org (last accessed: 4.6.2015).

Mind (2011). Mental Health Facts and Statistics. London: Mind.

O'Hagan, M. (2004). Recovery in New Zealand: lessons for Australia? *Australian e-Journal for the Advancement of Mental Health* **3** (1). http://www.familymentalhealthrecovery.org (last accessed: 4.8.2015).

Perkins, R. (2012). *Why a Recovery College?* http://www.cnwl.nhs.uk (last accessed: 22.6.2015).

Reeves, A. (1999). *Recovery: A Holistic Approach, Gloucester.* http://www.workingtorecovery.co.uk (last accessed: 27.5.2015).

Roberts, G. & Wolfson, P. (2004). The rediscovery of recovery: open to all. *Advances in Psychiatric Treatment* **10**, 37–49.

Rose, D. (2001). *Users' Voices: The Perspectives of Mental Health Service Users on Community and Hospital Care.* London: The Sainsbury Centre for Mental Health.

Shepherd, G., Boardman, J. & Slade, M. (2008). *Making Recovery a Reality.* London: Sainsbury Centre for Mental Health.

Shepherd, G., Boardman, J., Rinaldi, M. & Roberts, G. (2014). *ImROC Briefing Paper 8: Supporting Recovery in Mental Health Services: Quality and Outcomes.* https://www.imroc.org (last accessed: 15.8.2016).

Slade, M. (2009). *Personal Recovery and Mental Illness: a Guide for Mental Health Professionals.* Cambridge: Cambridge University Press.

Smith-Merry, J., Freeman, R. & Sturdy, S. (2011). *Implementing Recovery: an Analysis of the Key Technologies in Scotland.* http://www.ncbi.nlm.nih.gov (last accessed: 3.6.2015).

South London & Maudsley NHS Foundation Trust and South West London & St George's Mental Health NHS Trust (2010). *Recovery is for All. Hope, Agency and Opportunity in Psychiatry. A Position Statement by Consultant Psychiatrists.* London: SLAM/SWLSTG.

Thornicroft, G., Tansella, M. & Law, A. (2008). *Steps, Challenges and Lessons in Developing Community Mental Health Care.* http://www.ncbi.nlm.nih.gov (last accessed: 20.5.2015).

Unzicker, R. (1989). On my own: a personal journey through madness and re-emergence. *Psychosocial Rehabilitation Journal* **13** (1), 71–77.

Warner, R. (2009). Recovery from schizophrenia and the Recovery model. *Current Opinion in Psychiatry* **22** (4), 374–380.

Warner, R. (2010). Does the scientific evidence support the Recovery model. *The Psychiatrist* **34** (1), 3–5.

Woodbridge, K. & Fulford, K.W.M. (2004). *Whose Values? a Workbook for Values-based Practice in Mental Health Care.* London: The Sainsbury Centre for Mental Health.

# Chapter 8

# Occupational therapists delivering rehabilitation

*Hannah Chapman*

## Introduction

The words 'rehabilitation' and 'Recovery' are often used interchangeably without always being fully understood. As occupational therapists branch out into new and different settings in mental health, it is important to have a clear understanding of the two terms and how they correlate with occupational therapy in a variety of settings. This understanding can help to increase confidence and skills as a practitioner.

This chapter explains the term 'rehabilitation' within a context of Recovery, then uses a case study as an example of an occupational therapist working in a non-traditional setting. It goes on to explore the challenges and benefits of working in this setting and concludes by looking at implications for future practice.

## Key points

- Rehabilitation can be seen as the generic systems which function in order to support the personal journey of Recovery.
- There are strong historical links between rehabilitation and occupational therapy services; however, arguably our role in these services is to ensure an occupational focus is maintained.
- Rehabilitation outcomes can be easier to measure than Recovery-related outcomes; however, systems can be put in place to ensure outcomes are measured to satisfy all stakeholders.
- With shifts in policy and a competitive climate, occupational therapists may be called upon to demonstrate their value across a range of diverse settings.
- Maintaining an occupational focus can turn difficult generic tasks into meaningful opportunities.

# Defining rehabilitation in the context of Recovery

Recovery-focused practice is increasing in the field of mental health, with some describing it as the 'new mantra for mental health' (Lal 2010, p. 82). Contention around the meaning of the term 'Recovery' (as easily confused with 'recovery' as in 'cure') has arisen. As services shift towards Recovery, there can be seen to be a move away from more traditional terminology and practice surrounding 'rehabilitation' as a whole.

It has been agreed (see Chapter 7) that 'Recovery is not an intervention and professionals cannot "do" Recovery "to" people' (Government of South Australia 2012, p. 8). However, rehabilitation 'is the process and the tools that practitioners utilise and provide to people to assist in their Recovery journey' (Government of South Australia 2012, p. 9).

Therefore although the focus is increasingly on Recovery, as practitioners our role to empower and support people can sometimes be rehabilitative in nature. For, 'while Recovery is owned by and unique to each person, mental health rehabilitation services that are Recovery-oriented play an important role in creating environments that facilitate and support a person's own personal Recovery journey' (Government of South Australia 2012, p. 6).

The word 'rehabilitation' has a number of associations across different sectors within health and social care, e.g. drug rehabilitation, vocational rehabilitation and functional rehabilitation. So within a mental health setting, what exactly is it that we are hoping to achieve and what is the difference between achieving rehabilitation and achieving Recovery? The answers to these questions may be difficult to define and the examples below may help to increase clarity.

Traditionally mental health rehabilitation has been seen as intensive support for a small number of people experiencing mental illness and can be defined as 'specialist assessment, treatment, interventions and support to enable the recovery of people whose complex needs cannot be met by general adult mental health services' (Joint Commissioning Panel for Mental Health 2012, p. 6). The focus here appears to be on the 'specialist' nature of rehabilitation, whereas Recovery can be deemed to be more universal in nature.

Viewed in comparison to physical illness, the distinction may be easier to see. For instance, there are many physical health conditions which people may need to recover from, but without needing specialist support or rehabilitation as such conditions do not significantly affect their daily living. (For example, a person may sustain a knee injury and be able to self-manage using a brace or crutches. In other cases, the person may need rehabilitative physiotherapy if their function has been significantly decreased.)

The task for individuals and practitioners is to recognise this distinction and the need for further intervention – which, as occupational therapists, we may well understand to be related to occupation and a person's ability to engage in occupations with or without the need for a structure of support around them.

## Box 8.1: Case study

The following case study aims to show how Recovery and rehabilitation interlink within an occupational therapy context in a non-traditional setting. The study is based on coordinating a local authority's mental health rehabilitation service. A position was advertised as 'mental health rehabilitation service coordinator' on the local authority website and required a qualification in social work, psychology, mental health nursing or occupational therapy, as well as experience in managing services and staff teams. Although the service had a history of being coordinated by a range of professionals it had a strong link to occupational therapy in particular, as an occupational therapist had a key role in setting the service up.

The role itself entailed managing teams in the delivery of a rehabilitation service to people experiencing mental illness. This included a 24-hour staffed rehabilitation unit, group homes in the local community and floating support in private homes. The floating support element included staff supporting people to meet their rehabilitation goals within their own homes or community, for instance spending a few hours per week supporting with shopping, household activities or accessing social groups.

As a non-health service, the programme was largely funded by the government's Supporting People programme and required the regular provision of statistics to demonstrate that the service was meeting predetermined Supporting People outcomes. Besides local authority service, many similar schemes exist in private, third and housing sectors, and provide competition to similar statutory services. Many housing associations, for example, now have a support service specifically aimed at mental health provision. In a similar way many mental health charities are taking on commissions for the 'floating support' roles which previously would have been carried out in the statutory sector.

People using the service described in this case study were under secondary mental healthcare as defined in the *Mental Health Measure* (Welsh Government 2010) and had to have care coordinators in order to access the service. Such access could start at any point within the service, but it was designed to follow a pathway taking each individual from leaving hospital, to the rehabilitation unit, on to a group home, then eventually to his/her own accommodation (still with support from staff if needed).

Individuals accessing the service were supported to draw up their own support plans, which would include individual occupational aspirations. For those living in shared accommodation, however, there were also generic 'rehabilitation' activities in which all were encouraged to take part, e.g. cleaning, shopping and house meetings. These were transferred to support plans.

Staff in the teams were classed as support workers or senior support workers and not specifically linked to an occupational therapist. Staff feedback identified the need for a clearer understanding of the term 'rehabilitation', particularly within the context of providing outcome-based statistics to Supporting People and working consistently as a team. This led to a staff training programme, designed to explore the meaning of Recovery and rehabilitation and to introduce basic occupational therapy theory, i.e. occupational balance, occupational analysis and some theory on approaches. The training was designed to allow staff to draw on their own rich experiences within the service, linking these to the meeting of funding requirements and to the process of supporting individuals to meet their own goals.

To understand the key concepts, a diagram was built up throughout the training session so that staff had a visual reference for future use (see Figure 8.1). It was a simple diagram but staff found it useful as a point of reference to demonstrate where their roles fitted in and what the different terms meant.

Alongside the training, a recovery measurement scale was developed; service users could use it by themselves or together with staff, to identify their own aims and milestones and keep track of their attainments or progress towards attainments. With service users' permission, these could also be used as evidence for Supporting People records and statistics.

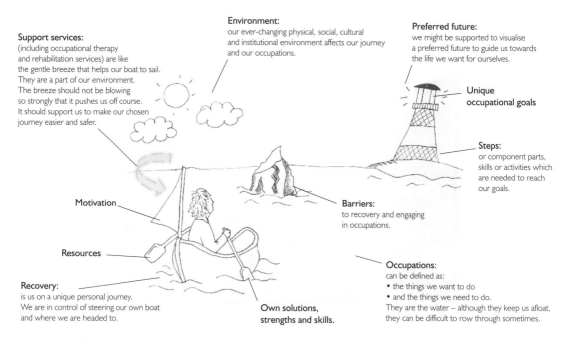

*Figure 8.1: Diagram used to illustrate the relationships between occupation, recovery and rehabilitation*

# Understanding rehabilitation and Recovery in this setting

One of the main purposes of the training described in Box 8.1 (above) was to explore the inter-relation of Recovery and rehabilitation and how to shift to a Recovery focus whilst maintaining a rehabilitation setting. The staff in the team were seen to be part of the rehabilitation process, and their skills, training and approaches were all part of the 'system' of rehabilitation. This meant that many staff felt strongly about acting consistently as a team so that each staff member was working towards supporting people to do things for themselves and regaining skills and confidence.

The consistent nature of this approach, however, could be seen at times to be in juxtaposition to the unique client-led nature of Recovery. For example, there were times when a compensatory approach (e.g. online shopping to avoid anxiety related to public spaces) was deemed appropriate to support someone to carry out an occupation that was more important to them, such as being able to provide healthy meals to their children. In terms of rehabilitation, the onus was no longer on the functional process – going shopping – but on the larger occupational aspiration related to a person's personal perception of Recovery.

This called for staff to maintain a delicate balance, that of carrying out tasks relating to their rehabilitation roles whilst also keeping in mind the very personal hopes and ambitions of Recovery personal to each client, bearing in mind that these could change within a given period of time.

Both staff and management found that rehabilitation was simpler to measure as it was largely tangible, so it was easy to identify key generic milestones. Recovery, however, was much more abstract, and therefore harder to measure, as it was very much dependent upon the thoughts, feelings and experiences of the individual clients.

# Challenges of being an occupational therapist in this setting

As this service was not labelled specifically as an occupational therapy service, it brought certain challenges in terms of practice – particularly for a worker being an occupational therapist working in isolation in a non-health setting.

## Overlap of roles

One of the first challenges was that the role of the rehabilitation support workers often overlapped, and occasionally even conflicted, with the role of the support workers employed by the Community Mental Health Team (CMHT). Each service user not only had a support plan through the rehabilitation service, but also had a care and treatment plan through their care coordinator.

This meant that management and staff had to be proactive in ensuring that regular contact was kept with colleagues in the CMHT. For instance, the rehabilitation team may have set up a graded plan for a service user to attend his/her hospital appointments independently by bus, but then found that a well-meaning health colleague may have been taking out another client by car and offered this particular user a lift.

## Being the landlord

Another key challenge was that the service was housing-orientated. This meant that the rehabilitation service was essentially acting as landlords as well as being a support service. If people failed to keep up their tenancy agreement or breached house rules then they could be subject to eviction. Obviously having to tell someone that they are at risk of being evicted from their home can have an impact on the therapeutic relationship.

Some similar, but larger, organisations in the private sector have overcome this problem by having tenancy managers in separate teams, so that the therapeutic and landlord positions are assigned to different people. Where this is not possible due to staffing levels, some teams find it useful to ensure that the 'tenancy' conversation is undertaken by a staff member who has less face-to-face contact, for instance a senior manager.

Another challenging aspect was balancing the support to the individuals against the available resources, i.e. in this example, the supply of housing. As the service was housing-related and a step-down pathway had been established, the 'reward' to people for having achieved certain goals was the reality that they would have to pack up their things and move on to a new home. For some this was an exciting opportunity but for others it was an exhausting process both physically and mentally. When setting occupational goals surrounding accommodation, the limitations because of housing availability are a real barrier. However, barriers are encountered in any setting!

## Managing a non-occupational therapy team

When managing a non-occupational therapy team, a frequent challenge was how to explain to staff the reasons for taking certain actions. For instance, as mentioned previously, all service users were asked to take part in group/essential rehabilitation tasks such as cooking and cleaning, but there were occasions when this rule needed to be adapted for individuals for therapeutic purposes. Another example is the use of professional judgement to assess whether some individuals might need additional support to begin with (e.g. lifts in the car in order to ensure that their confidence to reach a more long-term goal was not knocked initially), and this judgement being offset by the risk of it being viewed by others as preferential treatment.

A further challenge was to ensure that all staff were engaged with people's support plans, so that they were acting consistently in line with rehabilitation principles. In a 24-hour service, when management are not always on hand, it can be very easy to slip into habits of 'doing for' people rather than supporting them to do for themselves. Incorporating support plans and rehabilitation practice as regular topics into supervision helped to ensure that staff maintained a constant awareness of their requirements.

## Professional identity

Working in the setting described earlier (Box 8.1) threw up a number of challenges:

### Additional assessments and measures

It was apparent that there was scope and opportunity to implement a number of occupational therapy-based assessments and outcome measures. However, issues included lack of funding to access the measures, and placing additional unnecessary stress and anxiety on service users by adding extra assessments on top of those required by the service providers. Therefore, the challenge here was not to see how occupational therapy tools could 'fit' into the service, but finding ways of combining the two. This was done by developing measures that were service user friendly and occupationally focused which also incorporated the measures needed for Supporting People's outcome recording. In this context it meant having the confidence to move beyond using solely occupational therapy-specific outcome measures so that the funding body could also be satisfied without causing duplication for the client.

### Demonstrating outcomes

Increasingly, as more services are commissioned out, occupational therapists will have to work in a way that demonstrates measureable outcomes to a number of audiences ranging from the client to the funding body. It is possible that, as Supporting People aim to work towards enabling people, occupational therapists could in future use such occupation-focused systems to influence the processes.

### Maintenance of standards as an occupational therapist

It is essential to be aware of anything which may be useful to a professional within a non-occupational therapy team, and awareness needs to be coupled with sufficient assertiveness to ensure that opportunities are not missed.

In a role that requires a professional qualification, occupational therapists have the right to ask for Continuing Professional Development (CPD) as this helps them to maintain their registrations. Regarding the case study (Box 8.1), this issue was taken on immediately after qualifying so this aspect felt particularly pertinent, especially as peers were taking on rotation roles and being supported through preceptorship programmes. This was raised at interview stage and, on the offer of employment, it was agreed that clinical supervision sessions with a health occupational therapist would take place. Once in post, occupational therapy-related assessments and training were discussed in management supervision and negotiated on a case-by-case basis.

### Identity and future of the profession

As a professional, working in isolation like this has the potential to cause a crisis of confidence. If occupational therapy is viewed as a profession in its adolescent stages (Turner 2011) then this can be an age where identity is crucial, but can also be an age of risk taking. Within this setting, the risk of not always feeling an 'identity' of occupational therapy was taken in order to try to ensure the best possible outcome for service users. For example, many generic tasks related to management had to be taken on, including finances and staff rotas, which had potential to cause a crisis of identity. Maintaining an occupational therapy identity whilst managing staff meant taking on these tasks to try to create an environment where staff as well as service users could thrive.

# Benefits of being an occupational therapist in this setting

Although working in isolation in a non-traditional setting can cause a certain amount of identity-related anxiety, it can also be argued that there are a number of benefits for the professional and for the service users.

## More than just rehabilitation

As occupational therapy is often seen as 'central to mental health rehabilitation' (Killaspy et al. 2014, p. 39), the setting appeared to lend itself to occupational therapists' skills and ideas. Occupational therapy, however, is more than just rehabilitation (Friedland 1988) and for this reason having an occupational therapist in this role was able to give added value. By focusing on clients' unique individual occupations, rather than solely a standard set of rehabilitation activities, people were supported towards Recovery by giving their rehabilitation programme unique meaning. This helped to increase motivation levels and participation from service users.

By focusing on the bigger picture of occupations, by default, occupational therapists are able to identify the other goals achieved in order to meet funding requirements. For instance, one of the Supporting People outcome headings is 'feeling safe'. A service user may not identify feeling safe as a goal in itself, but may identify living in a certain area of town, away from previous negative connections and dangerous temptations, as a goal.

In addition, although it was mentioned in the previous section that the role also entailed acting as a landlord and having difficult conversations with people, arguably an occupational therapist is well placed to do this. Although telling somebody that they are at risk of losing their tenancy is difficult, it is also an opportunity to review where that person is headed and what he/she hopes to achieve. For many, the behaviours that caused them to risk a breach of tenancy were either a cry for help or a need for change in either the individual or his/her environment. Through use of occupational analysis, keeping up a tenancy agreement can be seen as an integral part of, or step towards, their chosen occupations. Through problem solving and recognising the barriers presented by certain behaviours, plans could be made. In this way, conversations about at risk tenancies were turned around from a negative experience into opportunities to feel positive, find solutions, and eventually to move forwards.

## Occupational analysis and care plans

The client group using the service all had care coordinators and a care plan (see Chapter 1). One complaint of the Care Programme Approach (CPA) is that many service users do not feel in control or aware of their care plan (Mind 2009). Occupational analysis in this setting can offer an excellent opportunity to help clients to engage with their support plans (through which the service was being commissioned).

The reason for referral as outlined on the care plan was often only one or two lines, e.g. 'to regain skills and confidence in a 24-hour staffed setting with a view to independent living'. With these broad goals, occupational analysis skills could really come into play. By working with each client to discover what 'independent living' meant specifically to them, occupational analysis skills could be used to determine the skills and steps needed to participate in these occupations. For instance, many service users viewed 'living independently' as having their own place. By breaking this down, the concepts of applying for benefits, paying for bills and cooking on a budget could be explored. This in turn helped to increase motivation to gain these skills within the described setting.

Use of care plans also meant keeping regular contact with care coordinators to ensure overlap did not occur, as mentioned earlier. Working within a model of occupational therapy by considering the care plan as part of a person's institutional environment ensured that this overlap, or any conflict, was minimised.

## Freedom of role

Practising in a non-traditional setting can also lend itself to more variation and freedom. For instance, it was identified that often by the time people have reached the stage where they are accessing a rehabilitation service, they have had to tell the story of their illness a number of times; this can lead to their becoming stuck in the problem, or defined by their illness. Solution-focused techniques were used to adapt the assessment process. Redefining assessment questions, to have more of a solution focus, allowed for the opportunity to concentrate on strengths and empowerment. In addition, '[s]olution-focused conversations allow the client to carry out their own occupational analysis through describing in detail what they will be doing when life is going well' (Ghul 2012, p. 7). This means that much of the work for the following support plans is thought through already by the service user. In this way, although the essential service requirements for initial assessment were met, an occupational focus could also be given.

In addition, groupwork could be run in accordance with the demand of the client group and observations from staff. Service users had the opportunity to access groups externally through the local authority and third sector. However, sometimes people stated that they felt more at ease exploring some topics in their home environment where relations were already comfortable. So long as resources could be found within budget, then the nature, timing and topics of groupwork could be as flexible as needed. This allowed for them to be designed specifically as a mechanism to support people's occupational aspirations. In some cases clients were also helped to build up their confidence to attend groups in the community, where this was needed in their care plans.

It can be argued that it is this freedom from walking the same trails that other professionals have trod beforehand that allows new trails to be made (Wackerhausen 2009). Being in a setting without occupational therapy systems that had already been set up allowed for creativity and inventiveness by using clinical reasoning to develop new ways of working.

## Cross-sector working

The role also allowed for relationships to be built across sectors. As a service commissioned by health, links were built with care coordinators in order to enable strong partnership working. As there were no other occupational therapists in the service, clinical supervision was carried out by an occupational therapist who worked for the local CMHT. This led to an added benefit: increased understanding of the view of the care coordinators, as well as ensuring consistent practice across health and social care.

In addition, the role entailed working closely with housing providers as people moved on from the service, and establishing sustainable links in the community and third sector so that people were able to build up their lives outside of the service.

These relationships are particularly pertinent as many of the other services provided 'competition' to the rehabilitation service. Therefore it was useful not only for supporting service users, but also from a professional point of view. Although the post under discussion was permanent, at the time of writing the entire service has been disbanded due to local government cuts. Therefore the knowledge of other Supporting People funded projects, and how occupational therapy can fit into them, is crucial as, increasingly, contracts move away from the statutory sector.

# Conclusion

As our climate becomes more competitive and with implementation of new legislation, e.g. the Social Services and Wellbeing Act (Welsh Government 2014), many services (including rehabilitation services) are more likely to be carried out by other sectors and with an increased focus on outcomes. As occupational therapists we may need to become more familiar with adjusting our skills to other settings, to justifying our added value, and to showing how we support service users to take control of measuring their own outcomes.

The Royal College of Psychiatrists is promoting a national policy to continue to invest in rehabilitation services (Killaspy & Meier 2010), highlighting that the disinvestment in local services has led to increased out-of-county placements which not only cost more, but more importantly can have a detrimental effect on recovery by moving service users away from their own community.

It could be said that there continues to be a role for occupational therapists in rehabilitation services, but that it may become more diverse in nature as they move away from traditional NHS settings. It has already been established that the Recovery ethos fits very well with occupational therapy and we are well placed as a profession to find ways to combine the two.

If occupational therapists are brave enough to tread new paths then there is scope for them to continue to shape the rehabilitation services of the future, helping to ensure that such services are both Recovery- and occupation-focused. However, therapists will need to ensure that they are working towards the aspirations of occupation and Recovery and not towards the goals of the system of rehabilitation itself. The tangible outcomes that can be achieved through rehabilitation do put occupational therapists in an excellent position to demonstrate to funding providers the benefits of engaging occupational therapists.

# Useful resources

- Ghul, R. (2012). *Mental Creating Positive Futures. Solution Focused Recovery from Distress*, eds. R. Ghul, L. Duncan and S. Mousley. London: BT Press.
- Government of South Australia (2012). *The Framework for Recovery-oriented Rehabilitation in Mental Health Care*. Adelaide: SA Health.
- Joint Commissioning Panel for Mental Health (2012). *Guidance for Commissioners of Rehabilitation Services for People with Complex Mental Health Needs*. http://www.jcpmh.info
- Welsh Government (2014). *Social Services and Wellbeing Act.* Cardiff: Welsh Government.

# References

Friedland, J. (1988). Occupational therapy and rehabilitation: an awkward alliance. *American Journal of Occupational Therapy* **52** (5), 373–380.

Ghul, R. (2012). 'Introduction' in *Creating Positive Futures. Solution Focused Recovery from Mental Distress,* eds. R. Ghul, L. Duncan and S. Mousley. London: BT Press.

Government of South Australia (2012). *The Framework for Recovery-oriented Rehabilitation in Mental Health Care*. Adelaide: SA Health.

Joint Commissioning Panel for Mental Health (2012). *Guidance for Commissioners of Rehabilitation Services for People with Complex Mental Health Needs.* http://www.jcpmh.info

Killaspy, H., Marston, L., Green, N., Harrison, I., Lean, M., Cook, S., Mundy, T., Craig, T., Holloway, F., Leavey, G., Koeser, L., McCrone, P., Arbuthnott, M., Omar R.Z. & King, M. (2014). Clinical effectiveness of a staff training intervention in mental health inpatient rehabilitation units designed to increase patients' engagement in activities (the Rehabilitation Effectiveness for Activities for Life [REAL] study): single-blind, cluster-randomised controlled trial. *Lancet Psychiatry* **2** (1), 3–48.

Killaspy, H. & Meier, R. (2010). A fair deal for mental health includes local rehabilitation services. *The Psychiatrist* **34** (7), 265–267.

Lal, S. (2010). Prescribing Recovery as the new mantra for mental health: does one prescription serve all? *Canadian Journal of Occupational Therapy* **77** (2), 82–89.

Mind (2009). *Personalisation in Mental Health: Breaking Down the Barriers. A Guide for Care Coordinators*. London: Mind.

Turner, A. (2011). The Elizabeth Casson memorial lecture 2011: Occupational therapy – a profession in adolescence? *British Journal of Occupational Therapy* **74** (7), 314–322.

Wackerhausen, S. (2009). Collaboration, professional identity and reflection across boundaries. *Journal of Interprofessional Care* **23** (5), 455–473.

Welsh Government (2010). *Mental Health Measure.* Cardiff: Welsh Government.

Welsh Government (2014). *Social Services and Wellbeing Act.* Cardiff: Welsh Government.

# Chapter 9

# Roles in vocational rehabilitation

## Sarah Mead

## Introduction

I came into vocational rehabilitation in the UK quite by accident. The year I graduated as an occupational therapist many rotational posts were cut in my area. Coupled with this, and very ironically, it was hard for me initially to find a health and social care employer who would accommodate my mild physical disability. So I began to search more widely for roles that would encompass the spirit and values of occupational therapy, outside of health and social care. I had heard of emerging role occupational therapy, but never experienced it, so I sought advice from my university and they were incredibly helpful. Since qualifying, I have worked in two roles in relation to vocational rehabilitation, with an additional role in adult social care occupational therapy. In this chapter I aim to convey the challenge of the role and the type of work involved. I love vocational rehabilitation and I hope you will too, when you hear just how made for occupational therapists it is!

## Key points

- The occupational therapist's involvement in vocation/employment areas of a person's life has always been a key concern; it has, however, been provided in a wide variety of shapes and models of service delivery over the years.
- The third/voluntary sector is increasingly being commissioned to provide this type of service.
- Occupational therapists employed in vocational rehabilitation posts do not necessarily have 'occupational therapist' as their designation.
- Occupational therapists have all the essential skills and more for these roles.

# What is vocational rehabilitation (VR) and why do we need it?

Vocational rehabilitation is a combination of complex therapeutic interventions that enable clients to return to or gain work (Waddell et al. 2008, DWP 2004). The term 'work' itself has various interpretations and definitions, some only encompassing paid work, others more expansive and including voluntary work and childcare (COT 2009). As a vocational rehabilitation occupational therapist, your definition of work will very likely be constrained by the service you work for, depending on whether or not the service favours paid employment outcomes. In the current economic climate in the UK, the cost of unemployment is often headline news. Figures vary widely, but are often quoted as being in the tens of billions. The cost of unemployment is not just that of paying out benefits, but also the loss of potential revenue from potential tax payers who are not working. In addition, there is the cost of the health impacts of not working. Statistics show that long-term unemployment is bad for your health, with higher mortality and illness, and increased healthcare needs, including mental health issues, occurring in this group of people (Waddell & Burton 2006).

But if people are unwell, surely they cannot work? It is interesting to note Holmes' perspective on post-Second World War health services in the UK, as he held that work was potentially toxic to those who were already unwell (Holmes 2007). Today it is openly acknowledged that work can have negative effects on those who were not previously unwell (HSE 2014). Many of us have experienced the effect a negative working environment or experience can have on the mental health of friends and loved ones, and as health professionals, we ourselves are not immune to this. The Health and Safety Executive (HSE) highlighted that the majority of stress-related illness occurred in health professions or teaching roles (HSE 2014). Anecdotally, as a vocational rehabilitation occupational therapist, I have worked with health and social care professionals as clients many times. Ideas about work and ill health or disability have changed over time (Holmes 2007), and it is now thought that some work can be therapeutic, or even life lengthening, promoting physical, cognitive and emotional stimulation as well as having social inclusion benefits, making workers feel part of our society in the UK today (COT 2009, NHS 2015a, Waddell & Burton 2006).

# What is the experience of occupational therapists working for the vocational rehabilitation industry in the UK today?

A survey of OT News from January 2006 to May 2015 shows that there are some 60 articles related to vocational rehabilitation practice, guidelines and national policies, with over a third specific to mental health, a third updating on government policy and service changes and the rest related to physical and learning disabilities. The College of Occupational Therapists (COT) actively supports vocational rehabilitation occupational therapists via:

- Specialist Section Work (COT) who host regular Continuing Professional Development (CPD) events

- Hosting vocational rehabilitation posters, presentations and workshops at the COT annual conference

- Online CPD resources such as *Work Matters* for occupational therapists wanting to learn more about vocational rehabilitation (COT 2011)

- Research regularly reported in the *British Journal of Occupational Therapy* (BJOT).

This is clearly an active domain for occupational therapists in the UK, but where are vocational rehabilitation occupational therapists employed in the UK today? The vocational rehabilitation industry is very broad, covering physical disability, learning disability and mental health and across statutory, private and third sectors. In some ways it is difficult to quantify, because it is so widely spread and integrated into every sector (see Figure 9.1). Those new to the idea of vocational rehabilitation may not be aware of how established it is for occupational therapists in the UK.

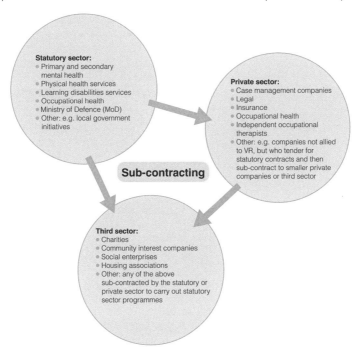

*Figure 9.1: An example of the broad range of the vocational rehabilitation industry in the UK today.*

It is clear to see that for vocational rehabilitation, there are many opportunities for occupational therapists both in the statutory and third sector. It is clear that parts of the statutory and third sector specialise in mental health, but as we shall see, occupational therapists who work with other client groups are often addressing mental health issues as part of their therapeutic work. A very small sample of occupational therapists working in vocational rehabilitation was interviewed during April 2015. These included:

- A consultant occupational therapist at strategic level working for COT/NHS/third sector charity
- Two independent occupational therapists working with employers – ergonomic and vocational rehabilitation consultant
- An occupational therapist working for a community interest company as an employability officer
- One specialist occupational therapist within secondary mental health.

As with generic mental health work, vocational rehabilitation occupational therapists often do not have occupational therapist within their job title. In my vocational rehabilitation roles, I was titled Employment Support Officer and Work & Learning Coordinator. As with many vocational rehabilitation occupational therapists, I was working as an emerging role occupational therapist. An emerging role occupational therapist is defined as an occupational therapist who is working in a setting where there is currently no occupational therapy role established (COT 2006). Guidance on working in new and diverse roles is available from the College of Occupational Therapists (COT 2015a), who have also set up a network of occupational therapists with interest in this domain.

## So why vocational rehabilitation occupational therapy?

Because vocational rehabilitation occupational therapy isn't a straightforward, traditional pathway in the UK, occupational therapists seem to gravitate to it from very different starting points (as I found in my research when interviewing other vocational rehabilitation occupational therapists). Gerard was naturally drawn to vocational rehabilitation, with an interest in productivity, wanting to work holistically across the physical, social and mental health spectrum. For Veronica (independent) and Carol (mental health occupational therapist) it was their pull towards client-centred working that led their interest. They felt that clients were wanting to return to work, but resources were not available. They took the lead as occupational therapists to address work-focused goals, bringing the vocational services to the clients within their own service or indeed creating vocational services to address client needs. Zoe was drawn to occupational therapy because of vocational rehabilitation, after working for the government's condition management programme, part of 'Pathways to Work' which has now ended in England, Wales and Scotland (Nice & Davidson 2010). She loved it so much that she went on to train as an occupational therapist and has gone back into a vocational rehabilitation emerging role in the third sector. Margot began her career in Australia, where vocational rehabilitation is much more embedded into occupational therapy culture and is a very traditional alternative to working in health and social care. There is also substantial evidence that occupational therapists are increasingly working in occupational health (Bright *et al.* 2011, Cookson 2014, Lonnergan & Wick

2013, Williams 2015). Occupational therapists in vocational rehabilitation seem determined to retain their occupational therapy identity, using occupational therapy with entrepreneurial and marketing skills, to ensure that occupational therapy has a voice in this growing industry.

# The vocational rehabilitation and occupational therapy processes

I am often asked if emerging roles fit into the occupational therapy process. My answer is 'yes, depending on the role'. It is not a case of fitting the vocational rehabilitation role into occupational therapy; rather, the vocational rehabilitation role *is* already occupational therapy. It is often a question of language, perspective and skills of the person in that role. In my experience of working in emerging roles, we can have a team of people from multiple professional backgrounds doing the same role using similar and different skills. Sounds familiar doesn't it? Multi-disciplinary teams, inter-professional teams, generic roles: these are all terms we are familiar with in traditional practice. Each practitioner may describe the role in their own terms, particular to their profession, or describe them in the generic terms of their employer.

We can explore the idea of language and perspective by looking more closely at the vocational rehabilitation and occupational therapy process and how they mirror each other. Vocational rehabilitation is a progressive pathway with a pre-vocational stage where the client is preparing, exploring and considering vocational options, and an active vocational stage where the client is engaging actively with vocational rehabilitation activities to find work or return to current employment.

Ross (2007, p. 120) succinctly outlines the vocational rehabilitation process in a linear diagrammatical form which includes referral, initial interview/assessment, pre-vocational phase, worksite visit, return to work plan, intervention, evaluation and discharge. She goes into some detail about each stage and if you want to find out more, this is a very accessible format. Ross (2007) acknowledges that different vocational rehabilitation services will vary slightly from this pattern. Figure 9.2 gives an indication of the elements of the vocational rehabilitation and occupational therapy processes. Using Ross (2007) as a starting point, I have added elements from my own vocational rehabilitation experience and that of the interviewees to this process.

As we can see in Figure 9.2, vocational rehabilitation maps very easily on to an occupational therapy process and in fact the approaches used in vocational rehabilitation and occupational therapy can both be seen as rehabilitative (relearning skills, learning new skills) and compensative (adaptations/ reasonable adjustments to physical, environmental or cognitive elements to facilitate task/activity completion). Some of the terminologies are different, but the skills used can be the same. It is my belief that occupational therapists have particular skills to offer vocational rehabilitation in the domains of functional assessment, activity analysis and grading. With our evidence-based knowledge of assessment and treatment planning, occupational therapists are in prime position to produce cost-effective and sustainable vocational rehabilitation outcomes.

**141**

**Vocational rehabilitation process**

**Occupational therapy process**

1   Vocational rehabilitation referral for job retention

Occupational therapy referral for inpatient preparing to return home

**2**                **Initial interview/assessment**

**3**   Pre-treatment phase:
- Client considering information provided by occupational therapist

- Client considering options for vocational rehabilitation
- Client considering options for treatment

**4**   Vocational action planning with client:
Treatment planning with client:

**Client-centred goal setting**

**5**   Action plan implementation
Intervention

*Pre-vocational phase:*
*Pre-home discharge phase:*

- Groundwork for vocational rehabilitation
- Client receiving vocational training and/or learning coping skills/techniques relevant to work setting
- Functional Capacity Evaluation (FCE) and Transferable Skills Analysis (TSA)

- Groundwork for ADL rehabilitation
- Client receiving early stages occupational therapy input, re-training in ADLs, learning coping skills/ techniques relevant to home setting
- Functional assessment and activity analysis

Work hardening, increasing work activity and difficulty

Grading, increasing ADL activity tolerance and difficulty

*Vocational phase:*
*Home discharge preparation phase:*

**6** • Worksite visit, liaison with employer, support workers, mentors
- Discussion/negotiation of reasonable adjustments to the work environment and work tasks to facilitate return
- Job task analysis and observation
- Job coaching in work

- Home visit, liaison with family members/carers
- Discussion/negotiation of home ADL routines and environmental adjustments/adaptations required to facilitate return home
- ADL assessment in the home
- Rehabilitation activities in the home

- Return to work plan formulated
- Supported return to work (VR worker visiting, possibly giving in-work support)
- Vocational rehabilitation specialist to review progress
- Observational assessment
- Job coaching, vocational rehabilitation plan and reasonable adjustments re-negotiated as required

- Home discharge plan formulated
- Supported discharge home (carers/family in place, giving support)
- Occupational therapist visit to review progress
- Observational assessment
- Possible further rehabilitation or adaptation re-negotiated as required

**7**   Return to work achieved
Home discharge achieved

**8**                 Evaluation

**9**             Discharge from service

*Figure 9.2: The vocational rehabilitation and occupational therapy processes.*

With reference to the Functional Capacity Evaluation (FCE) and Transferable Skills Analysis (TSA), these are global terms for vocational rehabilitation assessments that focus on workplace function and skills respectively. This is similar to global terms in occupational therapy such as kitchen or wash/dress assessments that focus on function in ADLs. As with occupational therapy functional assessments, there are many examples of FCE and TSA across the range of standardised and non-standardised. An FCE enables the vocational rehabilitation specialist to assess the functional abilities of the client in the work setting, and this in turn, for example, enables them to 'develop a treatment program, to measure the physical abilities of patients before and after a rehabilitation program, to modify a rehabilitation treatment, to evaluate whether an injured worker can work, and to determine when he/she can return to work' (Chen 2007, p. 121).

A TSA tool enables the vocational rehabilitation specialist to help 'individuals identify their transferable skills to assist in career exploration and the job search' (Liptak & Shatkin 2011, p. 1). Transferable skills, here, are identified as 'portable skills that people take from one life experience to another', gained from and transferable across 'a wide variety of activities engaged in at work, at play, in the community, and with family and then transferred from one task to another' (Liptak & Shatkin 2011, p. 2). This model of thinking is surely the 'bread and butter' of the occupational therapist, as we assess our clients' strengths and enable our clients to use those strengths to move forward in areas of need or reduced capacity.

# Vocational rehabilitation models and approaches

As we know, occupational therapy models serve to guide us in our work, giving us an occupational system for clinical reasoning and intervention planning (Bryant et al. 2014). Frames of reference are the concepts behind the models, 'providing a conceptual foundation for practice' and approaches are the means by which we put the theory of the model into practice (Bryant et al. 2014, p. 43). In my vocational rehabilitation practice, I have not been permitted to use a formal occupational therapy model. Having spoken to other occupational therapists working in emerging roles I find this can often be the case. Nevertheless, my processes for assessment and treatment planning followed Model of Human Occupation (MOHO) concepts (Kielhofner 2008). I found the model useful and logical to frame my vocational rehabilitation practice and my CPD. What encouraged me was the MOHO's specific attention to vocational rehabilitation in the form of its Worker Role Interview (Braveman et al. 2005), and Work Environment Impact Scale (Moore-Corner et al. 1998) assessments. Both of these assessments have good evidence to support their use in mental health (Lohss et al. 2012, Williams et al. 2010). Although I was not permitted by my services to use standardised work-focused assessments, I created a home-grown initial interview based on MOHO principles, and this gave me a structure for my clinical reasoning, rooted deeply in occupational therapy principles.

A survey of the 20 or so OT News articles (2006 to 2015) concerned with mental health vocational rehabilitation, and of the five interviewees, showed that some of the following models, were used to support vocational rehabilitation treatment planning:

- MOHO (Kielfhofner 2008)
- Individual Placement and Support model (IPS) (Drake *et al.* 2012)
- Stages of Change Model (Prochaska & DiClemente 1984)
- Canadian Model of Occupational Performance (CMOP) (CAOT 2015)
- Stepped-care model of delivery (Bower & Gilbody 2005)
- Health Belief Model (Janz & Becker 1984).

The same survey, combined with interviewees and my own clinical choices for vocational rehabilitation, reveals a variety of approaches being used:

- Biopsychosocial approach
- Parachute approach (Bolles 2010)
- Cognitive Behavioural Therapy-based (IAPT 2011)
- SMART (specific, measurable, achievable, realistic and timed) goals approach
- Ergonomic approach
- Compensatory approach
- Rehabilitative approach
- Client-centred approach
- Bio-mechanical approach
- Narrative reasoning approach.

If we are looking for specific vocational rehabilitation models of practice, this can be more complex to understand from our occupational therapy perspective, because different professional areas can hold very different definitions of the concept of model. For example, a wider view of models is proposed by the National Institute for Health Research (NIHR) in its report *Economic Evidence Around Employment Support* (Wilkins *et al.* 2012). They use a 'fluid definition of "model" to include any documented approach, pilot or scheme, relating to supporting people with mental health illness or learning disability in employment' (Wilkins *et al.* 2012, p. 3). Rather than a model to support the formulation of clinical reasoning, this appears to be a definition for models of service. I feel it is important to make this distinction, especially if we wish to retain our HCPC registration as occupational therapists working in diverse settings. Retaining our HCPC occupational therapist registration comes with the expectation that we will be able to evidence our occupational therapy practice and CPD. Our occupational therapy clinical reasoning and intervention planning will be informed by clinical models that are concerned with these aspects. Our clinical reasoning and interventions may be bounded or even constrained by the service models within which we are working.

Wilkins *et al.* (2012) have done extensive research on vocational rehabilitation services and the economic evidence (or lack of it) to support their implementation. They reveal a huge variety of schemes and services related to vocational rehabilitation in the UK in the 21st century, including supported employment, sheltered workshops, schemes funded by DWP and JCP, charities, private companies, such as football clubs, healthcare services and local government. This is an extensive piece of work, useful not only for exploring the cost effectiveness of potential services, but also for providing us with a list of so many vocational rehabilitation opportunities for occupational therapists.

As for occupational therapy clinical models, vocational rehabilitation service models will also have fundamental frames of reference, congruent with their approaches to vocational rehabilitation. One of these is the concept of 'train and place' versus 'place and train' (Drake *et al.* 2012). Train and place models of service 'assume that the individual benefits from some form of training, instruction, or practice in a protected but artificial setting before entering a competitive work role' (Drake *et al.* 2012, p. 24). Whereas place and train models of practice are based on the principle that it is inefficient to try to train someone prior to establishing them in a work role, because specific learned skills are not necessarily transferable from one job to another (Drake *et al.* 2012).

If we categorise the service models in the NIHR report (Wilkins *et al.* 2012), a pattern begins to emerge. Some types of service may feature in either 'train and place' or 'place and train' models, depending on how they are conceived.

## Box 9.1: Train and place vs place and train – vocational rehabilitation service models

### Train and place

- Supported employment (physical and learning disabilities and mental health)
- Sheltered workshops (Remploy, Able and Willing) – workplace specifically tailored to suit the abilities of its disabled workforce
- Local initiatives between community and business (e.g. football clubs such as Brighton & Hove Albion's project 'Albion in the Community')
- Clubhouse model – often within a mental health service – practice for interview techniques, experience of different job roles within a supportive setting
- VR within day centre services
- IAPT employment support model – encompassing CBT therapy with specific employment support (either in-work support or promoting clients' self-advocacy at work)
- Employment preparation – social enterprises
- Employment support for the unemployed
- Employment support for those already working (job retention)
- Using personal budgets to buy VR support.

**145**

**Place and train**

- Individual placement and support model (severe and enduring mental ill health)
- Supported employment (physical and learning disabilities and mental health)
- Sheltered workshops (Remploy, Able and Willing) – workplace specifically tailored to suit the abilities of its disabled workforce
- Workstep and Supported Permitted Work – Job Centre Plus funded employment support schemes
- Volunteering support initiatives – local and national schemes
- Work experience placements – via schools, employment support services, local initiatives
- Employment support for the unemployed
- Employment support for those already working (job retention)
- Using personal budgets to buy VR support
- Access to Work – central government grants for equipment and support (clients have to be in employment or about to start working before they become eligible).

# Individual placement and support: 'place and train' – the debate for occupational therapy

You will notice that the IPS model features in the place and train list (Box 9.1). Individual placement and support has become very popular in the UK, with many mental health services implementing it (Bones 2013, McGall & Hilditch 2013, Parkin 2014, Young 2014). This model for supported employment has much evidence to support it, including randomised controlled trials carried out in the US, where the model was developed (Drake *et al.* 2012). Individual placement and support has been mainly used in relation to finding employment rather than job retention (retaining current employment). Individual placement and support places itself firmly in the place and train area of vocational rehabilitation. It has eight principles upon which the model of practice is based and upon which any service wishing to use it will be evaluated and rated. Rating is completed using the IPS Supported Employment Fidelity Scale (Drake *et al.* 2012, p. 137) (see Box 9.2).

Box 9.2: The features of the IPS Supported Fidelity Scale

**1. Competitive employment:**
seeking voluntary, sheltered or any unpaid work is discouraged.

**2. All clients who express an interest are eligible:**

the client will be accepted whatever their condition or stage of their illness.

**3. Supported employment and mental health services are integrated into a team:**

interestingly, some occupational therapists have successfully used elements of IPS when it has not been possible to implement the whole model, specifically when it has not been possible to integrate the supported employment service into the mental health service (Waghorn et al. 2011).

**4. Client-centred goals**

**5. Benefits advice personalised to the client**

**6. Rapid job search:**

no lengthy pre-employment assessment, treatment, training or counselling.

**7. Development of employment opportunities:**

employment specialists build up an employment network with local employers.

**8. Time unlimited and individualised support:**

this is potentially a difficult requirement to meet, given the funding and time constraints of NHS services at the present time.

Adapted from: Drake, R.E., Bond, G.R. & Becker, D.R. (2012). *Individual Placement and Support: an Evidence Based Approach to Supported Employment.* New York: Oxford University Press.

## Pre-employment training and IPS

Individual placement and support strongly advocates that pre-employment training is not efficient or effective. Furthermore, IPS proponents believe that social skills learned in pre-vocational settings do not transfer into work settings for people who have severe and enduring mental health problems (Drake et al. 2012, Waghorn et al. 2009). However, this view, as noted in Waghorn et al. (2009), appears to stem from an article written in 2006 by Kopelowicz et al. The article, a critical review, seeks to examine the use and efficiency of social skills training for people who have a diagnosis of schizophrenia. The article does not indicate that the findings are generalisable to other clients who have severe and enduring mental health problems other than schizophrenia.

For clients who do have schizophrenia, the article states, their learning of social skills is impaired or has been interrupted before adult social skills have been acquired. Therefore these clients will have a significant social skills gap. Kopelowicz et al. state that '[r]epeated practice or overlearning is essential to ensure assimilation and durability of interpersonal skills' (Kopelowicz et al. 2006, p. 14). They state that studies over the preceding three decades showed discouraging results for transferring learned social skills into clients' environments. However, they also state that 'the more alike the training and natural environments, the more likely the behaviors will be used in everyday life' (Kopelowicz et al. 2006, p. 14) and that more recent studies have shown that when this is the case, it increases the likelihood of social skill transfer to everyday life settings. I would therefore argue that the transferability of social skills into a work setting may depend on the skills of the occupational therapist or vocational rehabilitation specialist.

As occupational therapists we are particularly skilled at analysing activities, including elements of social skills required, and at incorporating this into a graded client-centred rehabilitation plan, regularly reviewed with the client, to support them to achieve their goals. The article does not state that the principle of social skills training mapped into real life experiences means that paid employment is the only work outcome (an IPS model condition). Opportunities to practise social skills in a work environment and to receive the rewards therein are therefore not solely the domain of paid competitive work. For some clients, paid competitive work will be the ultimate or only goal; for others, voluntary work, work placements or apprenticeships may be part of the vocational rehabilitation journey or indeed their ultimate goal. As an occupational therapist, I feel that occupational therapy principles are based on the fundamental belief that skills are transferable. When we consider a client's occupational strengths and needs we are analysing what strengths (skills) they have that can be used to help them address their occupational needs as part of our treatment planning. I also feel that occupational therapy is based on the principles of train-place-train: we begin rehabilitation after assessment, using a graded approach, often in a controlled setting, before putting the client into a live situation, be it bathing or a walk in the community, and we then follow this up with further rehabilitation (or training to use adaptations/compensatory techniques) to increase exposure or strength or stamina in more challenging situations, until a client has reached their intended goal.

## Train and place – pre-vocational training and volunteering – evidence and experiences

Although the evidence for the use of IPS is strong, this doesn't necessarily negate the use of other forms of vocational rehabilitation. I wonder how well IPS would work for clients who have mental health problems combined with more complex disabilities such as learning disabilities or brain injury or stroke, or indeed physical disabilities or life limiting health conditions. In my experience as a vocational rehabilitation occupational therapist, many of my clients who had physical or learning disabilities had varying degrees of mental health problems at some time, and at times over half my caseload in primary care mental health comprised clients who had physical disabilities or health conditions. Clients with complex conditions have required a carefully graded treatment plan to bring them close to the competitive job market or back to their current employment. In addition, there are some circumstances where it may not be possible for clients to gain employment in the paid competitive job market, such as forensic mental health, or to immediately return to their current employment, e.g. for someone who has had a recent inpatient admission. In both cases, clients will need a carefully graded treatment plan to enable them to find new or retain their current employment. Probyn and Barnhouse (2012) stated that a quarter of inpatient acute admissions required employment advice or support, and Szerezla (2009) emphasises the benefits of patients being encouraged to discuss employment issues early in the admissions process.

A survey of *OT News* provides much practice-based evidence of mental health occupational therapists using train and place and pre-vocational methods to work with clients, where a hospital, charity or social enterprise provides in-house training. This included vocational preparation, voluntary work and sometimes paid work for patients/clients (Chester 2009, Coxon 2008, Crispin 2011, Gumaste 2009, Hadley 2013, McMorris 2010, Meredith 2011, Robertson 2011, Szerezla 2009). It is extremely important for any occupational therapist involved in vocational rehabilitation to be confident about advising clients on disclosure of a disability or health condition. The addition of a forensic history increases this even further (Meredith 2011, Paden & Bradford 2014). There is much good advice on mental health disclosure from organisations such as Time to Change (TTC 2015), Rethink (Rethink 2015a) and Mind (Mind 2011) and on disclosure of criminal convictions (Nacro 2015, Rethink 2015b).

Overall, more occupational therapy research in the area of pre-vocational training and voluntary work would be helpful for occupational therapists who are considering the best vocational rehabilitation models and approaches to use with their specific client groups and services in mental health. It appears that many occupational therapists support the use of voluntary work as a rehabilitative environment or as a goal unto itself, and feel strongly that it can have positive benefits for mental and physical health (Baldotto 2009, Black & Living 2004, Hawkins 2008, Meredith 2011). In addition, the NHS (NHS 2015b) and the Institute for Volunteering Research (IVR) (IVR 2015) provide links to much research in the field of the benefits of volunteering for mental health across the lifespan.

# Employment support in primary mental healthcare

Initially opened to patients of working age, Improving Access to Psychological Therapies (IAPT) services were, in part, created to address the growing issues of sickness absence due to mental ill health. These services are principally based on the use of CBT for clients who have mild to moderate depression, anxiety and phobias. In my experience as a vocational rehabilitation occupational therapist, the IAPT services in different geographical areas can have very different names e.g. 'Brighton & Hove Wellbeing Service', 'Time to Talk', 'Health in Mind' (no connection to the charity Mind), which can be confusing for clients (and sometimes for health professionals too!) as they do not necessarily initially understand that this is an NHS service. However, as regards the effectiveness of CBT alone to address employment issues and mental health, this has been questioned (Cameron 2012). Improving

Access to Psychological Therapies now uses employment support or advice services in conjunction with its CBT treatment: '[t]he IAPT programme's introduction of link employment support workers can be seen as an acknowledgement that CBT intervention alone may be insufficient to produce positive work outcomes' (Cameron 2012, p. 462).

Improving Access to Psychological Therapies services now serve the whole of England (IAPT 2015), and with evidence to support employment advice/support services within them, opportunities for vocational rehabilitation in this domain are increasing. A review of the pilot employment service for IAPT (Gov.uk 2013) revealed the success of the Employment Advisors (EAs). Upon first reading, we may wonder what role an occupational therapist could have within an employment advice service, but having read the report, and from my own experience, it is clear that 'advice' covered much more than providing information. The employment services develop client-centred action plans to address low confidence levels, gaining new insights into experience and feelings about work, gaining advice on employment rights, learning CV and interviewing skills, negotiating with the employer, exploring changing jobs or staying in the current job. In my service, we took a holistic view of work, to encompass voluntary work, education or theory associated training as vocational rehabilitation. Day (2014) also has experience of working for an employment support coordination service within IAPT, mainly working with job retention clients. Day's service used activity analysis, grading, analysis of job demands, impact of the job on health, exploration of the work environment (Day 2014). The Gov.uk review of IAPT employment services identified that the clients 'seeking the support of EAs had more complex needs' (Gov.uk 2013, p. 3); in the IAPT service world, this would mean clients who are in the moderate range of mental health problems rather than mild or severe and enduring. Surely this indicates a gap for vocational rehabilitation occupational therapists to fill. Overall, the evidence seems to indicate that the best outcomes are for IAPT clients to receive therapy and employment support to achieve the best employment outcomes for the client (Cameron 2012, Gov.uk 2013).

# Assessments and tools for vocational rehabilitation

It would not be possible to list all the assessments and tools available to a vocational rehabilitation occupational therapist. We have seen previously that some occupational therapy models already have vocational rehabilitation assessments in place, with evidence to support their use behind them. A survey of the 20 or so *OT News* articles (2006 to 2015) concerned with mental health vocational rehabilitation, and of the five interviewees in my own survey, found that some of the following assessments and outcome measures were used to support vocational rehabilitation treatment planning:

- Goal Attainment Scale (GAS) (Turner-Stokes 2009)
- Worker Role Interview (Kielhofner 2008)
- Canadian Occupational Performance Measure (COPM) (CAOT 2015)

- Outcome Star by Triangle Consulting Social Enterprise Limited (TCSE Ltd 2015)
- HSE-based risk assessments (HSE 2015)
- The pain self-efficacy questionnaire (Nicholas 1989)
- Hospital Anxiety and Depression Scale (HADS) (Zigmond & Snaith 1983)
- The fear-avoidance beliefs questionnaire (Waddell *et al.* 1993)
- Functional Capacity Evaluation (Matheson 2015)
- Home-grown assessments and outcomes measures based on principles of models above, but adapted to fit the service
- Transferable skills analysis tool (Liptak & Shatkin 2011)
- Wellness Recovery Action Plan (WRAP) modified for work (Copeland 1997)
- Eisenhower's Urgent Important Matrix (Coaching Tools 2015).

In my work as a vocational rehabilitation occupational therapist, I developed a transferable skills analysis tool based on theory from Liptak and Shatkin (2011) and Oswald *et al.* (1999). Together with this, I used a Wellness Recovery Action Plan (WRAP) modified for work (Copeland 1997), and tools like the Eisenhower's Urgent Important Matrix (Coaching Tools 2015), alongside the service scores for GAD7 anxiety and PHQ9 depression scales (IAPT 2011). Whatever tools you decide to use in your vocational rehabilitation practice, it is important to remember that your clinical decisions and treatment planning will need to be realistic for today's job market in the UK. A sound knowledge of government guidelines and benefits systems and fundamental employment law principles will enable you to effectively support your client into work. Resources can be found via COT Specialist Section Work (COT 2015b), Citizens Advice Bureau (Citizens Advice 2015) and Gov.uk (Gov.uk 2015).

# Occupational therapy vocational rehabilitation, future strategies for the UK

I ended my interviews with occupational therapists currently working in vocational rehabilitation by asking them: how would you like occupational therapy in vocational rehabilitation to develop in the future in the UK? Who better to ask than those who are working in the field today? I had a variety of responses, but they were all inter-connected:

Occupational therapists should be promoting occupational therapy in vocational rehabilitation expertise to stakeholders more:

- Occupational therapy in vocational rehabilitation should be integrated into occupational therapy and health services more
- Increasing our leadership in health and social care and commissioning in the UK as occupational therapists

- Increasing COT support and drive for occupational therapy in vocational rehabilitation
- Occupational therapists should be highlighting examples of good occupational therapy in vocational rehabilitation practice whenever they can.

Occupational therapists should be promoting to each other the contributions they can make to health, work and wellbeing:

- Teaching occupational therapy in vocational rehabilitation at university for under-graduate and post-graduate students
- Demonstrating to occupational therapists and occupational therapy students the individual contribution occupational therapists can make to vocational rehabilitation
- Ensuring that occupational therapists understand that occupational therapy in vocational rehabilitation is core occupational therapy in action
- Promoting vocational rehabilitation as a core skill for occupational therapists
- Using occupational science to frame our vocational rehabilitation practice.

Occupational therapists should be developing more occupational therapists in vocational rehabilitation opportunities in the UK:

- Demonstrating to students how they can work in this sector in the UK, even if the job doesn't have 'occupational therapist' or 'occupational therapy' in the title
- Ensuring that occupational therapists and occupational therapy students understand what the vocational rehabilitation industry is in the UK today – the different sectors, public, private and third sector
- Occupational therapists should also work more with disadvantaged groups in vocational rehabilitation, not just those who have health conditions, e.g. homeless people, long-term unemployed people, single parents
- Ensuring that vocational rehabilitation services take an early intervention approach – not waiting until clients are at risk of losing their jobs or have already lost them.

## Conclusion

During the course of this chapter, I have attempted to highlight some of the key issues faced by occupational therapy vocational rehabilitation in the UK. This is not an exhaustive exploration, but I hope it will serve to interest and excite occupational therapists about the wonderful opportunities and challenges that occupational therapy vocational rehabilitation can give us. I continue to promote the role of occupational therapist in vocational rehabilitation in my work as a practitioner, supervisor and lecturer and I am proud of the vocational rehabilitation occupational therapists who work hard to carve out their role in this emerging industry in the UK, using their clinical expertise, client-centred approach and leadership skills to promote our profession.

# Useful resources

- www.career-lifeskills.com
- www.citizensadvice.org.uk
- www.thecoachingtoolscompany.com
- www.cot.co.uk
- www.gov.uk/government
- www.ivr.org.uk
- http://jist.emcp.com
- www.ncbi.nlm.nih.gov
- www.mind.org.uk/media
- www.nacro.org.uk/resettlement-advice-service
- www.nhs.uk/Livewell/mentalhealth
- www.nhs.uk/Livewell/volunteering
- www.onetcenter.org
- www.rethink.org/living-with-mental-illness
- www.roymatheson.com

# References

Baldotto, J. (2009). The therapeutic benefits of volunteering and fundraising for service users. *OT News* **17** (2), 18.

Black, W. & Living, R. (2004). Volunteerism as an occupation and its relationship to health and wellbeing. *British Journal of Occupational Therapy* **67** (12), 526–532.

Bolles, R. (2010). *What Colour is your Parachute?* Berkeley: Ten Speed Press.

Bones, K. (2013). Taking the IPS approach. *OT News* **21** (5), 34–35.

Bower, P. & Gilbody, S. (2005). Stepped care in psychological therapies: access, effectiveness and efficiency. *British Journal of Psychiatry* **186** (1), 11–17.

Braveman, B., Robson, M., Velozo, C., Kielhofner, G., Fisher, G., Forsyth, K. & Kerschbaum, J. (2005). *Worker Role Interview (WRI) Version 10.0*. http://www.cade.uic.edu/moho (last accessed: 10.1.2016).

Bright, J., Bracher, M. & Stafford, K. (2011). Complementary professions? Occupational therapy and occupational health and the emergency services. *OT News* **19** (3) 30–31.

Bryant, W., Fieldhouse, J. & Bannigan, K. (eds) (2014). *Creek's Occupational Therapy and Mental Health,* 5th edn. Oxford: Churchill Livingstone Elsevier.

Cameron, J. (2012). Supporting workers with mental health problems to retain employment: users' experiences of a UK job retention project. *Work* **42** (4), 461–471.

Canadian Association of Occupational Therapists (2015). *Canadian Model of Occupational Performance.* https://www.caot.ca (last accessed: 15.4.2015).

Chen, J.J. (2007). Functional capacity evaluation & disability. *Iowa Orthopaedic Journal* **27**, 121–127.

Chester, P. (2009). Real work opportunities. *OT News* **17** (10), 42–43.

Citizens Advice (2015). *Basic rights at work.* https://www.citizensadvice.org.uk (last accessed: 15.11.2015).

Coaching Tools (2015). *Coaching Tools 101: the Urgent Important Matrix – What is it and How to Use it!* https://www.thecoachingtoolscompany.com (last accessed: 3.6.2015).

College of Occupational Therapists (2006). *Developing the Occupational Therapy Profession: Providing New Work-based Learning Opportunities for Students.* https://www.cot.co.uk/ (last accessed: 21.5.2015).

College of Occupational Therapists (2009). *Specialist Section – Work (COTSS Work) Occupational Therapy in Vocational Rehabilitation: a Brief Guide to Current Practice in the UK.* https://www.cot.co.uk/ (last accessed: 15.5.2015).

College of Occupational Therapists (2011). *Work Matters: an Online Learning Resource.* http://www.cot.co.uk (last accessed: 2.4.2015).

College of Occupational Therapists (2015a). *New Roles for the Profession.* https://www.cot.co.uk (last accessed: 1.4.2015).

College of Occupational Therapists (2015b). *Specialist Section – Work (COTSS Work): Supporting People to Remain in, Return to, or Obtain Work is a Key Function of Occupational Therapy.* https://www.cot.co.uk (last accessed: 30.11.2015).

Cookson, K. (2014). Occupational therapy in occupational health – is it working? *OT News* **22** (4), 28–29.

Copeland, M.E. (1997). *WRAP and Recovery Books.* http://www.mentalhealthrecovery.com (last accessed: 5.5.2015).

Coxon, C. (2008). Getting a foot in the revolving door. *OT News* **16** (10), 22.

Crispin, D. (2011). Turning over a new leaf. *OT News* **19** (12), 32.

Day, C. (2014). Working well. *OT News* **22** (6), 41.

Department for Work and Pensions (2004). *Building Capacity for Work: a UK Framework for Vocational Rehabilitation.* London: DWP.

Drake, R.E., Bond, G.R. & Becker, D.R. (2012). *Individual Placement and Support: an Evidence-based Approach to Supported Employment.* New York: Oxford University Press.

Gov.UK (2013). *Evaluation of Employment Advisers in the Improving Access to Psychological Therapies Programme.* https://www.gov.uk (last accessed: 13.3.2015).

Gov.UK (2015). *Your Rights at Work and Trade Unions.* https://www.gov.uk (last accessed: 1.12.2015).

Gumaste, D. (2009). Vocational skills training with a new medium secure forensic service. *OT News* **17** (10), 26–27.

Hadley, L. (2013). Planning the future. *OT News* **21** (9), 35.

Hawkins, S. (2008). Volunteering improves health and wellbeing, study finds. *OT News* **16** (10), 6.

Health & Safety Executive (2014). *Stress-related and Psychological Disorders in Great Britain 2014.* http://www.hse.gov.uk (last accessed: 25.2.2015).

Health & Safety Executive (2015). *Interactive Tools.* http://www.hse.gov.uk (last accessed: 3.6.2015).

Holmes, J. (2007). *Vocational Rehabilitation.* Oxford: Wiley-Blackwell.

*Improving Access to Psychological Therapies (2011).* The IAPT Data Handbook:

*Guidance on Recording and Monitoring Outcomes to Support Local Evidence-based Practice.* http://www.iapt.nhs.uk (last accessed: 1.5.2015).

*Improving Access to Psychological Therapies (2015). Regions.* http://www.iapt.nhs.uk (last accessed: 3.12.2015).

Institute for Volunteering Research (2015). *Welcome to IVR's Evidence Bank.* http://www.ivr.org.uk (last accessed: 15.11.2015).

Janz, N.K. & Becker, M.H. (1984). The health belief model: a decade later. *Health Education Quarterly* **11** (1),1–47.

Kielhofner, G. (2008). *Model of Human Occupation: Theory and Application,* 4th edn. Philadelphia: Lippincott, Wilkins and Williams.

Kopelowicz, A., Liberman, R.P. & Zarate, R. (2006). Recent advances in social skills training for schizophrenia. *Schizophrenia Bulletin* **32** (S1), S12–S23.

Liptak, J.J. & Shatkin, L. (2011). *Transferable Skills Scale, Administrator's Guide*, 2nd edn. Indianapolis: JIST Works.

Lohss, I., Forsyth, K. & Kottorp, A. (2012). Psychometric properties of the Worker Role Interview (version 10.0) in mental health. *British Journal of Occupational Therapy* 75 (4), 171–178.

Lonnergan, D. & Wick, C. (2013). Occupational therapy in occupational health. *OT News* 21 (10), 22–23.

Matheson, R. (2015). *The Matheson FCE Model.* http://www.roymatheson.com (last accessed: 15.4.2015).

McGall, J. & Hilditch, M. (2013). Working your way to recovery. *OT News* 21 (9), 46.

McMorris, C. (2010). Developing a forensic employability pathway. *OT News* 18 (10), 28.

Meredith, R. (2011). Vocational rehabilitation within a forensic service. *OT News* 19 (7), 26.

Mind (2011). *Managing and Supporting Mental Health at Work: Disclosure Tools for Managers.* https://www.mind.org.uk (last accessed: 12.9.2015).

Moore-Corner, R.A., Kielhofner, G. & Olson, L. (1998). *Work Environment Impact Scale (WEIS) Version 2.0.* http://www.cade.uic.edu/moho (last accessed: 10.1.2016).

Nacro (2015). *Disclosing Criminal Records to Employers.* https://www.nacro.org.uk (last accessed: 12.9.2015).

National Health Service (2015a). *Returning to Work after Mental Health Issues.* http://www.nhs.uk (last accessed: 1.5.2015).

National Health Service (2015b). *Should I Volunteer?* http://www.nhs.uk (last accessed: 12.11.2015).

Nice, K. & Davidson, J. (2010). *Provider-led Pathways: Experiences and Views of Condition Management Programmes.* https://www.gov.uk (last accessed: 1.6.2015).

Nicholas, M.K. (1989) *Pain Self-efficacy Questionnaire (PSEQ) in Self-efficacy and Chronic Pain*. Paper Presented at the Annual Conference of the British Psychological Society. St. Andrews.

Oswald, F., Campbell, J., McCloy, R., Rivk, D. & Lew, P. (1999). *Stratifying Occupational Units by Specific Vocational Preparation* (SVP) (Human Resources Research Organization and National Center for O'NET Development). http://www.onetcenter.org (last accessed: 4.6.2015).

Paden, S. & Bradford, S. (2014). To disclose or not to disclose. *OT News* 22 (9), 28–29.

Parkin, C. (2014). Using the Individual Placement and Support model. *OT News* 22 (9), 38–39.

Probyn, J. & Barnhouse, J. (2012). Employment works. *OT News* 20 (9), 36–37.

Prochaska, J.O. & DiClemente, C.C. (1984). *The Transtheoretical Approach: Crossing Traditional Boundaries of Therapy,* 1st edn. Homewood: Dow Jones/Irwin.

Rethink (2015a). *Discrimination and Mental Illness – Equality Act 2010 – disclosure.* https://www.rethink.org (last accessed: 12.9.2015).

Rethink (2015b). *Criminal Convictions – How and When to Tell Others*. https://www.rethink.org (last accessed: 12.9.2015).

Robertson, C. (2011). First steps to work. *OT News* 19 (6), 22.

Ross, J. (2007). Occupational Therapy and Vocational Rehabilitation, 1st edn. Chichester: John Wiley & Sons.

Szerezla, L. (2009). Inpatient vocational group. *OT News* 17 (3), 31.

Time to Change (TTC) (2015). *Telling My Manager: Talking about Mental Health Problems at Work.* http://www.time-to-change.org.uk (last accessed: 12.9.2015).

Triangle Consulting Social Enterprise Limited (TCSE Ltd) (2015). *Outcomes Star: an Evidence-based Tool for Supporting and Measuring Change.* http://www.outcomesstar.org.uk (last accessed: 3.6.2015).

Turner-Stokes, L. (2009). Goal Attainment Scaling (GAS) in rehabilitation: a practical guide. *Clinical Rehabilitation* 23 (4), 362–370.

Waddell, G. & Burton, A.K. (2006). *Is Work Good for Your Health and Wellbeing?* Norwich: Stationery Office.

Waddell, G., Burton, A.K. & Kendall, N.A.S. (2008). *Vocational Rehabilitation: What Works, for Whom, and When?* London: Stationery Office.

Waddell, G., Newton, M., Henderson, I., Somerville, D. & Main, C.J. (1993). A Fear-Avoidance Beliefs questionnaire (FABQ) and the role of fear-avoidance beliefs in chronic low back pain and disability. *Pain* **52** (2), 157–168.

Waghorn, G., Lloyd, C. & Clune, A. (2009). Reviewing the theory and practice of occupational therapy in mental health rehabilitation. *British Journal of Occupational Therapy* **72** (7), 314–323.

Waghorn, G., Stephenson, A. & Browne, D. (2011). The importance of service integration in developing effective employment services for people with severe mental health conditions. *British Journal of Occupational Therapy* **74** (7), 339–347.

Wilkins, A., Love, B., Greig, R. & Bowers, H. (2012). *Economic Evidence around Employment Support, National Institute for Health Research*. http://www.ndti.org.uk (last accessed: 20.10.2015).

Williams, A., Fossey, E. & Harvey, C. (2010). Sustaining employment in a social firm: use of the Work Environment Impact scale v2.0 to explore views of employees with psychiatric disabilities. *British Journal of Occupational Therapy* **73** (11), 531–539.

Williams, J. (2015). An OT in occupational health. *OT News* **23** (3), 38–39.

Young, K. (2014). Employment and recovery. *OT News* **22** (5), 42.

Zigmond, A.S. & Snaith, R.P. (1983). The Hospital Anxiety and Depression Scale (HADS). *Acta Psychiatrica Scandinavica* **67** (6), 361–370.

# Chapter 10

# Occupational therapists delivering assistive technology

Clare Weale, Amie Witherspoon and Karen Bradshaw

## Introduction

This chapter aims to provide the reader with an insight into how assistive technology (AT) can be utilised in the mental health field to provide support and reassurance to service users and carers and to promote independence. It discusses the ethical issues relating to assistive technology use and the role of occupational therapists in assessing for AT. Some case studies are provided as examples to demonstrate the positive impact assistive technology can have on the lives of those with mental health conditions and their carers.

## Key points

- Assistive technology has an important role to play in a holistic care plan.

- It can help to reduce isolation, increase compliance with medication, reduce carer stress, support with routines and provide a modern method of accessing support services which, many feel, does not have the stigma associated with it that traditional methods do.

- Assistive technology is currently under-utilised and there is significant disparity in knowledge amongst occupational therapists.

- The unique knowledge and assessment skills of occupational therapists make them ideally placed to lead in this field and develop holistic services and robust assessment tools.

## Assistive technology: definitions

The World Health Organisation (WHO) defines assistive technology (AT) as, '[a]n umbrella term for any device or system that allows individuals to perform tasks they would otherwise be unable to do or increases the ease and safety with which tasks can be performed' (WHO 2004, p. 10).

The most commonly recognised form of assistive technology is Telecare, which the Telecare Services Association defines as:

> support and assistance provided at a distance using information and communication technology. It is the continuous, automatic and remote monitoring of users by means of sensors to enable them to continue living in their own home, while minimising risks such as a fall, gas and flood detection and relate to other real time emergencies and lifestyle changes over time.
>
> (Telecare Services Association 2016)

Many of these sensors can also be used as stand-alone devices, being linked up to a pager to alert an on-site carer as opposed to alerting a monitoring centre via a community alarm.

Assistive technology also includes stand-alone devices which do not raise an alarm, but can prompt or remind users to complete certain tasks or to avoid something which could pose a danger.

A newly coined term within the assistive technology arena is Technology Enabled Care Services (TECS), which refers to the use of telehealth, telecare, telemedicine, telecoaching and self-care in providing care for people with long-term conditions that is convenient, accessible and cost-effective. Telehealth refers to the remote monitoring of physiological data that can be used by health professionals for diagnosis or condition management. Examples of telehealth devices include blood pressure monitors, pulse oximeters, spirometers, weighing scales and blood glucometers. It is often used in the treatment of long-term conditions such as Chronic Obstructive Pulmonary Disease (COPD), Coronary Heart Disease (CHD) and diabetes.

Telehealth can also cover the use of information and communication technology for remote consultation between health professionals or between a health professional and a patient, e.g. providing health advice by telephone, videoconferencing to discuss a diagnosis or capturing and sending images for diagnosis. The terms 'telemedicine' or 'telecoaching' are sometimes used to describe these interventions.

# Policy and background

The 2005–2008 spending review introduced a preventative technology grant providing £80 million over two years to assist local councils to provide alarm technology to 160,000 vulnerable older people (Audit Commission 2004). The government pledged to provide initial investment, coordinate demand to ensure industry growth and raise awareness and knowledge amongst those commissioning telecare services and those who would benefit from them.

Subsequently, the Department of Health announced the Whole System Demonstrator, the world's largest Randomised Controlled Trial (RCT) of telecare and telehealth (DoH 2011). The trial ran from 2008 to 2012 and involved 6,000 people across sites in Kent, Newham and Cornwall. The results of the study indicated that, if used correctly, telecare and telehealth can deliver a 15 per cent reduction in A&E visits, a 20 per cent reduction in emergency admissions, and a 14 per cent reduction in bed days. The study suggests that at least 3 million people in the UK with long-term conditions and/or social care needs could benefit from using telecare and telehealth.

Following on from this, the Department of Health launched the *3 Million Lives* programme (NHS England 2014) to promote use of telecare and telehealth, aiming for at least 3 million people in the UK to benefit from these interventions over a five-year period. This has since been superseded by the TECS programme at NHS England (2015) which will focus on delivering a set of practical tools and resources to provide support and guidance on how to commission, procure, implement and evaluate so as to maximise the value of these types of solutions and services.

# Political context

The recognised drivers of telecare are:

- The demographics of the global aging population
- The focus on wellbeing and the prevention agenda for health
- Carer responsibility
- Digital inclusion agenda
- Social inclusion agenda (mental health).

National policy drivers have mainstreamed the requirement for knowledge of telecare in job competencies whilst simultaneously incentivising the private sector to invest in telecare innovation. This two-pronged approach has resulted in a mushrooming of new devices and new suppliers. In a rapidly evolving sector it is critical to keep up to date with innovation and participate in the collaborative network.

# Ethical issues

Assistive technology can offer many benefits; however, there is also potential for it to be misused. An ethical framework, originally developed by Beauchamp and Childress (1994), has been widely adopted to illustrate the ethical issues relating to assistive technology. This framework comprises four key principles (described in Box 10.1).

**Box 10.1: Four key principles of an ethical framework for assistive technology**

**Autonomy**

This refers to respecting a person's right to make their own choices relating to independence and day to day activities.

**Beneficence**

This refers to working for the benefit of the individual. The prime reason for implementing assistive technology should be to support or help the person.

**Justice**

This refers to fairness in access to services or technology, taking into account diversity and individual differences and seeking not to disadvantage one population group in favour of another.

**Non-maleficence**

This is the principle of 'doing no harm'. We need to consider if implementing a piece of assistive technology could potentially cause more harm than good. Some equipment could have the potential to further confuse or distress a person and other equipment, GPS (Global Positioning System) devices, for example, have the potential to be intrusive if used incorrectly; therefore, it is important that a balance is achieved between ensuring someone's safety and invading their privacy (NHS England 2015).

Adapted from Beauchamp and Childress (1994).

# The telecare team

A multi-disciplinary team (MDT) approach is essential when working with AT. The members of the team aim to address the issues with technology so may be different from the conventional MDT. Traditionally, over the last ten years, telecare coordinators, suppliers and developers have worked closely with care managers/social workers to identify the best solution for the person, looking at what adjustments may be made to ensure the equipment delivers the intended purpose. The multi-disciplinary approach to the provision of assistive technology and telecare remains critical to arriving at a successful outcome, and consequently this chapter has been developed and written with other professional representatives from this sector.

The MDT has often forgotten the role of the occupational therapist in the assessment process. The occupational therapist is essential in ensuring the robustness of the assessment and applying the technology in the occupational domains. Occupational therapists need to apply their usual approach to assessment and implementation in this area. The occupational therapist is ideally skilled to undertake work in the field of assistive technology and telecare as their primary role or as part of their occupational therapist role: there is a great opportunity here for occupational therapists to lead in this field and develop holistic services.

The success of equipment not only depends upon assessment, but also the support required during and after its installation. This is often quite sophisticated equipment made to look simple and it requires a good introduction to the customer, correct programming, and then regular review followed by adjustment (if required). Some items of equipment need the person to be 'coached' in their use and how to achieve optimum impact from them.

# Choosing the equipment

There are thousands of devices on the market, all claiming to aid people who may have physical disabilities, cognitive impairment or be generally vulnerable. However, experience has shown that many of these devices do not always deliver as initially perceived. With this in mind, it is imperative to get to know the equipment, understanding how it works, and what conditions it works best in or with. Understanding battery life is essential (as we all know with mobile phones how frustrating it is when we need to use it and the battery is flat).

Many suppliers will provide support in choosing equipment or installing it but do bear in mind that they do have 'bottom lines' to meet. There are independent show houses or rooms like the Disability Living Foundation (DLF). There are also several excellent events each year which showcase existing equipment but also new innovative kit.

Traditionally, telecare has involved extra equipment put into someone's home and linked to a monitoring centre. As the market is growing, this is likely to change to using the client's existing technologies like smart phones and tablets, mainstream apps and systems like skype, WhatsApp, etc. The monitoring may not be done by a specific call centre but by friends and family, or even condition-based support groups/clinics, etc. This will help remove the 'stigma' often associated with having pendants etc. and will truly embrace the idea of assistive living and technology enabled care services. The evidence base is growing – for example, the ongoing Assistive Technology and Telecare to Maintain Independent Living at Home for People with Dementia (ATTILA) study (King's College London 2016) which aims to find out if telecare can safely extend the time people with dementia can continue to live independently in their own homes, and whether this is cost effective.

# Emergence of telehealth

Telehealth is an area where there will be a large increase in usage of equipment/devices/gadgets. We have seen the surging market around health bracelets in the consumer area which will contribute to the acceptance of devices to assist with health conditions.

Already in the area of cognitive impairment there are devices to assist with people being out in the community, apps on phones or tablet devices that can help monitor anxiety levels, look at motivation (and how this can be increased), as well as prompting functions to increase compliance to routines. Equipment might aim to support independent living, supply reassurance, assist in routine management, or prevent social isolation. It may take the form of: lifestyle monitoring; pendant alarm; community alarm; sensors within the home; social media; TV-top box. Box 10.2 shows how various clinical concerns could be addressed with various technical options. The key with any new technologies is to ensure the person understands the benefits of the device, how it can add value to their life, and what is entailed in optimising its use.

Box 10.2: Illustration of how various clinical concerns could be addressed with various technical options

**Independent living**
- Trial independent living with lifestyle monitoring and managed environmental risks.

**Reassurance**
- Pendant alarms, environmental sensors

**Support with routines**
- Devices which alert
- Calendars
- Mobile phones
- Apps.

**Health**
- Apps
- Monitoring devices
- E-support groups.

**Wellbeing**
- Mood recording devices or apps
- E-support groups
- Virtual counselling and support – visual and audio.

**Social integration**
- Social medical media
- GPS devices
- Navigation and environmental prompting devices.

# Assessment approaches to the provision of AT/ telecare in health and social care

As with most emerging areas of clinical practice, occupational therapists began to work with clients without an established standardised assessment tool or practice to draw upon, but using observations, previous experience and understanding of different models of practice. Historically, telecare required for use in the community was assessed for by a social worker or requested via a referral form from a social care provider. The service provider triaged referrals and gathered more data from their environmental visit. The analysis of the suitability of the equipment was determined from technical functioning requirements of the system.

The assessment of need and determining of the suitability of a device as part of a clinically reasoned process differs from selecting an item out of a catalogue or from just reading the information in a referral form. Consequently, in a new area of practice, it is essential to research into the models of provision and to review literature on occupational therapy interventions in assistive technology.

Occupational therapists offer an essential contribution to multi-disciplinary interventions for the prescription of sensory impairment equipment, digital communications aids or environmental controls. Many devices are typically standalone and do not sit within services which offer monitoring and response. The additional social care support element, and the funding associated with telecare as part of the care package provision in the social care model, means the recommendation is for a charged-for service in some circumstances. Equipment is provided free of charge on long-term loan arrangements for aids and adaptations provided within the funded care package, but not when devices are provided as preventative measures.

It is therefore necessary to understand the application of digital assistive technology for use in the home linked to telecare or remote monitoring platforms. It is important to understand how to devise an appropriate assessment to identify equipment or solutions likely to have effective outcomes not only in terms of wellbeing but in ways where their impact on care packages can be measured.

Consequently, it is necessary to use forums and networks to learn about how the equipment is assessed for and provided in local authorities. Through this contact it is possible to get informal supervision, compare knowledge of products and collaborate to devise appropriate assessment tools, as well as access to the undocumented evidence base. Through collaborative working with other members of the MDT it is possible to benchmark practice and ensure that the standard of clinical practice is, as far as possible, aligned with current good practice and evidence which is currently undocumented or captured in scientific studies.

# New way of working

Fortunately, policy has now caught up with practice and we have the Care Act (UK Parliament 2014). This new legislative guidance has a significant impact on current and future practice and broadens the scope of provision. It has now been made explicit in the Act that people with mental health needs and their carers are eligible for assessment and services to receive support that arises as a consequence of impairments from various long-term conditions.

In the past, occupational therapy service provision in adult social services was primarily to meet the needs of persons with physical disabilities and cognitive impairment to support with equipment provision and major adaptation to promote independence and reduce the need for personal care packages. Inherent in the Act are the principles of wellbeing and supporting independence. Needs are to be identified using the strengths-based approach to the assessment.

Interventions are intended to prevent, reduce or delay the need for packages of care and support for all local people. The strengths-based approach to assessments dictates a client-centred practice is to be adopted. Additionally, the assessment of need is more holistic and incorporates the provision of services to adults of working age, and considers support to access opportunities for engagement in employment and social inclusion, linking with drives around promoting health and socio-economic wellbeing. Finally, outcomes (of the process of the assessment and the intervention itself) are to be measured against wellbeing indicators shown in Boxes 10.3 and 10.4. Boxes 10.3 and 10.4 detail the eligibility criteria and outcomes of wellbeing. Although the guidance and legislation does not provide a supporting assessment framework, this structure impacts upon the assessment. Simultaneously the legislation gives rights to carers to have their needs assessed too. Consequently, the person cannot be assessed in isolation.

## Box 10.3: Eligibility criteria for services

### 1. Needs

The adult's needs arise from or are related to a physical or mental impairment or illness.

### 2. Outcomes

As a result of the needs, the adult is unable to achieve two or more of the following:

- Managing and maintaining nutrition
- Maintaining personal hygiene
- Managing toilet needs
- Being appropriately clothed
- Maintaining a habitable home environment
- Being able to make use of the home safely
- Developing and maintaining family or other personal relationships
- Accessing and engaging in work, training, education or volunteering
- Making use of necessary facilities or services in the local community including public transport and recreational facilities or services
- Carrying out any caring responsibilities the adult has for a child.

### 3. Wellbeing

As a consequence of not being able to achieve two or more of these outcomes, there is, or is likely to be, a significant impact on the adult's wellbeing, in the following specified areas:

- Personal dignity (including treatment of the individual with respect)
- Physical and mental health and emotional wellbeing
- Protection from abuse and neglect
- Control by the individual over day-to-day life (including over care and support provided and the way it is provided)

- Participation in work, education, training or recreation
- Social and economic wellbeing
- Domestic, family and personal relationships
- Suitability of living accommodation
- The individual's contribution to society.

*Note*: Local Authorities' Care Act (2014) duties on meeting needs relate to unmet eligible needs, i.e. needs that are not being/will not be met by carers, families, friends, individuals' local and community support network, existing universal/community-based services/facilities/resources. The Act fundamentally promotes supporting individuals to manage their needs, e.g. through changes to lifestyle and more importantly through provision of information advice and guidance/signposting.

## Box 10.4: Carer eligibility

### 1. Needs

A carer's needs meet the eligibility criteria if the needs arise as a consequence of providing necessary care for an adult.

### 2. Outcomes

The effect of the carer's needs is that any of the following specified circumstances apply to the carer.

(a) The carer's physical or mental health is, or is at risk of, deteriorating.

(b) The carer is unable to achieve any of the following outcomes:

- carrying out any caring responsibilities the carer has for a child
- providing care to other persons for whom the carer provides care
- maintaining a habitable home environment in the carer's home (whether or not this is also the home of the adult needing care)
- managing and maintaining nutrition
- developing and maintaining family or other personal relationships
- engaging in work, training, education or volunteering
- making use of necessary facilities or services in the local community, including recreational facilities or services
- engaging in recreational activities.

**3. Wellbeing**

As a consequence there is, or is likely to be, a significant impact on the carer's wellbeing. 'Wellbeing' is a broad concept. It is described as relating to the following areas in particular:

- Personal dignity (including treatment of the individual with respect)
- Physical and mental health and emotional wellbeing
- Protection from abuse and neglect
- Control by the individual over day-to-day life (including over care and support provided and the way it is provided)
- Participation in work, education, training or recreation
- Social and economic wellbeing
- Domestic, family and personal relationships
- Suitability of living accommodation
- The individual's contribution to society.

*Note*: Under the Care Act (2014), carers' eligibility for State support is dependent on whether as a consequence of being unable to achieve any of the above outcomes, there is, or there is likely to be, a significant impact on the carer's wellbeing, i.e.:

- The carer's needs impact on at least one of the areas of wellbeing in a significant way, *or*
- The cumulative effect of the impact of a number of the areas of wellbeing means that they have a significant impact on the carer's overall wellbeing.

# Using telecare to support therapeutic interventions and rehabilitation

The use of unmonitored devices in care management for people with mental health problems has primarily been around supported medication management and the provision of digital medication dispensers or reminder systems. The monitoring aspect of telecare support and reablement strategies could be applied to enable recovery for some individuals to gain confidence with managing their medication.

Consideration could be given to developing care models of recovery and reablement for people being discharged from acute mental health hospitals to support transition to independent living. The services are used especially to promote confidence, reduce anxiety and to support with routine and time management. These are all services that support the recovery of ordinary lives (COT 2006).

Anxiety and issues with community access can be improved with the application of locating technology. Locating technology has been used (with client consent) to support with managing relapses in conditions where there is a need for timely intervention. Locating technology is applied to support with managed community access which requires supervision for forensic service users.

# Other applications of technology enabled care services in mental healthcare and condition management

The use of apps for mood monitoring is essential for the management of wellbeing and good mental health. This should be increasingly promoted as part of preventative health strategy. It should be considered as part of general health maintenance and health promotion as the use of wearable technologies is marketed in the mainstream to support with weight management and exercise monitoring.

In terms of care delivery, as an intervention, the ongoing monitoring of mood enables care to be more bespoke and moves away from crisis management. Crisis management in mental healthcare services is traumatic for the persons concerned and burdens the acute services unnecessarily. Timely care and access to care at the convenience of the service user is encouraged and being supported by the use of websites such as The Big White Wall (2016).

Telephone helplines have been providing counselling support services for many years and these concepts are being applied to web-based services. The use of multi-media and social media chat rooms is broadening the accessibility of care delivery platforms. The web-based services which are emerging are useful in that these services can work to provide interventions as well as deliver preventative care at more convenient times. Furthermore, having the option to take up care via telecoaching or video conferencing can facilitate more discretion and sensitivity in the method of delivery. It may be helpful to some individuals who feel unable to deal with the stigma of mental ill-health. The use of written text to communicate is also beneficial where people with mental health problems may have sensory loss and find it difficult to communicate by telephone. Telecoaching and the use of online cognitive behavioural therapy and other psychological interventions are making this type of care more accessible and affordable to the population at large. Consequently, more mixed interventions may be available, providing choice in care options where drug therapy may be being routinely resorted to without consideration of other treatment options.

Appointment reminder software and text messaging services in telehealth are supporting with long-term condition management and reducing the issues around missed appointments. From the perspective of the NHS, savings are being achieved from reducing the number of appointments missed and creating efficiencies around rescheduling missed appointments.

Having strategies around promoting technology enabled services will be essential to the development of more contemporary and inclusive care pathways. The fragmented use of devices is providing evidence that technology as simple as sending a text message linked to a clinical triage is effective at delivering efficiencies. Emerging web-based services also have the potential to meet the needs of various service user groups, making care more inclusive and accessible. There is scope to create technology enabled care services to assist with promoting psychological wellbeing, long-term condition management, and the delivery of therapeutic care, all of which have vast potential if utilised strategically with consideration and input from clinicians.

There follows a selection of case studies to illustrate the use of assistive technology (Boxes 10.5, 10.6, 10.7, 10.8 and 10.9).

## Box 10.5: Case study – reassurance and carer support

Mr H is an 85-year-old gentleman with advanced dementia who lives with his wife. He has switched on the gas cooker several times, regularly leaves taps running, wanders around the house at night and has wandered out of the house several times when Mrs H has popped to the local shops.

Mrs H is suffering from significant carer stress as she has to constantly supervise Mr H to ensure that he is safe. She gets very little sleep as Mr H is very disorientated to time and tends to wake up often throughout the night. Mrs H reported that she was struggling to cope and was considering moving Mr H to a nursing home which wasn't what either of them wanted.

A lockable gas valve with its own key safe was provided in the kitchen so that Mr H would be unable to switch on the gas. The plugs in the bathroom and kitchen sinks were replaced with magiplugs so that, should Mr H forget to switch off the taps, the magiplug would automatically drain the water, preventing a flood. A memo-minder was positioned by the front door to discourage Mr H from going out by playing a message (recorded by his wife) asking him to go back inside when he walked towards the door.

The equipment has now been in place for over a year and there have been no incidences of Mr H leaving the house unsupervised and, as a result of the lockable gas valve and magiplugs, no incidents of the gas being left on, or flooding.

Mrs H reports feeling much less stressed and says that she now does not have to worry about Mr H so much. The social worker involved reports that Mrs H is looking much brighter and is coping much better. Mr H has been able to remain living at home with his wife, which is where both of them wished for him to remain as long as possible.

## Box 10.6: Case study – video calling

Mrs B is a 78-year-old lady who has severe arthritis and poor mobility, resulting in her not being able to get out of the house very often. Since her husband died a year ago, she has become increasingly socially isolated, often feeling very lonely and low in mood. Mrs B has been offered the opportunity to attend day centres but she did not wish to take this up. She has a big family but many of them do not live locally so Mrs B isn't able to see them as often as she would like to.

Mrs B's family felt that it would be useful for her to have a computer or tablet so that they could keep in touch with her more easily; however, having never used a computer before, Mrs B was not keen on this idea. Mrs B enjoys watching television so a set-top box with a simple remote control was installed which enables video calling via her TV. Mrs B's family can now video call her whilst she is sitting in the comfort of her armchair and she only has to worry about pressing one button to answer the call.

Mrs B is now able to see and speak with her children, grandchildren and great-grandchildren on a regular basis. This has greatly improved her mood and reduced her feelings of isolation.

## Box 10.7: Case study – reassurance, telecoaching

Mrs J is a 38-year-old single parent. Since the breakdown of her marriage 18 months ago, Mrs J has become increasingly withdrawn and depressed. She has very limited family support and feels very isolated and lonely. She has had previous involvement with the Community Mental Health Team during a period of crisis and is looking into local volunteering opportunities to reduce her social isolation.

Mrs J's psychiatrist issued her with a login for an online community, accessible via her computer or an app on her phone. People who are anxious, low in mood, and finding it difficult to cope can support and help each other by sharing what's troubling them, guided by trained professionals. The resource is available 24 hours a day and is completely anonymous so she can express herself freely and openly. There are professionally trained guides online at all times to assist members and ensure their safety.

Mrs J reports that her mood has improved and she feels she now has an outlet to discuss what's troubling her. She feels she is generally coping much better with the stresses in her life and finds it reassuring to know that there are people there 24 hours a day to provide reassurance and support if she is having a particularly difficult day.

## Box 10.8: Case study – medication prompting

James, a young man in his early 20s, with a learning disability, needed prompting with medication. He wanted as much independence as possible, attended day services, and enjoyed spending time with friends. If he missed his medicine his deterioration was quite rapid. The option of a medicine prompting device was explored, but this was too cumbersome for his lifestyle.

As his mobile phone was something he used in his everyday life and had with him wherever he was, this was used. It was set up for three alarms at set times each day with a very specific ring, so he would identify the ring with tablet taking. This has been successful for over three years and as he upgrades his phone he re-programs it each time.

## Box 10.9: Case study – taking medication

Mrs W was 90 years old and had had a fall. She had visual impairment and was not able to differentiate her tablets. She had some dexterity issues as well so used to have her tablets put in bowls to be taken, but she often forgot and also didn't necessarily see all of them to get them out. A medicine dispenser linked to a community alarm was provided. Each dose was timed and when she was due to take them she tipped the box onto a saucer and could take the tablets. If she was late taking them it would alert her for ten minutes and then after this period rung out to the monitoring centre who telephone prompted her and rang her daughter to let her know to check. She volunteered on Tuesdays at a local cancer centre and one of her doses was due at a lunchtime. That Tuesday lunchtime dose was kept out of the box and she took those tablets with her on that day after being prompted by the carers in the morning. A note was put on her record at the monitoring centre to say ignore the alert for Tuesday lunchtimes.

Mrs W was able to go on holiday following her reablement period and she took her dispenser with her. She loved it so much that the staff on the holiday wondered why her handbag was so heavy every day – she explained that she had the dispenser in there as she did not want to leave it in the hotel room in case it got stolen. Mrs W used the device for three years, until she passed away. It enabled her to remain independent with medication management and gave her family great reassurance.

# Useful resources

- AT Dementia: https://www.atdementia.org.uk
- NHS England Technology Enabled Care Services: https://www.england.nhs.uk/ourwork/qual-clin-lead/tecs
- Telecare EPG: http://www.telecare-epg.co.uk
- Telecare Services Association: https://www.tsa-voice.org.uk

# References

Audit Commission (2004). *Implementing Telecare: Strategic Analysis and Guidelines for Policy Makers, Commissioners and Providers.* London: Audit Commission.

Beauchamp, T.L. & Childress, J.F. (1994). *Principles of Biomedical Ethics.* Oxford: Oxford University Press.

Department of Health (2011). *The Whole System Demonstrator (WSD) Programme is the Largest Randomised Control Trial of Telehealth and Telecare in the World.* http://www.gov.uk

College of Occupational Therapists (2006). *Recovering Ordinary Lives: The Strategy for Occupational Therapy in Mental Health Services: A Strategy for the Next Ten Years.* London: COT.

King's College London (2016). *The Assistive Technology and Telecare to Maintain Independent Living at Home for People with Dementia (ATTILA) study.* http://www.kcl.ac.uk (last accessed: 13.2.2016).

NHS England (2014). *Sir Bruce calls for Support for Technology Enabled Care Services Programme.* http://england.nhs.uk (last accessed: 13.2.2016).

NHS England (2015). *Technology Enabled Care Services Resource for Commissioners.* http://england.nhs.uk (last accessed: 13.2.2016).

Telecare Services Association (2016). *What is Telecare: How can Telecare Help You?* https://www.tsa-voice.org.uk/ (last accessed: 13.2.2016).

The Big White Wall (2016). *About the Big White Wall.* http:www.bigwhitewall.com (last accessed: 13.2.2016).

United Kingdom Parliament (2014). *The Care Act.* London: TSO.

World Health Organisation (2004). *Ageing and Health Technical Report, Volume 5: A Glossary of Terms for Community Health Care and Services for Older Persons.* http://www.who.int (last accessed: 13.2.2016).

# Chapter 11

# The child and adolescent primary mental health work role

Robert Kirkwood

## Introduction

Child and Adolescent Mental Health Service (CAMHS) Primary Mental Health Workers (PMHWs) work within community settings with non-mental health specialist professionals, children and young people, and their families. Principally, they provide specialist mental health expertise in the form of advice, consultation and training to professionals, and direct assessment and treatment to clients. This chapter sets out to describe the CAMHS PMHW role: the background to the role's instigation and development; the practical aspects of what the role involves from my own experience and perspective, and the role's suitability (or otherwise) as a future role for occupational therapists considering the field of mental health with children, young people and their families.

There are similarly titled primary mental healthcare roles based within adult services. However, this chapter focuses solely upon the CAMHS primary mental health work role. Equally, this chapter does not touch upon the IAPT (Improving Access to Psychological Therapies) roles that have been developed within CAMHS and within adult primary care mental health services to promote early intervention. That role is described more fully in Chapter 18.

Throughout the chapter I touch upon my own experience as a part-time CAMHS PMHW, and contrast it with my other part-time role as a clinical specialist occupational therapist within CAMHS.

## Key points

- CAMHS Primary Mental Health Workers provide early intervention in the field of mental health and emotional wellbeing with children, young people, their families and universal children's services.
- The Primary Mental Health Worker role is a specialist role, positioned predominantly within the NHS, which requires a professional qualification as well as mental health experience.

**173**

- The Primary Mental Health Work model focuses upon three main areas: consultation for other practitioners/workers; clinical intervention for children, young people and families; and providing mental health training.

- Occupational therapists are well placed to use their existing skills and knowledge to work with children, young people and families in community contexts through the Primary Mental Health Work role.

# Background

The NHS Health Advisory Service's (HAS) report entitled *Together We Stand* (DoH HAS 1995) delivered the first major review of child and adolescent mental health services in the UK a little over 20 years ago. This review highlighted a significant disparity in CAMHS staffing and models of practice. Across the board, the report highlighted a service gap between primary care services and CAMHS. Fundamentally, the NHS based services set up to respond to child and adolescent mental health were seen as difficult to access and in need of a significant overhaul to improve their accessibility.

In response to this service gap, *Together We Stand* outlined a 4-tiered model of CAMHS, which was subsequently implemented nationwide through the *Every Child Matters* agenda (Department for Education and Skills 2004). The model sought to create clear partnerships between services (both statutory and non-statutory with a child and young person focus), supporting health promotion and early intervention initiatives. It asserted that all children's services held a mandate to support child and adolescent mental health, not just the specialist Child and Adolescent Mental Health Services per se. Describing the 4-tiered model, Tier 1 services were conceptualised as being provided by non-mental health specialist practitioners including teachers, health visitors, general practitioners (GPs) and youth services. Tier 2 services were to be provided by specialist CAMHS clinicians in community and primary care settings, to act as a bridge between the interface of Tier 1 and Tier 3. Tier 3 services (commonly referred to as CAMHS) provided a multi-disciplinary service, offering specialist intervention for more complex, severe and persistent disorders. Tier 4 CAMHS services were those providing highly specialist assessment and treatment through, for example, child and adolescent inpatient settings or community based crisis response teams (DoH 2009).

At Tier 2 level, the NHS Health Advisory Service's report proposed the development of the CAMHS primary mental health worker role to support the mental and emotional wellbeing of children and young people through consultation within the primary care arena in contexts such as schools, medical practices and multi-agency forums as well as providing direct intervention (assessment and short-term treatment) with children, young people and families (Hickey *et al.* 2008, Williams 2011).

Crucially, the HAS report described the role of PMHW as operating at the primary-secondary care interface; supporting Tier 1 workers by increasing their ability to manage children and adolescents with mental health problems instead of predominantly relying on referrals to Tier 3 CAMHS. The report proposed that the PMHW would undertake clinical intervention with more complex cases and provide a triaging role to reduce the number of referrals that reached Tier 3 CAMHS. To achieve this, the primary mental health worker role was formulated as community-based rather than clinic-based. As PMHWs undertook this work, it was envisaged that the pathways between Tier 1 services and CAMHS would become more effective and efficient.

From this point, the PMHW role began to be implemented across health authorities in the UK. Initially, PMHW roles were recruited mainly from the mental health nursing profession. However, the net has since widened and there is evidence of PMHWs having been recruited from a wide range of regulated professions including nursing, social work, occupational therapy, arts-based psychotherapy and other allied therapies. This occurrence is illustrated by my own journey to becoming a PMHW. I myself applied for a CAMHS primary mental health position with no previous professional experience of CAMHS, although as a field of work, I had been seeking opportunities to get 'my foot in the door'. Having been working as a senior occupational therapist within an adult mental health inpatient setting for several years, the PMHW role was put to me by a more experienced occupational therapist colleague as a useful way of getting into CAMHS as there were no occupational therapists working within CAMHS in my locality at that time.

# Service structure for CAMHS primary mental health workers

Several models have emerged over the years in terms of framing where PMHWs are situated within a service structure and how they are organised at an operational level. In some regions, PMHWs can be found embedded within CAMHS Tier 3 multi-disciplinary teams, effectively operating an 'outreach' model into the community from their Tier 3 base. In others, PMHWs are linked specifically to an associated locality network of schools (both primary and secondary) and are most likely to have a work base situated within one of the schools. There are also PMHW teams that are situated within NHS Trusts alongside, yet separate from, CAMHS Tier 3 services, with separate line management.

Each of these models holds its own strengths and weaknesses. The recommendation that the location of mental health workers for children and young people should be made more diverse to improve access and reduce stigma, such as those based in schools (DoH 2004), is to be weighed against the professional and clinical support gained from being based within a multi-disciplinary mental health team (MacDonald et al. 2004). My own experience has been mixed. When I first took up my PMHW position, I was working within a discreet PMHW team, independently line managed but embedded within the wider CAMHS directorate. After a couple of years, the PMHW team was dissolved through service restructuring which led to each PMHW being repositioned into their own locality's CAMHS teams. In my specific context, several localities were served by one Tier 3 CAMHS service and so three PMHWs (including myself) were repositioned into that service, but each working in a different geographical area. This created the opportunity for us to reform as a virtual team to support each other and manage the referrals that were passed from the CAMHS referral triaging pathway to us as PMHWs.

The example of restructuring described above will no doubt resonate with the experience of many occupational therapists who have worked within occupational therapy departments that have subsequently been dismantled in favour of multi-disciplinary models of team working within mental health services over the last 15 years.

As a final word on the 4-tiered CAMHS model, it is worth noting that the National CAMHS Review (DCSF 2008), initiated by the government's *Children's Plan* (DCSF 2007), highlights a move away from the 4-tiered model of CAMHS, towards the framing of services as *universal*, *targeted* and *specialist* to reflect the greater integration between services for children that is being widely promoted. However, there remains a degree of dissonance between these two models in terms of how services are structured and it is my personal experience that both models are often articulated in the language and descriptions that services and practitioners use. I feel that it is fair to say that the 4-tiered model is still the main view held by Tier 1 (or universal) practitioners within children's services. Figure 11.1, reproduced from *CAMHS in Context* from the National CAMHS Workforce Programme (Nixon 2010), merges the well-known CAMHS tier-based pyramid with the universal, targeted and specialist service categories.

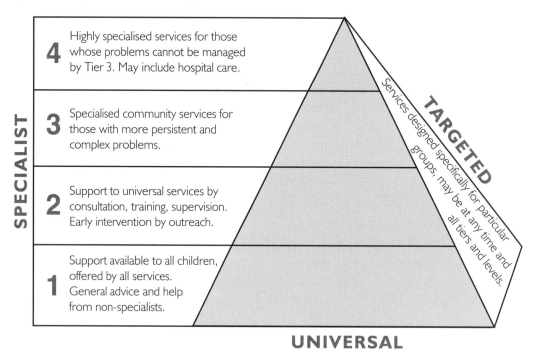

*Figure 11.1: Integrated CAMHS service model (Nixon 2010).*

# What a PMHW role involves

Principally, the role of the PMHW combines three strands: consultation-liaison with primary care workers; direct and joint clinical work with children, young people and families; mental health training and promotion to primary sector workers (Hickey *et al.* 2008). A key issue for PMHWs is finding the balance across the provision of these three strands within their work. This balance varies from service to service and is often dependent upon how PMHW roles have arisen, pressures being placed upon the PMHW based upon the needs of the wider CAMHS service and the skill sets of the individual practitioners. From my experience of working within one service, the balance to aim for was always presented to me as 60 per cent consultation and 40 per cent direct work with additional training needs facilitated by all PMHWs through a rolling training programme. However, PMHWs operating in different localities have tended to work in varying ways, depending on the needs and experience levels of the Tier 1 practitioners they have built working relationships with within their locality. Below, the three strands of the PMHW role are discussed in turn. The terms 'child' and 'young person' are used interchangeably.

# Consultation

The strategic goal of PMHW consultation is to provide an early, preventative intervention that meets the needs of clients before their difficulties escalate, thus reducing the number of cases that may potentially become more complex and require a referral to Tier 3 CAMHS. At the same time, it aims to up-skill Tier 1 practitioners who, through the consultation process, gain increased knowledge and confidence regarding strategies to support low risk mental health issues in their community setting. In a practical sense, the term 'consultation' describes the process by which a child or young person's case is presented to and discussed with the PMHW by a Tier 1 practitioner such as a school nurse, teacher, Special Educational Needs Coordinator (SENCo) or GP, because the difficulties that the child or young person is experiencing have been flagged by school staff or other workers involved with that young person. The PMHW may be contacted by the primary care practitioner on an ad hoc basis or through scheduled consultation slots, either in person or over the phone. In the initial discussion, the PMHW will invariably want to gain a history of the presenting problem as well as information regarding the child's family background and developmental history if possible. The PMHW may suggest a possible formulation for the young person's mental health needs and will, along with the consultee, think about the most appropriate ways to meet these needs within the young person's context whilst also agreeing who may be involved in this process.

As with any CAMHS intervention, understanding the child's context (and that of their family) is critical to determining whether the roots of the presenting mental health issues are developmental, predisposed, familial (systemic), socially triggered or, as is most often the case, a combination of these. To do this, the PMHW will be considering a range of possible factors influencing the presenting behaviour – parenting styles; attachment issues; signs of neurodevelopmental influences; symptoms of low mood or anxiety; psycho-social factors. The PMHW will also be assessing the level of risk associated with the behaviours (for example, deliberate self-harm (DSH) or child sexual exploitation). Again, understanding the context plays a key part in determining levels of risk. If the PMHW knows the school well, for instance, they may also be taking into consideration how effective the school's pastoral structure is and whether the school has been providing appropriate support to the child. This example demonstrates how essential it can be for the PMHW to have a good grasp of their own locality or 'patch': what resources are available locally in terms of voluntary and community sector services and projects (which may well pop up and then disappear over a period of time due to limited funding streams); whether the neighbourhood that the young person is living in is deprived or not; how schools have responded to the needs of other young people that the PMHW may have worked with. Using this knowledge, the PMHW can be more effective in directing young people to the appropriate support services.

Based on my own experience, another key function of consultation is to help manage and contain the levels of concern held by Tier 1 professionals such as school staff as they deal with young people whom they may consider to be at significant risk. Appropriate discussion of risk management strategies and providing containment for professional anxiety are skills regularly employed by PMHWs. For example, a teacher may be very worried that a young person has deliberately self-harmed. However, understanding the context of each individual case, such as the severity and frequency of the Deliberate Self-Harm, where it occurs, what the young person gains from their DSH, will inform the risk assessment and the recommended response. Tier 1 professionals may feel that eliciting this level of information in an appropriately sensitive way is beyond their skill-set. This situation is a good example of when a consultation may lead to the need for direct assessment of the young person by the PMHW. In turn, it becomes an opportunity for the direct session to be conducted jointly with the consultee (if the young person agrees) to potentially further the consultee's knowledge of the young person's needs whilst also promoting the safe sharing of information which, time and again in my experience, leads to increased and more robust support for the young person.

## Clinical intervention

As indicated above, direct PMHW intervention with a young person and their family functions most effectively when it arises from initial consultation with a Tier 1 professional. In this way, the PMHW already has a link person in Tier 1 to liaise with and give feedback to. So if, at any time in the consultation process, the PMHW feels that meeting the child and/or family to undertake a more in-depth mental health assessment is necessary to gain a clearer understanding of the issues, this will be arranged. The PMHW's initial assessment may then lead to further treatment sessions by the PMHW or signposting to other support networks. It may just as readily lead to simple feedback to the family and/or the initial consultee with ideas and strategies to better support the child within their existing contexts. When direct intervention from a PMHW is provided, it will commonly be intended to be short-term. If during further treatment sessions, the PMHW feels that there are issues of a mental health nature that are more complex, severe and persistent, they are likely to refer the case back to CAMHS Tier 3 for consideration.

As a PMHW, my own direct work with children and young people varies considerably. In terms of initial assessment, I will make contact with either the young person (dependent upon their age) or their parent/guardian, introducing myself and my role and making initial inquiries about the situation. I will want to find out where the child or parent would prefer to meet, at home, at school, or at another community venue. Some young people prefer to meet at home. This may be due to concern about receiving awkward questions from peers. Other young people may prefer to meet at school, especially if they are reluctant for their family to be involved or are at an age where they are seeking a greater level of independence. Other young people may wish to meet in young people's centres, away from both home and school. Equally, I may suggest this myself if I sense a reluctance to meet at home or school. I have also been asked by parents to meet at home without the child present to discuss their concerns more candidly.

Depending upon how the case has reached me, the young person or family may be ambivalent or even resistant to engaging with me, or CAMHS at all. I find that young people who are school refusing can often be reluctant to meet a practitioner such as myself at home. If I feel I have undertaken a thorough enough assessment over the phone, based upon that information, I may decide that the best way forward initially, is to hold a meeting at the school (for example) with the family and school represented. In such cases, I put a great deal of thought into how I position myself in the meeting. At times I have felt it most appropriate, and beneficial for the young person, to take on a position of being the young person's advocate towards the parent and/or school. At other times, I mediate between the family and school to reach a better understanding of each other's views and to establish an action plan for both the school and family to undertake.

When the assessment process highlights the need for further intervention for presenting issues which I feel are, on the one hand deemed to be more severe or complex than would be safe to stay solely within Tier 1, but on the other hand do not meet the criteria for Tier 3, I may offer some therapeutic sessions. Obviously, the young person's presenting problem is the main determinant for deciding which treatment approach to use. However, the skill set of each individual PMHW, in terms of which therapeutic modes they have gained the appropriate level of knowledge and experience to use, also comes into play. In this sense, the PMHW often needs to have at least a basic understanding of a range of treatment modes in order to either use these within the sessions themselves or to know enough to establish what specialist treatment the young person or family may need. The National Institute for Health and Clinical Excellence (NICE) clinical guidelines serve as a useful benchmark to guide evidence-based practice. For example, the low intensity treatment given to an 8-year-old presenting with excessive hand washing and other obsessive compulsive related traits will differ in many respects from the treatment offered to a 16-year-old with low mood and poor self-esteem who is engaging in deliberate self-harming. Similarly, work with a parent to manage their child's Attention Deficit Hyperactivity Disorder (ADHD) related behaviours will differ from strategies given to a parent of a teenager presenting with social withdrawal and refusing to attend school.

Many CAMHS practitioners, including PMHWs, will have gained further qualifications in additional therapeutic treatments or have attended sufficient short-term courses to feel confident enough to use these concepts within their practice. Cognitive Behavioural Therapy (CBT) is a clear example of this within my own practice. I am not a qualified CBT practitioner. However, over the years I have attended enough workshops and short courses exploring aspects of CBT to allow me to feel confident in using the concepts within my practice. It has also given me the awareness to recognise when I need to refer someone for CBT when the issues appear too entrenched to be overcome through low intensity work. Similarly, I have gained a good grounding in sensory processing theory through my occupational therapy training and subsequent workshops, courses and supervision. However, I do not hold any formal qualifications in Sensory Integration (SI). This does not stop me from regularly supporting teachers in schools to reframe the 'naughty' child that they are consulting with me about, through a sensory lens. Other therapeutic modes that I and other PMHWs may draw upon as a knowledge base to inform our practice include: Solution Focused Therapy (SFT); Motivational Interviewing (MI); attachment styles; Neuro-Linguistic Programming (NLP); systemic psychotherapy.

In a later section I touch upon an issue that relates closely to this matter of gaining additional training in other therapeutic modes, namely, how does my core occupational therapy training govern my PMHW treatment sessions? I shall explore this later, but anecdotally, whilst attending an extended course to learn behavioural activation and graded exposure techniques from a CBT perspective a couple of years ago, I and several other occupational therapy-registered practitioners in the room were surprised by the degree of overlap between core occupational therapy theory and what was being taught to us, albeit from a different perspective. This served as a timely reminder to me of my need to assertively integrate my occupational therapy core training into my own practice more explicitly.

## Training

The third strand of the PMHW role is the delivery of training to Tier 1 colleagues. The training PMHWs provide can benefit Tier 1 professionals in several ways. I have discussed the benefit of joint sessions with Tier 1 colleagues above, in terms of sharing clinical reasoning and developing practice-based knowledge. PMHWs in many areas also provide formal training opportunities for Tier 1 staff. By providing workshops centred around key mental health related topics, Tier 1 staff can either gain or renew their knowledge in key areas that they may encounter regularly in their own settings. This in turn is expected to build their confidence in recognising or identifying mental health related issues as they arise within their own setting, responding to and managing the issues they are dealing with, and helping them to assess levels of risk appropriately – not minimising distress or reacting inappropriately to certain challenging behaviours.

In a more general sense, training programmes support both the promotion of mental health and an evidence-based response to mental and emotional distress at a Tier 1 level. It helps to foster greater awareness and acceptance of issues that children and young people are likely to experience as well as building stronger links between the tiers.

The topics included in the PMHW training programme that I and my colleagues are involved in delivering include: mental health awareness; depression and suicide; anxiety; attachment; early brain development; deliberate self-harm. Based on my experience, one dilemma that has arisen from such a training programme is the occasional indication from Tier 1 colleagues that, having been on specific training, they know all they need to know without the need for further consultation with Tier 2 or 3 practitioners, or even to facilitate subsequent in-house training based upon what they have learnt. Our response to this rare situation is to reassert the need for professional guidance as evidence-based practice changes over time, and to emphasise the need to work together to build rather than erode links across the tiers in order to better support our young people.

In terms of mental health promotion, primary healthcare principles that focus upon community-based intervention (Koch & Kralik 2006) have developed internationally as recognition of the perceived effectiveness of preventative and promoting measures within public services has increased over a number of years (Raeburn & Rootman 1998). The drivers for this increase are manifold. Politically, the need for financial savings has led to a greater investment in health promotion strategies. From a workforce perspective, developing a broader professional capacity to promote mental health reduces reliance upon specialist services for the more tailored work which specific responses to illness episodes necessitate. Both PMHW and occupational therapy embrace the mental health promotion agenda within their core values. Primary mental health work has reflected this through the very development of the role, and occupational therapy, through its recognition that mental health promotion often champions the link between meaningful occupations or activity and positive mental wellbeing. Therefore, mental health promotion can be framed as a component of PMHW training that can potentially be embedded in every aspect of the role.

## Primary mental health work and occupational therapy

Before we look more closely at the commonalities between PMHW and occupational therapy, it is important to briefly explore the PMHW role from a governance perspective. The Association of Primary Mental Health Work and Training (CAMHS) (www.pmhw.org.uk) offers its members a professional network supported by regional hubs and a national conference. However, the association does not hold governance powers in the same way that other registered governing bodies do, such as the British Association of Occupational Therapists (BAOT). This is largely due to the fact that the title 'Primary Mental Health Worker' is not a protected professional title and there are currently no education and training programmes that lead to registration as a primary mental health worker in the UK. This all leads to a good degree of variation in how the role is interpreted across UK services. Essentially, for me as a PMHW, what this means is that in terms of practice and governance, as well as NHS Trust operational policy, the professional duties carried out through my PMHW role are in fact governed by the standards and codes of conduct outlined by the statutory regulating body and the professional body that I am associated to through my ongoing registration as an occupational therapist, namely the Health and Care Professions Council (HCPC) and the BAOT.

Given that my professional conduct is regulated through my occupational therapy affiliation, it stands to reason that I should be using my occupational therapy professional training and qualification as the bedrock for all my clinical practice. For, if I am not, it begs the question: 'what am I basing my clinical reasoning and decision-making upon?' From this stance, it becomes easier to critically evaluate where and how PMHW and occupational therapy practice converge.

In terms of its presence in CAMHS as a whole, occupational therapy provision has been steadily increasing over the last decade. However, there are still Tier 3 CAMHS services which do not have occupational therapists as part of their multi-disciplinary team. Personally, most of my CAMHS career has encompassed a split working week, working part-time as both a primary mental health worker within one locality CAMHS service for half the week and as a Clinical Specialist Occupational Therapist within another locality CAMHS service the other part of the week. Difficulties with juggling workloads aside, the split role across two very different CAMHS services has given me a good deal of insight into the overlapping nature of these different roles.

I have concluded that occupational therapists are well placed to use their existing skills and knowledge to work with children, young people and families in their own community contexts through the primary mental health work role. Two broad themes are outlined below that I feel best encapsulate a number of overlapping characteristics and concepts that unite occupational therapy and primary mental health work.

# Context and environment

Context and environment are central tenets within most occupational therapy models, from the Model of Human Occupation (MOHO) (Kielhofner 2008) to the Canadian Model of Occupational Performance (CMOP) (Townsend et al. 2002, Townsend & Polatajko 2007) and the Kawa Model (Iwama 2006). The systemic inter-relatedness of people as subsystems converging within specific but constantly changing contexts is a concept that most if not all occupational therapists should be able to connect with, in reference to their core training and subsequent practice. I have conveyed in previous sections, the importance of context to the role of the PMHW. Not only is context a key aspect of assessing what factors have led to a certain issue or presentation, it also plays a key role when considering how best to engage with a young person, their family and Tier 1 colleagues embedded in the community that surrounds them.

The importance of how PMHWs adapt to different contexts is reflected in Standard 9 of the National Service Framework for Children, Young People and Maternity Services (DoH 2004) which also recommends that the access to and location of mental health services for children and young people should be diversified in order to improve access and reduce stigma. This recommendation, central to the development of the PMHW role, also resonates with the values of client-centred practice that underpin occupational therapy (Parker 2006).

This holistic perspective of the client that unites occupational therapy practice models (Hemphill-Pearson 2008) is also clearly evident, from my perspective at least, in the approach that a PMHW takes toward intervention. The consultation for example, seeks to gain information pertaining to a range of factors across the psychosocial spectrum. It is a discursive process that uncovers details related to the child's wider context in order to paint as extensive picture as possible – a macro view as opposed to a diagnosis-led line of enquiry. This approach is continued through the assessment phase of direct work if undertaken, or through the action plans that come from school meetings.

## Doing 'with' not 'for'

The PMHW consultation and liaison roles are prime opportunities to work in partnership with the wider network. By primarily supporting the existing system around the young person to implement the necessary changes or interventions, the PMHW is allowing change to become more sustainable. This perspective can only be enhanced by a PMHW who is drawing from a professional theoretical underpinning (such as occupational therapy) that upholds the value of 'enabling' occupation as a core competency (Townsend *et al.* 2007). Primary mental health workers are in the business of supporting young people to engage in the activities and occupations they need to engage in, such as education, training on employment, as well as the activities and occupations they enjoy such as hobbies in order to enhance their social interaction. Primary mental health workers are often engaged with supporting young people to functionally manage their routines and to consider the impact of various lifestyle choices. Dunn's 'ecology of human performance' (Dunn *et al.* 1994) cites five types of interventions: establish/restore; adapt; alter; prevent; create. This has been a useful model through which to reflect upon my own interventions. I can safely say that each of these intervention types has been utilised in one way or another through my PMHW role, whether it is advising upon creating reduced timetables in schools, offering parents advice on supporting their children with worries at home or creating new opportunities through signposting to clubs or groups.

## Further thoughts to consider

In some authorities PMHWs are employed at Agenda for Change (AfC) Band 7 pay scale. Increasingly, NHS-based PMHW positions have been advertised at band 6 or even 5. Because PMHW is not a protected job title, recognised or regulated by statutory bodies in the same way that the role of occupational therapist is, for example, there is greater variation across the UK in how the title is used and what level of experience the practitioners in the role will have needed to demonstrate. I happen to have worked within a Trust that has, in the main, employed PMHWs at Band 7. Attempts to downgrade the role to a Band 6 have been opposed on the grounds that the levels of autonomy, self-directed working, skills and knowledge base, and risk management required for the role are commensurate with the expectations and specifications of an AfC Band 7 job description.

Developing formal career structures and effective career pathways for PMHWs, such as modular academic courses, has been mooted over the years but has not occurred yet. It would be wise for any occupational therapist thinking about a PMHW role to consider what other therapeutic practice knowledge they would bring to the role along with their occupational therapy core skills.

## Conclusion

This chapter has given an overview of the PMHW role, how it fits into the wider CAMHS structure and what the work entails at a practical level. I have suggested ways in which an occupational therapist's core skills and the value base of the profession would fit well within the PMHW role. I have spoken of my own experience of working as both a PMHW and a CAMHS occupational therapist. In summing up, I would like to leave the reader with an understanding that the PMHW role gives enough room for practitioners to apply our own clinical reasoning to the cases based upon our own professional backgrounds. On this basis, an occupational therapist should be able to successfully apply their theoretical knowledge to much of the PMHW's work, and to good effect. Further research into the effectiveness of the PMHW role in general is certainly needed. Moreover, exploration of the added value an occupational therapist brings to this role would be a welcome addition to this field of research.

# Useful resources

- The Association of Primary Mental Health Work & Training (CAMHS): http://pmhw.co.uk/
- http://camh.org.uk
- https://www.gov.uk including: Department of Education (2015). *Mental Health and Behaviour in Schools: Departmental Advice for School Staff.* London: TSO and Department of Health (2015). *Future in Mind: Promoting, Protecting and Improving our Children and Young People's Mental Health and Wellbeing.* London: TSO.
- http://www.youngminds.org.uk/http://camh.org.uk
- Lougher, L. (2000). *Occupational Therapy for Child and Adolescent Mental Health.* London: Churchill Livingstone.

# References

Department for Children, Schools and Families (2007). *The Children's Plan: Building Brighter Futures.* London: TSO.

Department for Children, Schools and Families, and the Department of Health (2008). *Children and Young People in Mind: the Final Report of the National CAMHS Review.* London: DCSF.

Department for Education and Skills (2004). *Every Child Matters: Change for Children.* London: Department for Education and Skills.

Department of Health (2004). *National Service Framework for Children, Young People and Maternity Services: The Mental Health and Psychological Wellbeing of Children and Young People.* London: TSO.

Department of Health (2009). *Children and Young People in Mind: the Final Report of the National CAMHS Review.* London: DoH.

Department of Health, Health Advisory Service (1995). *Together We Stand.* London: TSO.

Dunn, W., Brown, C. & McGuigan, A. (1994). The ecology of human performance: a framework for considering the effect of context. *American Journal of Occupational Therapy* **48** (7), 595–607.

Hemphill-Pearson, B.J. (ed) (2008). *Assessments in Occupational Therapy Mental Health*, 2nd edn. Thorofare NJ: Slack Incorporated.

Hickey, N., Kramer, T. & Gerralda, M.E. (2008). Is there an optimum model of practice for the newly developed child and adolescent metal health worker posts? *Journal of Mental Health Training, Education and Practice* **2** (4), 11–18.

Iwama, M. (2006). *The Kawa Model: Culturally Relevant Occupational Therapy.* Edinburgh: Churchill Livingstone, Elsevier.

Kielhofner, G. (2008). *Model of Human Occupation: Theory and Application,* 4th edn. Philadelphia, PA: Lippincott, Williams and Wilkins.

Koch, T., & Kralik, D. (2006). *Participatory Action Research in Health Care.* Oxford, UK: Blackwell Publishing.

MacDonald, W., Bradley, S., Bower, P., Kramer, T., Sibbald, B., Garralder, E. & Harrington, R. (2004). Primary mental health workers in child and adolescent mental health services. *Journal of Advanced Nursing* **46** (1) 78–87.

Nixon, B. (2010). *CAMHS in Context (Induction Package): Helping you to Achieve Better Outcomes for Children, Young People and Families.* London: National CAMHS Workforce Programme, National CAMHS Support Service (NCSS).

Parker, D.M. (2006). 'Implementing client-centred practice' in *Client-Centred Practice in Occupational Therapy*, ed. T. Sumsion, 2nd edn. Edinburgh: Churchill Livingstone, Elsevier.

Raeburn, J. & Rootman, I. (1998). *People-Centred Health Promotion.* London: John Wiley and Sons.

Townsend, E., Stanton, S., Law, M., Polatajko, M., Baptiste, S., Thompson-Franson, T., Kramer, C., Swedlove, F., Brintnell, S. & Campanile, L. (2002). *Enabling Occupation, An Occupational Therapy Perspective.* Revised edition. Ottawa: CAOT Publications, ACE.

Townsend, E., Beagan, B., Kumas-Tan, Z., Versnel, J., Iwama, M., Landry, J., Stewart, D. & Brown, J. (2007). 'Enabling: occupational therapy's core competency' in *Enabling Occupation II: Advancing Occupational Therapy Vision for Health, Wellbeing and Justice Through Occupation,* eds. E. Townsend and H. Polatajko. Ottawa, ON: CAOT Publications ACE.

Townsend, E.A. & Polatajko, H.J. (2007). *Enabling Occupation II: Advancing an Occupational Therapy Vision for Health, Wellbeing & Justice Through Occupation*. Ottawa, ON: CAOT ACE.

Williams, H. (2011). Is there a role for psychological wellbeing practitioners and primary care mental health workers in the delivery of low intensity cognitive behavioural therapy for individuals who self-harm? *Journal of Mental Health Training, Education and Practice* **6** (4), 165–174.

Chapter 12

# Enabling young people's participation in their mental health service

Katja Michel

## Introduction

This chapter explores an occupational therapist's role in leading the participation and patient experience agenda in Child and Adolescent Mental Health Services (CAMHS). It outlines the skill set and theoretical foundations occupational therapists have and how these lend themselves easily to influence services towards greater participation of service users in their mental healthcare and delivery. Not only, however, do occupational therapists possess skills and an understanding of the importance of meaningful participation for children and young people to enhance their recovery, but the author concludes that because of our professional beliefs and values, it is our duty to contribute to the creation of services that support young people in their participation in their care to achieve the right outcomes and invest in our future generation.

## Key points

- Occupational therapists have a sound theoretical foundation from which to create and promote opportunities for participation.

- Facilitating young people's active participation in their healthcare promotes their development of occupational roles, skills and identity.

- Supporting children and young people to shape and drive forward their goals and priorities for recovery is an inherent part of client-centred occupational therapy practice; this can place occupational therapists at the forefront of advocating for and influencing services to embed meaningful service user participation into everyday practice.

- Involving and collaborating with users of services helps to ensure a service is fit for purpose for the population it serves.

- Understanding the experiences of service users (the good, the bad and the ugly) enhances clinical practice and is a powerful reminder of the core ethical principles of occupational therapy.

# Background

Health and care policy changes over the last 12 years have been putting increasing emphasis on the importance of listening and responding to the experiences and views of the users of children and young people's health and care services. This draws on the United Nations Convention on the Rights of the Child, which outlines the right of the child to be listened to and involved in decisions that affect them and to be provided with information that is accessible and meaningful to them (UNICEF 2016). Based on increasing evidence of the benefits of service users' participation, it is now part of national policy to encourage service users to share their views and experiences. In this way, service users (together with service providers) can influence change (Department for Education and Skills 2004).

The revised edition of *Hear by Right* (Badham & Wade 2010), the *Quality Criteria for Young People Friendly Health Services* (DoH 2011), as well as the development of the *Children and Young People Improving Access to Psychological Therapies* (CYP-IAPT) programme (NHS 2016) have further driven forward the understanding of the importance of meaningful participation of children and young people in their mental health care. This has led to designated funding for many mental health services to focus on embedding the principles of participation and collaborative practice into service delivery and design.

Participation in mental health services takes various forms, and may range from: being given accessible information; being involved with adult initiated consultations on particular issues or care pathways where children and young people's views are taken into account when decisions are made; to adult initiated projects where final decisions are shared between participants (examples of these may be designing and reviewing information resources, designing clinical spaces and involvement in staff training and recruitment); to partnership participation where children and young people are supported and encouraged to initiate projects, set their priorities and work collaboratively with adults to influence and affect change.

Additionally, participation should be non-discriminatory; it should be voluntary and opportunities for participation should be given to all children and young people accessing mental health services regardless of their age, race, religion, (dis-)ability or socio-economic and educational factors (Badham & Wade 2010).

# How occupational therapy fits in

Core to our professional values is the client-centred ethos with which occupational therapists work and set goals to ensure those are meaningful for service users' recovery (Sumsion 2006). Working with children and young people inevitably takes into account their developmental stages and needs.

Occupational therapists in addition, have an understanding of how a mental health or developmental condition affects the person's participation in daily activities, their ability to make meaningful contributions to their social community and thus their ability to fulfill their social and occupational roles (Kielhofner 2008). Occupational therapists, through their training and practice, have skills and knowledge in facilitating groups and creating cohesive and respectful teams. They are trained to use a range of social and communication skills in order to engage with their clients and through listening skills are able to understand and respond to clients' experiences, views and opinions. Having an understanding of clients' interests, values and desires is important in occupational therapy practice to understand the motivation for clients' occupational engagement patterns (Kielhofner 2008). As occupational therapists, we frequently act as advocates for clients, whether this is to advocate for their ability and right to live in the community, or adaptations needed to enable a person to fulfil meaningful productive and social roles. Last but not least, occupational therapists focus on enablement and independence throughout their therapy to aid recovery (Stoffel 2011). This places occupational therapists in a unique position to understand the importance of and the requirements needed to enable children and young people to participate in their mental health care. Therefore, working with young people to enable and empower them to share and influence services is not a new concept but sits comfortably within occupational therapy theory and practice.

## Participation in practice

It is helpful to make a distinction between different areas and manners of participation. For the purpose of this chapter, I am referring to this as internal and external participation. It is, however, important not to exclude one in favour of the other, and as a therapist not only to take responsibility for the more direct (or what I have called 'internal') client-therapist participation, as both types are inter-dependent.

External participation comprises participation activities that happen outside the therapeutic work. This may be in the form of consultations, specific projects, or being part of a service user advisory group that reviews, advises and influences developments in the service and the wider community. Participants may be involved in outreach work, workforce training and recruitment and may have a role in monitoring and challenging areas of practice. They may review and produce information materials to ensure they are user-friendly, such as leaflets, posters and websites. Levels of external participation vary considerably, but there are resources available that can support young people and those working with them to monitor their involvement and influence, so they can ensure participation remains meaningful. A useful guide for this has been outlined by Badham and Wade (2010), and even decades earlier by Hart (1992) with his participation ladder. When embarking on the role of a participation worker, it is important to have a sound understanding of the levels and types of participation activities to understand their potential benefits and limitations so that the integrity of participation and that of the young people is not jeopardised. Using a consultation event as an example, several factors need to be considered and assessed prior to the event. These include: what are the objectives of the event and whose objectives are they; will the event allow young people's views and opinions to be truly listened to; and can they realistically be used to drive developments forward? Furthermore, it is also important to consider who will be attending and engaging with the event and whose voices and opinions will remain absent. For participation to be inclusive and representative of a diverse group of service users, it is vital to use a range of approaches and methods to seek out and engage with children and young people.

Internal participation is a less visible part of participation, which takes place within a therapist-client relationship. Since 2011, the main driver for enhancing internal participation in CAMHS has been the introduction of the national CYP-IAPT programme, which places significant emphasis on developing collaborative working practices and reaching shared decisions through in-session rating scales and outcome monitoring, throughout a young person's mental health treatment (Jones et al. 2015). The CYP-IAPT has created an increasing evidence base on the benefits of collaborative working on young people's recovery. Examples of collaborative practice include making shared decisions about medication regimes, setting shared goals and review these regularly together, as well as developing agreements about methods of communication between client and therapist, and frequency, location and timing of appointments. The aim is that the relationship is collaborative and therapy is 'done with' as opposed to 'done to' a young person.

# Benefits for children and young people

It has been established that about 50 per cent of all mental health conditions start before the age of 14 (Angermeyer et al. 2007), affecting a child's and young person's typical development of social, emotional and independent living skills, which are all important aspects of their preparation for adulthood. If, however, young people feel valued, they understand the systems and services that are supporting them, and they are able to influence and make decisions about the care they receive, their engagement and outcomes for recovery are more positive (Badham & Wade 2010). This undoubtedly will also shape their engagement with mental health services as adults and put them in a greater position of empowerment and choice.

From personal experience in this role, children and young people predominantly seek to participate for two main reasons: they have had negative experiences in their own care (or that of a sibling or a friend) and are striving to improve the service for others, whilst also having an opportunity to vent their dissatisfaction; or they have had positive experiences and want to give something back to the service. Therefore, being actively involved in participation projects and shared decision making in their own care enables young people to shape and develop the meaning they attach to their experiences of mental health care and their mental ill-health. Being involved meaningfully in influencing and contributing to decisions about the services they receive elevates young people's roles and status to becoming experts by experience. By talking about and sharing poor and difficult experiences with providers of services, young people can transform some of their experiences into meaningful changes and improvements. For example, young people can drive forward the development of accessible care plans so they have a greater understanding and role in decisions about their care. They may develop training resources or facilitate training workshops to bring their experiences closer to the staff who work with them, thus layering positive meaning on to often challenging and distressing experiences.

Being involved in projects that influence change also supports the development of social and independent living skills, as long as the right support by those who facilitate projects is available so young people are prepared and thus able to contribute how and when they can and wish to. Furthermore, being part of a group of young people with mental health conditions offers an opportunity for shared experiences for young people who, because of their mental health issues, frequently experience social isolation. Participation thus has the potential to positively affect self-confidence and offer a sense of belonging, both of which are widely acknowledged to be mental health promoting (Mental Health Foundation 2016). Not only does participation support the development of personal and inter-personal skills, but it also offers experiences that equip young people with insight and skills for adult life. For example, being part of an interview process gives a unique insight into the requirements of particular jobs, writing styles of applications and how decisions and staff appointments are made. This, therefore, puts young people in a more informed and potentially confident position when they apply for jobs themselves, creating a greater opportunity for successful vocational achievement. Additionally, children and young people who are active participants develop a greater understanding of wider issues that affect health and social care, such as health policies and commissioning. This in turn can lead to further motivation and opportunities to participate in issues affecting their community and wider society.

# Ensuring mental health services are fit for the people they serve

Health services benefit from service user participation, both in terms of service user satisfaction and reduction in complaints, appropriate use of services and attendance of appointments, length of treatment, and positive treatment outcomes (Badham & Wade 2010, Jones *et al.* 2015). But it also yields benefits on a much wider societal level. Young people who are empowered to challenge the status quo, who are aware of their rights and have experienced the benefits of their contributions, who have become confident and skilled in talking about their needs, experiences and priorities for change, are likely to become advocates for others in the future. They are creating opportunities to reduce the stigma of mental ill-health in their schools, families, communities, colleges and workplaces and therefore are contributing to wider positive changes in the understanding and treatment of mental health.

# Reflections on the role of participation worker – a privilege and a duty

It genuinely feels a privilege to have been part of embedding children's and young people's participation and to have created a forum for participation projects that have influenced and affected the way services are delivered. It has allowed me to gain an insight into how children and young people experience mental health services. Hearing and understanding the barriers that mental health systems and services create for young people, which prevent them from becoming collaborators in their care, has been invaluable. Not only has this experience been invaluable, but it has also allowed me to draw on my professional values and skills to create opportunities for social and vocational participation for young people. Being a small profession in a large organisation, it is not always easy to identify and pursue opportunities to promote our professional values and affect change for service users on a large scale. However, this role has provided opportunities to raise awareness and appreciation of occupational therapy in our service. Having been in an influencing role and sat at tables where strategic decisions are made has provided an opportunity to promote occupational therapy thinking and demonstrate our broad range of skills. It has provided a range of opportunities to build relationships with other stakeholders and organisations, which otherwise would most likely not have occurred.

Whilst it is humbling to observe the journeys of so many children and young people to becoming greater advocates for the services they need, it also has become clear that it is a duty for all health professionals to promote and facilitate meaningful participation of young people in their care and the service that they use. If mental health services strive to improve the mental health of their young service users, all of those working for the service need to understand the experiences of their population and work with them to improve and develop sustainable services for the future that ensure they are accessible, meaningful and suit the needs and vision of young people.

Although it is heartening to observe that meaningful participation in mental health services for children and young people is developing, there is still a way to go to embed its core principles into every element of service delivery. Due to conflicting interests and priorities between stakeholders, a risk of tokenistic participation (Hart 1992) remains. However, having a sound understanding of the principles of participation and how this relates to the pursuit of meaningful and productive occupational roles will help us stay on the right course and persevere. As occupational therapists we are aware of the risk of occupational discrimination that can occur for children and young people who are experiencing poor mental health, and this enables us to continue to see the bigger picture and work with integrity towards meaningful participation. We are skilled in understanding the needs of children and young people and factors that are preventing their full participation. This gives us a theoretical and practical foundation that can give confidence to persevere and advocate, and thus pursue, together with young people, their full participation in services. It enables us to create an environment and work towards systems that support successful participation on a larger scale.

If there was a job advert in the paper for the ideal candidate as a participation worker, essential requirements would be: being curious, being non-judgemental, having a motivation to get things right and an ability to persevere, being realistic but striving high, being politically astute and able to build relationships with a range of stakeholders, and having an ability to step back and let young people be the drivers for change.

# Useful resources

- Arbesman, M., Bazyk, S., & Nochajski, S.M. (2013). Systematic review of occupational therapy and mental health promotion, prevention, and intervention for children and youth. *American Journal of Occupational Therapy* **67**, e120–e130. http:// dx.doi.org/10.5014/ajot.2013.008359

- http://www.cypiapt.org/participtation.php

- Evidence-based co-design toolkit: http://www.kingsfund.org.uk/projects/ebcd

- Evidence-based practice unit – bridging research and practice in child mental health: https://www.ucl.ac.uk/ebpu/docs/publication_files/ebpubrochure2016

- Law, M. (2002). Participation in the occupations of everyday life, 2002 Distinguished Scholar Lecture. *American Journal of Occupational Therapy* **56**, 640–649.

- Nine priorities for participation: http://www.youngminds.org.uk/for_children_young_people/guide_to_mental_health_services/children_and_young_peoples_iapt/the_nine_priorities_for_participation

- Sustaining children's and young people's participation: http://www.myapt.org.uk/year-4/camhs-sustaining-participation-ebook/

# References

Angermeyer, A., Anthony, J.C. & Kessler, R.C. (2007) Lifetime prevalence and age-of-onset distributions of mental disorders in the World Health Organization's World Mental Health Survey Initiative. *World Psychiatry* **6** (3), 168–176.

Badham, B. & Wade, H. (2010). *Hear by Right – Standards Framework for the Participation of Children and Young People.* National Youth Agency http://www.nya.org.uk/our-services/hear-right/ (last accessed: 23.10.2016).

Department for Education and Skills (2004). *Every Child Matters: Change for Children.* London: TSO.

Department of Health (2011). *Quality Criteria for Young People Friendly Health Services.* London: TSO.

Hart, R.A. (1992). *Children's Participation – from Tokenism to Citizenship. UNICEF International Child Development Centre.* https://www.unicef-irc.org/publications/100/ (last accessed: 23.10.2016).

Jones, M., Law, D. & Wolpert, M. (2015) *Using CYP IAPT Feedback and Outcome Forms to Aid Clinical Practice – Key Messages.* London: CORC.

Kielhofner, G. (2008). *Model of Human Occupation: Theory and Application*, 3rd edn. Baltimore: Lippincott Williams & Wilkins.

Mental Health Foundation (2016). *How to Look After your Mental Health.* http://www.mentalhealth.org.uk (last accessed: 26.2.2016).

National Health Service (2016). *CYP-IAPT Principles In CAMH services. Values and Standards – Delivering With and Delivering Well.* CAMHS Press. https://www.england.nhs.uk/wp-content/uploads/2014/12/delvr-with-delvrng-well.pdf (last accessed: 23.10.2016).

Stoffel, V.C. (2011). 'Recovery' in *Occupational Therapy – a Vision for Participation*, eds. C. Brown and V.C. Stoffel Baltimore: F.A. Davis Company.

Sumsion, T. (2006). 'The client-centred approach' in *Client-centred Practice in Occupational Therapy: a Guide to Implementation,* ed. T. Sumsion, 2nd edn. Philadelphia: Churchill Livingstone, Elsevier.

UNICEF (2016). United Nations Convention on the Rights of the Child 1990. http://www.unicef.org.uk (last accessed: 14.1.2016).

# Chapter 13

# Working with families

Paula Conneely

## Introduction

This chapter aims to introduce the reader to Family Work in the context of current mental health practice. It makes specific reference to the evidence-based model Behavioural Family Therapy (BFT) and describes the key aspects of the model. The chapter provides an overview of the process of intervention and illustrates this further with a case study. In addition, the author reflects upon her own role as a Clinical Specialist working for the Meriden Family Programme and describes why she feels occupational therapists make good family workers.

*Note*: For the purposes of this chapter the word 'family' is to be seen in its widest sense. Many will perceive family as a biological concept (e.g. parent/child) whereas 'family work' as described in this chapter can include biological family, partnerships, sibling relationships, friends, those in shared accommodation – indeed any individual or groups of people that the service user defines as significant within their lives.

## Key points

- Current clinical guidelines clearly advocate the use of evidence-based family interventions for those individuals and their families experiencing psychosis, schizophrenia and bipolar disorder (NICE 2014, NICE 2016).
- Working with the whole family can lead to more positive outcomes for both the service user and their family members.
- Family work is an intervention which views the service user in a truly holistic manner. It is skills-based and activity driven with goal setting and occupational performance at its heart. As such, it is an intervention ideally suited to the occupational therapist.

## The family context

When asked to define occupational therapy, we often use quotations and descriptions which emphasise the concept of independence and its client-centred nature. For example, '[o]ccupational

**195**

therapy takes a whole-person approach to both mental and physical health and wellbeing, enabling individuals to achieve their full potential' (COT 2015, para. 1) and 'provides practical support to enable people to facilitate recovery and overcome any barriers that prevent them from doing the activities (occupations) that matter to them' (COT 2015, para. 2). Further, occupation relates to those practical and purposeful activities that enable individuals to live independently and have a sense of personal identity (COT 2015). While these statements are valid and define the nature of occupational therapy well, it could be suggested they fail to acknowledge the importance of family and friends in developing and maintaining a person's wellbeing. As human beings we function best within the context of family groups and communities.

> With hundreds of miles open to habitation, people still tend to build their houses close to the houses of other people. No matter the continent, no matter the culture, no matter the era, this is what we do. And to find an individual choosing to live completely alone in the world is so rare as to confirm that human beings need to live amongst each other; indeed we are compelled from within ourselves to group together. Humans are social animals; it is our nature to be so.
>
> (Yeatts 1997, para. 1)

For many individuals, family is of huge importance. Families can provide practical support, shelter, finance and a physical environment conducive to wellbeing. Equally they can provide the nurturing, cognitive and emotional support necessary for a person to flourish. By the same token, in the absence of family or community a person can fail to thrive. For family members themselves, having a loved one who experiences ill health can be a cause of huge distress which can in turn impact on that person's own physical and emotional wellbeing (Carers Trust 2012, Savage & Bailey 2004). A recent survey by CarersUK (2015) cited 84 per cent of carer respondents as 'worried about their own health', with 78 per cent reporting increased anxiety, and 55 per cent significant levels of depression. Sleep disturbance, financial concerns, difficulty within relationships and maintaining work roles were also highlighted as significant challenges, all of which have a clear and direct impact on both the family member and service user they support. It could therefore be suggested that a profession which prides itself on being holistic needs to truly address the importance of these social and familial frameworks and recognise the importance of working with clients in a whole-family context.

## Family and carer involvement across the lifespan

Within paediatric occupational therapy, authors such as Edwards et al. (2003) and Thompson (1998) advocate family-centred practice and cite the collaborative involvement of parents and caregivers as a means of improving outcomes for children. The implementation of home programmes is improved when collaboration takes place and carers are included in the treatment planning process (Ketelaar et al. 1998). Involving parents, carers and siblings is often seen as best practice, a way of maximising resources, and a means of ensuring that treatment regimens are embedded in the normal routines and everyday activities of the family.

When considering family and carer involvement in the care of older adults, the literature again advocates that family carers are involved as a matter of routine. Indeed, the current NICE Guidelines (2006, modified 2015) are entitled *Dementia: supporting people with dementia and their carers in health and social care*, a title which acknowledges the inherent need for clinicians to work with both parties to ensure effective clinical practice. Authors such as Graff *et al.* (2006) acknowledge the impact of dementia in terms of both the service user and carers' own wellbeing; promoting inclusion in the treatment process as a way of improving mood, quality of life, health status and caregivers' sense of control over life events. Carer inclusion further indicates a cost saving for older adult services (Graff *et al.* 2008) through the enhancement of daily functioning for both the individual experiencing dementia and their primary family carer.

Why then, if carer and family involvement is so integral to the wellbeing of individuals across the lifespan, is it so historically neglected within the field of adult mental health? One suggestion is the issue of confidentiality and how this applies to those adults of working age. Clarity around how information is shared with family and friends has often caused concern across a wide range of professional groups with many clinicians erring on the side of caution and falling back to the position of not sharing information – often resulting in carers and family members feeling uninvolved, excluded and lacking the information which enables them to take an active and informed role in their loved ones' care (Rethink 2006). Fortunately, guidance is becoming more readily available with professional bodies and organisations taking a more proactive and commonsense stance on confidentiality (RCP 2015). Furthermore, initiatives such as the 'triangle of care' (Carers Trust 2013) are actively seeking to develop services and promote collaborative practice in mental health – perhaps highlighting a shift in thinking over recent years.

# Family involvement and occupational therapy in adult mental health

One of the most significant mental health oriented documents produced by the College in recent years is *Recovering Ordinary Lives: the Strategy for Occupational Therapy in Mental Health Services 2007–2017: a Vision for the Next Ten Years* (COT 2006a). However, if you search this extensive document you will find no matches to the words 'family' or 'friends'. In addition, the word 'carer' seems to be used in a somewhat tokenistic manner, i.e. service user *and carer* involvement, working in partnership with service users *and carers*. No reference is made to the rationale behind these statements and the value of working with carers seems focused more on the benefits to services, i.e. training of students and quality feedback. The active involvement of carers and family members in clinical practice can often seem overlooked in the field of occupational therapy in adult mental health, an occurrence that can be seen to a degree in other fields of healthcare: the routine involvement of carers and families only in situations where it is seen as 'necessary' or in the best interests of the service user (particularly where there are issues around consent, capacity and informed choice, e.g. children's services, learning disabilities, dementia care). In addition, the term 'carer' is often misunderstood or unidentified within the field of mental health. Family members may not perceive themselves as adopting a caring role (e.g. preferring to identify themselves as a wife, husband, mother, father) and with adult service users often resenting the implication that they are 'cared for' by another.

In the document which supported the 2007–2017 strategy *Recovering Ordinary Lives: Results from Service User and Carer Focus Groups* (COT 2006b), a consultation group consisting of 11 mental health carers described their perceptions and experience of occupational therapists working in the field of adult mental health. Of these 11 carers, three described their family member having had access to occupational therapy, with the remaining eight feeling that access to an occupational therapist would have been extremely beneficial *for their loved one*. It would appear then in both literature and practice that an acknowledgement of the carer as an individual with needs and aspirations *in their own right* is rare, as is a true acknowledgement of the benefits of family-centred interventions in occupational therapy in adult mental health for both the service user and the wider family network.

What is clearly apparent from the literature is that adopting a whole-family approach can have a significant, positive impact on outcomes for the service user. This is referenced more fully in subsequent paragraphs. However, what is also clear from clinical practice and experience is the impact that family work can have on the self-care, productivity and leisure roles of the carers and family members themselves. There is clear evidence that the impact of a caring role can affect a person's own emotional and physical wellbeing, with family members often experiencing high demands, isolation and the associated stigma of mental health issues. In 2003, the mental health charity Rethink found that of 1,451 carers surveyed, 25 per cent reported moderate to significant impact on their mental and physical health, leisure activities, family relationships, financial circumstances and career progress (Pinfold & Corry 2003). In a more recent study of over 4,500 carers (CarersUK 2015), the figure rises to 84 per cent citing increased stress and 76 per cent concerned for their own health and wellbeing.

It may be suggested then that the benefits of adopting a whole-family approach are multi-faceted, with service users experiencing positive benefits in terms of their mental health, carers feeling more able to function in their caring role (with associated benefits for the service user), carers feeling more able to address their own needs – and, of course, all the associated financial benefits to healthcare services and the wider economy (Schizophrenia Commission 2012).

# What are family interventions?

Evidence-based family interventions have been in existence for many years. Indeed, much of the initial research on the use of family interventions in serious mental health conditions was published during the 1980s and early 1990s (Barrowclough & Tarrier 1992, Falloon 1985, Pharoah *et al.* 2010).

Over the decades, certain models have been well proven in terms of efficacy and outcome (Pilling *et al.* 2002, Pitschel-Walz *et al.* 2001), one of which is Behavioural Family Therapy (BFT). The BFT or 'Meriden' model is perhaps the most commonly used model of evidence-based family intervention in adult mental health services in the UK today, largely due to the Meriden Family Programme and their extensive cascade training programme which has been in existence since 1998 (Fadden & Birchwood 2002, Fadden 2006, Fadden *et al.* 2010, Fadden & Heelis 2011). The author is an occupational therapist who has been working with the Meriden Family Programme as a clinician, trainer and supervisor since its conception.

Behavioural family therapy is a psycho-educational approach originally developed by Professor Ian Falloon and colleagues (Falloon *et al.* 1984, Falloon *et al.* 1999). It is an extremely practical, skills-based intervention that usually takes 10 to 14 sessions to deliver. It provides information to the service user and their family about the service user's mental health and treatment, exploring the way that the issues and experiences affect each family member. The family also complete work on recognising early signs of relapse and develop a clear 'staying well' plan together. Behavioural family therapy focuses on promoting positive communication through the teaching of specific communication skills. These include active listening skills, being able to notice and express positive feelings, making requests and expressing more difficult feelings. A 6-step model of problem solving is also introduced to the family, with the overall aim of reducing stress within the family environment and enhancing family-based coping strategies. The needs of all family members are recognised, and individual family members are encouraged to identify and work towards clear personal goals. With this in mind, BFT promotes positive outcomes for the service user while simultaneously addressing the needs of all other family members involved.

The overall aims of BFT are increased understanding of the mental health problem and its impact, stress reduction and improved communication and problem solving skills within the family. Research over the past three decades has demonstrated that family interventions are effective in reducing stress for both service users and their families and significantly reduce relapse rates (Falloon 2003, Tarrier *et al.* 1988). The promotion of recovery in those people experiencing severe and/ or enduring mental health problems is clearly documented. The main focus of delivery has been around providing intervention to those families affected by psychosis or bipolar illness. Indeed, the National Institute for Clinical Excellence Schizophrenia guidelines (NICE 2014) recommend family interventions should be offered to 100 per cent of individuals with schizophrenia who have experienced a recent relapse. In addition, family education, support and intervention feature strongly in the NICE Bipolar guidance (NICE 2016). Although the research evidence base is strongest for those families experiencing psychosis or bipolar illness, the approach can be utilised effectively to help meet the needs of other families in contact with mental health services. In addition, there is growing support for using the approach with families experiencing stress in relation to long-term physical conditions.

# Overview of the therapy process

The BFT approach is not a package in which all components are delivered to all families. Rather, it is a formulation driven approach where sessions are based on the assessment of each individual family, and tailored to their specific needs. Equally, the pace and timescale of the support offered varies from family to family. In this collaborative approach, the therapist and family determine together what the agenda will be. Family work is generally offered in the family home unless the family have a preference for meeting elsewhere or the living environment makes it impracticable. This often makes it easier for family members who are pressured for time to attend and can help maintain engagement/reduce the likelihood of dropout. Box 13.1 shows the elements of a typical family intervention.

## Box 13.1: List of elements which a typical family intervention would draw from

- Engagement – Meeting with the whole family to discuss the benefits of family work and agreeing with the family that they are willing to try the approach
- Assessment of individual family members – Each member meeting with the therapist(s) to determine their individual knowledge, perceptions and experiences
- Assessment of family's communication and problem solving skills
- Formulation – Review of the assessment information on the family's resources, problems and goals
- Meeting with the family to discuss/plan how to proceed and establishment of regular family meetings
- Information sharing – Reaching a shared understanding of the diagnosis/experience and any treatments or interventions
- Early warning signs and relapse prevention work – development of 'staying well' plans
- Helping the family to develop effective communication skills
- Supporting the development of the family's problem solving skills
- Booster sessions
- Review and ongoing support or closure.

As mentioned previously, BFT usually consists of 10–12 sessions as a minimum. Alongside these clinical sessions, the family is encouraged to establish their own regular family meetings in the absence of the therapist. The rationale for this 'family time' is that it enables the family to start generalising new skills and integrating them into their daily lives. Meeting without the therapist enables the family to experiment with new roles such as chairperson and scribe and offers additional time as a family unit to reflect on learning, practise communication skills and, as the work progresses, offers a forum in which the family can meet to problem solve any issues that arise for them. It is then hoped that when the therapist disengages from the formal intervention, the family are able to maintain improvements over time and become less reliant on external facilitators or services to 'sort things out'. Families who have established their own family meetings have reported finding them very helpful, with some reporting they still use the technique many years after the clinical intervention has ended.

## Box 13.2: Quotes from family members who have engaged in BFT

Oh definitely yes there's no tension. I mean there used to be a lot of tension between A and me and my husband.
*(Family member, cited in Campbell 2004)*

… we talk about it, just look at things in a different way. When I want G to do something, or when I say something to G I say it in a different way, not in an argumentative way.
*(Family member, cited in Campbell 2004)*

It helped us an awful lot, even from understanding the medication to different aspects of the illness. They were really good meetings and it's the only time we were all together.

It gave us a chance to say things that we wouldn't normally say, especially negative feelings.

I could breathe a sigh of relief even though it's an illness but you know that you can get treatment and that others can start to understand what you've been through.

Thank you for all the time you have spent with us to help rebuild our lives.
*(Quotes from family members at post-intervention evaluation, unpublished)*

# Occupational therapists trained in Family Interventions (BFT)

Training in the model of BFT has been undertaken by the Meriden Programme since 1998. The programme has adopted a cascade model of training whereby clinicians trained and experienced in family work can then go on to train as trainers and supervisors in their local areas. The training is multi-disciplinary in nature and Meriden has trained over 5,300 family workers and 400 trainer/supervisors including training provision in Europe, Canada, Australia, Africa and Japan. Those who have availed themselves of the training are predominantly from the nursing profession; however all other professions are represented to varying degrees. Current Meriden figures report that just over 4 per cent of UK staff trained are occupational therapists (although this figure rises to 13 per cent of those trained in Nova Scotia, Canada). Interestingly, a number of senior management staff driving the implementation of family interventions within services are occupational therapists by background, not currently employed in 'traditional' or clinical posts.

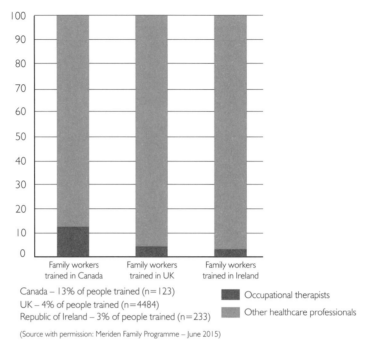

Canada – 13% of people trained (n=123)
UK – 4% of people trained (n=4484)
Republic of Ireland – 3% of people trained (n=233)

■ Occupational therapists
■ Other healthcare professionals

(Source with permission: Meriden Family Programme – June 2015)

*Figure 13.1: Graph showing percentage of BFT-trained occupational therapists.*

## Box 13.3: Case study – Peter

Dad, Peter, has a longstanding diagnosis of bipolar disorder which predated his marriage to Julie. They have two children, Neve (14) and Stephanie (17). Although having spent over 20 years in contact with mental health services, Julie had rarely had contact with professionals and the children had never spoken to anyone regarding their dad's health despite numerous admissions to hospital. Julie was in full-time employment as a care worker and Peter had not worked since studying fine art at university.

During the assessment process each family member was offered an individual interview. Each took the opportunity to describe how bipolar disorder had affected them personally. Julie talked of feeling excluded by services and of not really understanding her husband when unwell. She was 'at breaking point' following his recent admission to hospital and had given him the ultimatum that if things didn't change he would have to leave the family home. Peter himself spoke of feeling guilty, of feeling like he had let everyone down and that he had no 'connection' with his family any more. Both children spoke of feeling angry towards dad, that he wasn't 'helping himself' and that the stress was impacting on their schooling. All family members referred to feeling unsupported and that they had no one to talk to. In terms of identifying personal goals, Peter felt that time outside the family home was important and that renewing his interest in art would be helpful. Julie identified wanting to have more time to engage in hobbies (joining the gym, getting out to see friends) and the children both felt that having time out with friends, feeling less stressed at school/college and having a part-time job/regular income would be useful. Interestingly, all family members wanted more 'quality time' together, acknowledging that although they all lived in the same house, they rarely spent time together as a family.

Following the initial assessment period, a joint formulation session took place where we decided as a group what the aims of the intervention would be. Each felt that information would be key to developing a better understanding of Peter's experience. We decided we would look at bipolar disorder as a general topic and include specific information on medication and how low mood (in particular) affected Peter's ability to engage in daily routines. Each family member was also keen to look at staying well planning so they could better identify when Peter was becoming high/low and take preventative measures. Peter's last admission to hospital had been traumatic for the whole family and it was something they would rather not experience again.

The intervention as a whole took approximately 14 sessions to complete. Each session was of one-hour duration and took place at the family home. Stephanie attended alternate sessions due to college commitments, but the family fed back details to her of the sessions she was unable to attend. One of the first things to be established was the concept of family meetings which the family took to keenly. Outside our clinical sessions, the whole family took time out to meet as a family once a week. This was usually tied in to them eating a meal together, but also involved checking out how their week had been, practising skills learnt in the family sessions and completing homework tasks. Once established, the family reported that this was a really helpful way of connecting with one another and that it felt 'safe' due to having clearly defined boundaries and ground rules. Peter felt that it was helping to re-establish his relationship with the children and Julie found it a helpful forum in which to problem solve day to day issues (e.g. household chores, dog walking) which in turn alleviated her own stress. They were keen for this intervention to continue once the formal family work had concluded – something which is actively encouraged in family work.

Initial sessions focused on developing a better understanding of bipolar disorder. Peter, as an expert by experience, was able to describe to his family how it felt to experience the highs and crushing lows of his illness. Although the children in particular all had a 'text book' idea of bipolar from searching on the internet, they were able to talk openly and ask their dad questions about what it actually felt like to be manic/depressed, with the family worker facilitating this exchange. The family all stated that the depressive episodes were the most challenging to manage and the most frustrating for them.

Talking openly helped family members appreciate how difficult it was for Peter and that he couldn't just 'pull himself out of it', which in turn helped Peter feel less guilty that he was 'letting the family down'. Subsequent sessions focused on developing a staying well plan for Peter. Each family member contributed by identifying what they noticed prior to Peter becoming elated/depressed and a clear relapse signature was developed. In turn, each family member then identified how they would respond should they notice changes in Peter's health. A wide range of strategies were included, ranging from Stephanie offering to take dad out for a walk to take some photos/encouraging him to do some sketching, to Julie encouraging Peter to walk the dog with her each day, to Peter requesting to meet with his community psychiatric nurse and bringing his outpatient appointment forward (strategies graded from simple ones that the family could engage in independently/early on, to ones requiring a mental health service response).

Following the information sharing sessions, four sessions were dedicated to developing family communication skills. The first session consisted of encouraging the family to notice and comment upon the good things that were happening (expressing pleasant feelings).

**Example skill prompt sheet**

Expressing pleasant feelings

- Look at the person
- Say exactly what they did that pleased you
- Tell them how it made you feel.

© Meriden Family Programme 2015

In feedback, each family member felt this was helpful as their communication had become quite negative and critical over recent months. The second session focused on making requests and being able to clearly ask for what you want. Although a seemingly simple skill, Julie found this hard and acknowledged that she rarely asked for help or support – but often resented others for not helping out more. A clear rationale for using this skill was discussed, with Julie keen to begin practising the skill outside of sessions. The next two sessions were spent looking at active listening skills and being able to express more difficult feelings. Although listening skills posed little in the way of challenge to the family, expressing more difficult feelings was harder. Again, the rationale for the skill was explored and the family were able to acknowledge that *not* expressing difficult or unpleasant feelings often led to more conflict and stress in the long term.

Once the family felt that they were communicating more effectively, and this could be observed within the context of family sessions, time was spent looking at a 6-step method of problem solving.

*Example skill prompt sheet*

Problem solving/goal achievement

- Identify the problem/goal
- Identify potential solutions
- Advantages/disadvantages to each
- Decide on best solution
- Plan and implement
- Review.

© Meriden Family Programme 2015

During this time, the family were encouraged to develop the technique and apply it to issues/goals that impacted upon the whole family. As such, practice examples included the completion of household tasks (goal: to make sure the bathroom stays clean and tidy) through to planning a special occasion (goal: for the whole family to go out and celebrate Mum's birthday next month). In addition, the family were encouraged to use the problem solving method within their regular family meetings to problem solve issues as they arose. As such, many of the day-to-day unresolved issues that caused stress were dealt with in a 'fair' and family-oriented manner. This appeared to help on a number of levels. Peter felt he had more of a role in family discussions and decision making, Julie felt that she was no longer 'going round in circles' and the children felt that they had a voice and were involved, rather than 'Mum and Dad just telling us what to do and getting stressed out'.

Following completion of the family work, a final review session was held. Feedback from Peter was that he felt his relationship with Julie and the children was much improved and that they understood him more. Peter had managed to achieve his initial personal goal and was working part-time at a local charity shop. He was hoping to develop this further and begin a photography course at the local college the following September, having been successful in applying. Julie felt she understood Peter's illness more and acknowledged she had never appreciated how difficult it must be for him, especially when low in mood. She reported feeling more reassured that they could manage Peter's bipolar disorder more effectively as a family and was confident that she could act early should any symptoms of relapse appear. She also stated that she felt her relationship with mental health services was improved and that she no longer felt alone and unsupported. Feedback from both children was also positive, with each saying they felt they understood Dad's illness better, that they talked a lot more and felt like a 'normal family'. Stephanie had also achieved her goal of gaining part-time work at a local cinema.

# Why I believe occupational therapists make good family workers

I have always felt that occupational therapists make good family workers. Much of the underpinning theory of occupational therapy lends itself to seeing the 'bigger picture' and the service user as a whole. If we extend this whole to encompass those relationships around the person, family, friendships, community, then we are really able to view the person in context. Kielhofner's Model of Human Occupation (Kielhofner 2008) acknowledges the nature of dynamic systems and how we can influence domains both directly and indirectly. With this in mind, adopting a whole-family approach would seem a most natural thing for occupational therapists to do. Through positively influencing relationships and environment we can support both the individual and their family to build on strengths and maximise Recovery.

Occupation, as a core area of concern for occupational therapists, features strongly in family work with many of the goals that people set focusing on the domains of self-care, productivity and leisure. As a profession we acknowledge the importance of roles and routines, both of which are addressed within family work. The individual assessment schedule asks family members about their daily life pattern, asking 'what activities take up most of your time?' and 'are there any other things you would like to be doing? what prevents you?' alongside questions around where individuals spend their time and with whom. This information then feeds directly into goal setting for the family member, with specific activities clearly identified, implemented and reviewed within the context of the intervention. Families are asked to identify their own goals and aspirations and these commonly centre on everyday common tasks – things that can so easily fall by the wayside when the family is in chaos and doing their best to cope with the daily challenges of dealing with mental illness and distress. Maintaining daily routines, seeking role balance, regaining lost skills and seeking new, hopeful opportunities are all encompassed within family work. Goal setting and achievement are as core to family work as they are to the occupational therapy process.

The techniques used within evidence-based family interventions (BFT) are also readily accepted by occupational therapists who are familiar with the importance of 'doing'. Rather than simply talking about skills attainment, the family worker enables the family to try out and practise skills within the family work session. The rationale for a skill is explored, new or alternative skills are introduced (or revisited if the skills have been lost due to the impact of stress) and the family then demonstrate the skill in the session. Box 13.4 shows an example of this.

## Box 13.4: Example of process of session where the topic is 'listening skills'

- Family worker elicits the rationale for the skill of effective listening (e.g. 'How do you think listening more effectively would help you as a family?')

- Family worker explores current use of skill (e.g. 'Can you give me recent examples of when you felt able to listen to one another, or when you felt particularly listened to?')
- Family worker introduces the skill of 'active listening' using prompt sheets and material from the workbook
- Family worker requests that the family try out the new skill during the session using a specific exercise, with constructive feedback offered by both family members and family worker
- Family worker encourages the generalisation of the skill through encouraging the family members to use the skill outside sessions and use diary sheets
- Family worker reviews skill acquisition at subsequent sessions.

When training multi-disciplinary staff in family work, trainees often comment that they find the act of asking the family to practise a skill in their presence awkward or uncomfortable. This appears less so for occupational therapists who are accustomed to the use of activity as a therapeutic tool. Indeed, occupational therapists are often particularly enthused by the skills component of the BFT model, coupled with the 'simplicity' of the skills and their relevance in everyday lives.

I also find being non-affiliated with any other health profession or particular model of practice extremely beneficial, particularly when initially engaging with families. I have found families engage more readily with someone they perceive as an ally, a 'helping professional' who sees beyond diagnosis and medication. Equally, while we can draw from models and techniques such as Cognitive Behavioural Therapy (CBT) and mindfulness in our practice, they do not define us as a profession (I have often heard statements like 'it's the nurse's job to do the depots and manage the medication', 'the psychologist does all the talking therapies', 'if you need to talk about medication you need to speak to the psychiatrist'). As occupational therapists we 'wear many hats' and are perhaps able to select from this range more freely than some of the other professions. This flexibility can be seen to help avoid some of the stereotypes that influence how we are perceived by our service users and families. In addition, the stepping in and out of roles can prove a challenge to some, whereas I feel family work can be more readily incorporated into routine practice for many occupational therapists.

## Role reflection: my own role as a clinical specialist with the Meriden Family Programme

I have been working as a clinical specialist with the Meriden Programme for over 10 years now and feel that my role as an occupational therapist within the team is well established and recognised. I am passionate about the rationale for working with whole families and believe that acknowledging and including family members in mental health practice is essential, and yet often not done. I have confidence that working as part of a multi-disciplinary training team, which includes occupational therapy, enables us to engage with a much wider audience and reinforces the fact that psychological interventions are not purely the domain of certain professions. The core competencies involved in engaging with families and helping families develop strategies for wellbeing are not unique to any profession and yet lend themselves beautifully to that of occupational therapy. I appreciate that my role is unique, but having the time and capacity to work clinically with families, deliver training and supervision and also design and produce training courses and materials is hugely rewarding. I also appreciate that focusing purely on a family work agenda means that the role blurring, implementation issues and reality of caseload management are aspects I no longer deal with personally, although they are still issues affecting the clinical supervision I offer.

People often ask if my background as an occupational therapist impacts upon my current role, and yes, it does. The way that I approach my clinical work is heavily influenced by my occupational therapy roots, from assessment and formulation through to the practical activities we engage in during sessions (I have a particular passion for the communication skills and problem solving components of the model, as do many of the occupational therapists I encounter). During family work, the personal goals established by each family member inevitably relate to those occupations that hold most meaning to them, establishing daytime activities, returning to lost hobbies, studies or employment and regaining a more manageable balance in terms of life roles. The transparency of working with a whole family group enables me as a worker to gain a far better understanding of the physical, social and emotional environment in which the service user resides/interacts, and also a far greater understanding of the environment in which new skills and techniques are developed. For example, in previous roles where I have worked with service users in a group setting, skills practice outside sessions ('homework') has entailed individuals testing out skills on an unknowing and sometimes unreceptive audience. When the family members are supported to work together in developing skills, many of the barriers (such as awkwardness, lack of confidence and fear) are minimised.

Although training workers in BFT is a significant aspect of my role, helping people implement skills post-training is often the bigger challenge. Being able to identify and relate to some of the barriers clinicians face is always a benefit. As a trainer I still retain a clinical caseload and maintain my family work skills in a clinical setting. I feel that this is important, not only to 'practise what I preach' but to also demonstrate that occupational therapists can, and do, engage successfully in the role of family worker. Being able to provide vignettes and examples of the work I do brings the training I offer to life and, when there are fellow occupational therapists in the room, demonstrates the value that occupational therapy can bring to family work; and vice versa.

# Useful resources

- *Caring for Yourself* (self-help manual available www.meridenfamilyprogramme.com or https://www.rethink.org/resources/search?a=caring%20for%20yourself)

- Fadden, G. & Heelis, R. (2011). The Meriden West Midlands family programme: lessons learned over ten years *Journal of Mental Health* **20** (1), 79–88.

- http://www.meridenfamilyprogramme.com

- *MyCare* (available through Google Play or the Apple App store. Desktop version available at http://www.mycareapp.co.uk)

- http://www.nice.org.uk

# References

Barrowclough, C. & Tarrier, N. (1992). *Families of Schizophrenic Patients: Cognitive Behavioural Intervention*. London: Chapman & Hall.

Campbell, A.S. (2004). How was it for you? families' experiences of receiving behavioural family therapy. *Journal of Psychiatric and Mental Health Nursing* **11** (3), 261–267.

Carers Trust (2012). *Carers Trust Survey Briefing: Unpaid Carers Struggle for Years Without Support*. http://www.carers.org (last accessed: 5.1.2016).

Carers Trust (2013). *The Triangle of Care. Carers Included: a Guide to Best Practice in Mental Health Care in England*, 2nd edn. http:www.carers.org (last accessed: 5.1.2016).

CarersUK (2015). *State of Caring 2015 Report*. https://www.carersuk.org (last accessed: 24.10.2016)

College of Occupational Therapists (2006a). *Recovering Ordinary Lives: The strategy for Occupational Therapy in Mental Health Services: a Strategy for the Next Ten Years*. London: COT.

College of Occupational Therapists (2006b). *Recovering Ordinary Lives: Results from Service User and Carer Focus Groups*. London: COT.

College of Occupational Therapists (2015). *OT Helps You; What is Occupational Therapy?* http://www.cot.co.uk (last accessed 5.1.2016).

Edwards, A., Millard, P., Praskac, L. & Wisniewski, P. (2003). Occupational therapy and early intervention: a family-centred approach. *Occupational Therapy International* **10** (4), 239–252.

Fadden, G. (2006). Training and disseminating family interventions for schizophrenia: developing family intervention skills with multi-disciplinary groups. *Journal of Family Therapy* **28** (1), 23–38.

Fadden, G. & Birchwood, M. (2002). 'British models for expanding family psychoeducation in routine practice' in *Family Interventions in Mental Illness: International Perspectives,* eds. H.P. Lefley & D.L. Johnson. Westport, CT: Praeger.

Fadden, G. & Heelis, R. (2011). The Meriden West Midlands Family Programme: lessons learned over ten years. *Journal of Mental Health* **20** (1), 79–88.

Fadden, G., Heelis, R. & Bisnauth, R. (2010). Training mental health care professionals in Behavioural Family Therapy: an audit of West Midlands trainers' experiences. *Journal of Mental Health Training, Education and Practice* **5** (2), 27–35.

Falloon, I.R.H. (1985). *Family Management of Schizophrenia*. Baltimore: Johns Hopkins University Press.

Falloon, I.R.H. (2003). Family interventions for mental disorders: efficacy and effectiveness. *World Psychiatry* **2** (1), 20–28.

Falloon, I.R.H., Boyd, J.L. & McGill, C.W. (1984). *Family Care of Schizophrenia*. New York: Guilford Press.

Falloon, I.R.H., Held, T., Coverdale, J.H., Roncone, R. & Laidlaw, T.M. (1999). Family interventions for schizophrenia: a review of long-term benefits of international studies. *Psychiatric Rehabilitation Skills* **3** (2), 268–290.

Graff, M.J.L., Adang, E., Vernooij-Dassen, M.J.M., Dekker, J., Jönsson, L., Thijssen, M., Hoefnagels, W.H.L. & Olde-Rikkert, M.G.M. (2008). Community occupational therapy for older patients with dementia and their care givers: cost effectiveness study. *British Medical Journal* **336** (7636), 134–138.

Graff, M.J.L., Vernooij-Dassen, M.J.M., Thijssen, M., Dekker, J., Hoefnagels, W.H.L. & Olde-Rikkert, M.G.M. (2006). Community-based occupational therapy for patients with dementia and their care givers: randomised controlled trial. *British Medical Journal* **333** (7580), 1196–2002.

Ketelaar, M., Vermeer, A., Helders, P.J.M. & Hart, H. (1998). Parental participation in intervention programmes for children with cerebral palsy: a review of research. *Topics in Early Childhood Special Education* **18** (2), 108–117.

Kielhofner, G. (2008). *Model of Human Occupation: Theory and Application,* 4th edn. Baltimore: Lippincott Williams & Wilkins.

National Institute for Health and Clinical Excellence (2006, modified 2015). *Dementia: Supporting People with Dementia and their Carers in Health and Social Care.* London: National Institute for Health and Clinical Excellence. http://www.nice.org.uk (last accessed: 4.1.2016).

National Institute for Health and Clinical Excellence (2014). *Psychosis and Schizophrenia in Adults: Prevention and Management (CG178).* London: National Institute for Health and Clinical Excellence. http://www.nice.org.uk (last accessed: 4.1.2016).

National Institute for Health and Clinical Excellence (2016). *Bipolar Disorder: Assessment and Management (CG185).* London: National Institute for Health and Clinical Excellence. http://www.nice.org.uk (last accessed: 4.1.2016).

Pharoah, F., Mari, J., Rathbone, J. & Wong, W. (2010). 'Family intervention for schizophrenia', (Cochrane Review). *The Cochrane Library,* **12**.

Pilling, S., Bebbington, P., Kuipers, E., Garety, P., Geddes, J., Orbach, G. & Morgan, C. (2002). Psychological treatments in schizophrenia. I: meta-analysis of family intervention and cognitive behaviour therapy. *Psychological Medicine* **32** (5), 763–782.

Pinfold, V. & Corry, P. (2003). *Under Pressure: the Impact of Caring on People Supporting Family Members or Friends with Mental Health Problems.* London: Rethink.

Pitschel-Walz, G., Leucht, S., Bäuml, J., Kissling, W. & Engel, R.R. (2001). The effect of family interventions on relapse and rehospitalisation in schizophrenia – a meta-analysis. *Schizophrenia Bulletin* **27** (1), 73–92.

Rethink (2006). *Sharing Mental Health Information with Carers: Pointers to Good Practice for Service Providers.* London: Health Services Research Department, Institute of Psychiatry, Kings College London & Rethink.

Royal College of Psychiatrists (2015). *Carers and Confidentiality.* http://www.rcpsych.ac.uk (last accessed: 4.1.2016).

Savage, S. & Bailey, S. (2004). The impact of caring on caregivers' mental health: a review of the literature. *Australian Health Review* **27** (1), 103–109.

Schizophrenia Commission (2012). *Effective Interventions in Schizophrenia: the Economic Case.* http://mentalhealthpartnerships.com/resource/effective-interventions-in-schizophrenia-the-economic-case/ (last accessed: 24.10.2016)

Tarrier, N., Barrowclough, C., Vaughn, C., Bamrah, J., Porceddu, K., Watts, S. & Freeman, H. (1988). The community management of schizophrenia. a controlled trial of a behavioural intervention with families to reduce relapse. *British Journal of Psychiatry* **153** (October), 532–542.

Thompson, K. (1998). Early intervention services in daily family life: mothers' perceptions of 'ideal' versus 'actual' service provision. *Occupational Therapy International* **5** (3), 206–221.

Yeatts, Jr., H.W. (1997). *Simply Complicated: Understanding the Human Being.* http://www.threeleggeddragon.com (last accessed: 4.1.2016).

# Chapter 14

# Early intervention with psychosis: the occupational therapist's role

Jackie Parsonage

## Introduction

This chapter is written by an occupational therapist working with first episode psychosis, to provide real experience-based insights that help to further illustrate the role of the occupational therapist in this area. Reflecting a culture of evidence-based practice and the need to justify the added value of occupational therapy, where possible research, policy and relevant literature are included.

## Key points

- Early Intervention (EI) is an evidence-based health service model for the care and treatment of individuals suffering first episode.
- Occupational therapists can make a valuable contribution to the care provided by early intervention teams, as the philosophies of both are closely aligned.
- Early intervention services have a strong evidence base, in contrast to other mental health models, but more research into the added value of occupational therapy in this area is needed.

## Key terms

- Prodrome
- Duration of untreated psychosis (DUP)
- Recovery.

# What is early intervention?

Early intervention services are a specific and specialised mental health service that aims to support individuals during their first episode of psychosis and subsequent recovery. These services evolved from a belief that intervening in the early stages of psychosis could improve recovery to ordinary and meaningful lives. The pioneers of early intervention services even hoped to identify individuals in the prodromal stages of psychosis and prevent full psychosis developing. In practice, accurate early detection is improving through tools such as Comprehensive Assessment of At Risk Mental States (CAARMS), but remains difficult. As a result, EI services mostly focus on recovery following the first episode of acute psychosis rather than prodromal phases or at risk mental states.

# First episode psychosis

The onset of psychosis typically starts during a key stage of social and emotional development, typically between 14 and 35 years of age (Brown et al. 2003), but can start at any age. This is a significant period of transition for young people and is a time when they may be expecting to sit exams which affect further education choices and subsequent career options. Maturation is occurring at a very fast pace. At this stage of development individuals are transitioning from being children into adults (Chudleigh et al. 2011). There is an expectation of developing skills for more independent living and separation from the support given by parents. However, psychosis frequently disrupts this process of transition and can cause individuals to fall behind their peer groups and developmental milestones (Mackrell & Lavender 2004). They are subsequently further disadvantaged as they may encounter other political and social barriers to recovery (Harrop & Trower 2001).

## Box 14.1: Symptoms of the prodromal phase

- Reduced concentration and attention
- Reduced drive, motivation, anergia
- Depressed mood
- Deterioration in role functioning
- Sleep disturbance
- Anxiety
- Social withdrawal
- Suspiciousness
- Irritability.

# Prodrome

Prior to the onset of acute psychotic symptoms, there exists a period known as the prodromal phase (see Box 14.1). This phase is characterised by small and often subtle changes in an individual's mood and behaviour (Brunet & Birchwood 2010). Unfortunately these changes are not in themselves a clear predictor that an individual may develop psychosis, as many of the symptoms have parallels with behaviour associated with adolescent maturation (Brunet & Birchwood 2010). Following the prodromal stage comes the 'acute stage', sometimes referred to as the first onset of psychosis. Individuals may experience both positive and negative symptoms of psychosis at this stage. In one study, following up individuals after treatment found that 52 per cent recovered from symptoms but only 26 per cent recovered functionally (Wunderink et al. 2009). This is a finding regularly recorded in other relevant studies showing that functional recovery is consistently poorer than recovery from acute symptomology.

# Psychosis and the assessment of symptoms

Accurate assessment and understanding of psychosis is vital to the success of occupational therapy interventions. The following section is a brief guide to the important aspects of psychosis from an occupational therapist's point of view.

Firstly, 'psychosis' is a broad term used to describe a collection of mental health diagnoses involving a loss of contact with reality (Cardinal & Bullmore 2011). It may take the form of delusions and/or hallucinations without insight (Oxford University Press 1997). The term 'psychosis' includes schizophrenia, bipolar disorder, substance induced psychosis, schizo-affective disorder, and psychotic depression.

The nature of symptoms experienced by an individual can vary considerably from person to person. The specific combination of symptoms will have an impact on the way an individual's occupation is disrupted and consequently their experience of psychosis. For example, the individual who is experiencing paranoid delusions, and believes his communications are being bugged, may be unwilling to use a phone or the internet or go out in the community. Another may believe that he is a special messenger from God with a mission to fulfil, and consequently may be unwilling to engage in any activity that takes him away from his divine purpose. Yet another may believe she has special powers or can do anything, but may lack the capacity to make a real appraisal of her ability and try to engage in too many different occupations whilst being unable to do any of them to a sufficient level of competency.

Symptoms of psychosis are divided into two groups: positive and negative symptoms. According to Cardinal and Bullmore (2011) symptoms of psychosis include:

## Positive symptoms

**1.** Thought disorder: thought echo, thought insertion, withdrawal and thought broadcasting.

**2.** Hallucinations: these are vivid perceptions originating in the mind rather than being real; service users may describe hearing voices that give a running commentary on their behaviour, or individuals may see things that others cannot.

**3.** Delusions: beliefs that an individual has no reason to have, which are often culturally inappropriate, impossible or bizarre in nature. They may be of a persecutory nature.

**4.** Disorganised thinking and speech: a person's speech may be rapid, confusing, illogical and disjointed.

**5.** Catatonia: in more rare cases an individual might experience catatonia in which an individual may become mute, rigid or unresponsive.

## Negative symptoms

**1.** Apathy: loss of motivation to engage in activity or attend to basic self-care tasks.

**2.** Anhedonia: the loss of pleasure can affect all areas of life – even activities that were previously found to be enjoyable are no longer of interest.

**3.** Changes in affect: this is where emotions are blunted or incongruent. A person may say they are very happy but look sad or appear to make no emotional response where one would normally be expected.

**4.** Asociality: social withdrawal and decline in social performance.

**5.** Attention: difficulty with concentration.

**6.** Alogia: poverty of thought.

**7.** Avolition: this is where an individual may demonstrate a lack of planning, appearing more chaotic and disorganised than normally.

**8.** Anergia: reduced energy levels.

Recognition of the symptoms is important, but accurate assessment of the nature and pattern of each symptom, as it is experienced by the individual, is required for effective treatment planning (Bryant et al. 2014). To draw a parallel to physical healthcare, understanding the fine detail of psychotic symptoms is akin to knowing how long an individual can stand to perform a task or what range of movement they have. For example, it would be unhelpful for an individual who hears voices in response to anxiety in the work environment to be supported back to employment without ensuring an appropriately targeted care plan is in place to manage the specific situational stressors in the workplace.

Assessing the detail requires a sensitive but enquiring approach that asks questions about the nature and detail of the various psychotic symptoms. A therapist should expect the assessment to require a number of appointments to complete, as some individuals may need time to build trust and rapport before feeling safe enough to disclose distressing experiences.

The case study (Box 14.2) is an example of an individual suffering from a first episode of psychosis.

## Box 14.2: Case study 1

Kam is a 19-year-old man who was born in India and moved to the UK with his parents when he was seven years old. He did well in school and achieved his A-levels, consequently going to university. He started using cannabis when out with friends in his first year of university, and later also used it during assessment periods when he felt particularly anxious about achieving. He stated that he used it to help him relax. While he was in his second year of studies he started to struggle with sleep and he found it harder to concentrate on his studies, often staying up later to try to keep on top of his work. He became worried about passing end of year exams and received news that he had failed one of his assignments. Kam started to experience paranoia that his next door neighbours were part of a Russian conspiracy to harm him. He was arrested by the police for behaving bizarrely in a public place and later detained under Section 2 of the Mental Health Act (Ministry of Justice 1983/2007).

Kam laughed the first time he met the occupational therapist when asked about his experiences of becoming unwell. He struggled to remember some aspects of what had happened and the occupational therapist was able to prompt him using transcripts from his tribunal hearing. He could not believe that he had behaved in that way and repeated on a number of occasions that he was not the kind of person to behave like that.

Kam stated that he started to believe that the Russians must be altering his brain waves because he was struggling with his work and could not concentrate. He also talked about problems with the neighbours but frequently laughed, stating he had believed that they were spies from Russia. He said that at the time he had felt terrified. He described spending his time trying to work out what to do to protect himself, and how he began to think other people around him were also working for the Russians. At the time he did not know why they were focused on him.

**Questions**

- Which type of symptoms did Kam report experiencing?
- How would you describe his delusions?
- What were the possible triggers or early warning signs that Kam was becoming psychotic?

# The philosophy of early intervention services

The International Early Psychosis Association (IEPA) in partnership with the World Health Organisation (WHO) developed a consensus statement, detailing the vision and values for early intervention and recovery for young people experiencing psychosis for the first time (Bertolote & McGorry 2005). This statement provided a consensus view that guided service development and delivery. The five core values are: improving access to and engagement in care; promoting recovery of ordinary lives;

engaging and supporting families; raising community awareness; and teaching practitioners and community workers to provide more active care (see Box 14.3) (Bertolote & McGorry 2005). The philosophical standpoint of occupational therapy dovetails well with the ethos and values of early intervention services (Kupra *et al.* 2010, Lloyd *et al.* 2008).

## Box 14.3: Early Intervention Declaration jointly issued by the World Health Organisation and International Early Psychosis Association

**Values:**

- Respect of the right to recovery and social inclusion and support to the importance of personal, social, educational and employment outcomes.
- Respect of the strengths and qualities of young people with a psychosis, their families and communities, encouraging ordinary lives and expectations.
- Services that actively partner young people, their families and friends to place them at the centre of care and service delivery, at the same time sensitive to age, phase of illness, gender, sexuality and cultural background.
- Use of cost-effective interventions.
- Respect of the right for family and friends to participate and feel fully involved.

The importance of occupation to an individual's recovery and wellbeing is advocated by occupational therapists. The College of Occupational Therapists' own strategic vision for mental health stated that it considered occupational deprivation as a violation of human rights (COT 2006). The 2014 NICE guidelines for psychosis contain sections which correspond to the ethos of occupational therapy, i.e. offering support to regain occupation and employment, health promotion and psycho-education, peer support, and supporting carers. The aim is to promote Recovery, encourage the development of self-management, and prevent relapse (NICE 2014).

Occupational therapists are therefore well placed to contribute meaningfully to the occupational and functional recovery of individuals following the first onset of psychosis. The role of occupational therapists in early intervention services involves: 1) the specific assessment of how psychosis has impacted on the individual in all aspects of daily life; 2) the identification of barriers hindering a return to normal occupational activities; and 3) the creative, client-centred approach to goal setting and treatment that enables individuals to overcome barriers and return to valued occupations.

**Box 14.4: The Mental Health Policy Implementation Guideline (DoH 2001) recommendations**

- 5-year age entry criteria
- Specific interventions should be provided during the first three years following onset of psychosis
- Aim to reduce the duration of untreated psychosis to less than three months
- Maximum caseload ratio of one care coordinator to 15 clients
- For every 25,000 (depending on population characteristics), one team with:
  - total caseload 120 to 150
  - 1.5 whole time equivalent (wte)
  - other specialist staff to provide specific evidence-based interventions.

This chapter is written by occupational therapists working with first episode psychosis, to provide real experience-based insights that help to further illustrate the role of the occupational therapist in this area. Reflecting a culture of evidence-based practice and the need to justify the added value of occupational therapy, where possible research, policy and relevant literature are included.

# What do early intervention services look like?

Early detection service such as the Early Psychosis Prevention and Intervention Centre (EPPIC) (Australia), IRIS (http://www.iris-initiative.org.uk) (Birmingham) and OPUS (lonepetersen@mail.dk) (Denmark) have demonstrated success in their strategies. Further research has contributed to a supportive evidence base for the effectiveness of this approach.

In 2001 the UK Government released the policy implementation guide which identified that individuals experiencing their first onset of psychosis should have access to specialist treatment and intervention provided by specifically commissioned early intervention teams (DoH 2001). Despite this, it took over ten years to see services established across the UK.

The policy implementation guideline made recommendations for the key components of early intervention services and advocated a dedicated specialist team. Three models emerged from the recommendation (Dodgson & McGowan 2010). The three key early intervention service models are:

**1.** The stand-alone service model – seen as the gold standard model. The team consists of specialist staff working together from a centralised location.

**2.** The 'hub and spoke' model – a lower cost compromise on the stand-alone model. It consists of a small centralised core of professionals (management and expertise) who link in to smaller satellite services, often based within mental health teams, with one or two early intervention professionals delivering care.

**3.** The CMHT service model – one or two professionals identified to work with first episode psychosis within a larger mental health community team.

This led to wide variation across the UK with different health bodies commissioning different models of early intervention. In 2014 a new set of NICE guidelines was introduced with specific requirements of early intervention services including waiting time targets, and other time related treatment targets. It also made specific changes to the referral criteria. This has served to improve parity across services around core elements of the service provided.

# What does an early intervention team look like?

The early intervention approach is particularly multi-disciplinary. Staffing typically includes an administrator, a staff grade doctor, nurses, occupational therapists, a psychiatrist, a psychologist and social workers. Some services may also include an activity coordinator, an employment specialist, a family therapist, and/or a research assistant/assistant psychologist. In more creative approaches to service provision, students and volunteers may also be recruited to the staff team.

It is common practice for the nurses, occupational therapists and social workers to work as care coordinators. In some areas there are specific occupational therapy posts, but this is not the norm across the UK. Often, occupational therapists have a mixed role, as both care coordinator and occupational therapist, and have to juggle the sometimes conflicting demands of this dual role.

# What might the care pathway look like?
## Referrals

In earlier aspirational models of early intervention there was a focus on working with those with at risk mental states and those experiencing a prodromal episode of psychosis. Referrals were taken from youth centres, schools and youth justice teams. Consequently such services engaged in significant community outreach work. However, the evidence for prevention of psychosis at prodromal stage remains inconclusive and many services are not commissioned to do this work (Marshal & Rathbone 2011).

Referral of those experiencing first episode of psychosis may come from GPs, A&E departments, children and adolescent services, psychiatric home treatment teams or other mental health services. Referrals are usually screened for suitability against the service criteria. Typical early intervention service referral criteria for the last ten years included four criteria: individuals should be between 14 and 35 years of age; should be experiencing a first episode of psychosis; should not have received mental health treatment for psychosis previously; should live within a defined locality with a local GP. Early intervention services have now been asked to accept all first episodes of psychosis irrespective of age, following recent NICE guideline changes. In addition to this, all referrals meeting the suitability criteria for EI services must be assessed and treatment initiated within a 14-day window.

# Assessment

Following referral it is usual for an initial assessment to be conducted by one or two of the qualified members of the team. This assessment is usually about establishing the match between the individual's needs and the service criteria, but is also frequently the start of the engagement process (see Box 14.5 for areas covered in the assessment). In many cases, service users may be too unwell to cope with completing more comprehensive assessments such as adult health and social needs assessments, those carried out by occupational therapists or similar more detailed psycho-social-related assessment. Consequently assessment is an ongoing process that continues after an individual is accepted by an early intervention team.

## Box 14.5: What should an assessment include?

1. What signs and symptoms of psychosis are being experienced?

2. What is the history of their presentation? – with particular reference to potential trigger events, and establishing the length of the prodromal phase.

3. What is the person's insight and understanding of their experience of their illness?

4. Is there a history of drug or alcohol misuse?

5. What is the current housing situation and what impact does that have on mental health and wellbeing?

6. What is the social situation? – including current and historical nature, and quality of friendships.

7. What is the education and employment history?

8. What family support is available to the individual experiencing psychosis? – include family history of psychosis, understanding of mental illness.

9. What are the risks this person poses to themselves and others?

10. Is there sufficient capacity to engage with a treatment plan?

# Treatment

Early intervention teams aim to work intensively in partnership with service users to improve recovery, support a more rapid remission of symptoms, lower distress and ease the burden on the family. They also aim to reduce the risk of severe adverse events and the consequence on life, such as criminal record, violence, self-harm or abuse (NICE 2014). The NICE guidelines for psychosis identify an evidence-based timeframe for specific interventions within the first three years following the onset. Professionals working in this area should ensure that they have read this document and take this into consideration when working in partnership with individuals.Partnership working enables the professional to work with the individual to identify an individualised treatment package that meets his/her specific and individualised needs. The various components that may be included in a treatment package are:

1. **Psycho-social education** – to improve an individual's understanding of the experience of psychosis, including promotion of understanding of potential triggers and learning of self-protection strategies to prevent further relapse. Delivery methods may include individual, groupwork or a combination of the two.

2. **Activity groups** – focused on meeting with peers and developing peer support. Activities may be focused on leisure or social interests. Groups focus on wellbeing, not on diagnosis. Examples include: 'bend it without breaking' – the sessions include discussion about issues such as gratitude, hope, zest, activity and exercises; they last for two hours, run weekly, are manual-based. Other examples include: pottery groups run at a local arts centre, an 'act group' based on mindfulness.

3. **Skills-based groups** – focusing specifically on skill development such as a work skills group or preparing to live alone groups (focused on life skills such as budgeting, avoiding isolation etc.).

4. **Physical health interventions** – some medications are associated with weight gain and other effects on physical health. Interventions must now include regular health monitoring and may also include health promotion, tailored exercise advice from a sports technician, sports focused groups, use of personalised budget funding to pay for gym memberships. Physical health is now a key target area for early intervention services (NICE 2014).

5. **Employment and educational support** – For the young people accessing early intervention services this is commonly their area of highest priority. The evidence-based Individual Placement and Support (IPS) model may be used to get those who are job-ready back into employment (Bond 2004). Tailored support may still be required to plan a phased return to educational or work settings.

6. **Talking therapies** – The NICE guidelines for first episode psychosis (2014) recognise the importance of Cognitive Behavioural Therapy (CBT) and access to talking therapies. Specifically, all individuals should be offered 10 sessions of psychosis-specific CBT starting in the first three months of referral to the service. There has been a growing recognition that individuals may need support to deal with past trauma and/or the trauma caused by experiencing psychosis. There is also evidence to suggest that CBT can help with the management of positive symptoms such as psychosis, delusions and hearing voices.

7. **Housing support** – some people may need housing advice and signposting to appropriate services. In a small number of cases service users may need additional support to access housing services. This is particularly prevalent in areas of housing shortages such as London.

8. **Family support** – all EI services must now provide up to 10 sessions of family intervention to families of individuals experiencing psychosis for the first time. Some services may have a family therapist or specific family worker, otherwise groups or individual support from care coordinators may be offered to meet this target. Additionally, carers should be offered a carers assessment and may be signposted to local branches of national carer support groups such as Rethink.

9.  **Medication and mental health review** – regular meeting with a psychiatrist to review mental state and prescription of medication. This should include providing information about medication and managing issues regarding compliance.

10. **Relapse prevention** – individuals should be supported to understand their own relapse signatures, and be supported to develop a relapse prevention plan. This can also include advanced decisions about their care should they become unwell.

11. **Care coordination** – to provide individual support and direction during the recovery process.

12. **Occupational therapy** – focusing on occupational aspects of recovery, including regaining meaningful occupation.

## Discharge

The length of time a person may receive input from early intervention services, before discharge to GP or transfer to alternative mental health services, varies and is dependent on local commissioning arrangements. Typically, services offer between two and five years. The general consensus is that five years is regarded as the ideal, as research suggests that five years is the critical period for relapse following first episode. Therefore, it has been argued that a longer period of support to prevent relapse will reduce the likelihood of further relapse in the future. The recent NICE guidelines suggest that those who have not yet made a full recovery should be offered the opportunity to continue work with early intervention services (NICE 2014).

The prospect of discharge can often be a very difficult and unsettling time for service users. General mental health teams and GPs often have less time than the more resourced early intervention teams. As a consequence, individuals familiar with early intervention services may struggle to adjust to a decreased level of support. It is essential that individuals are prepared in advance of discharge to avoid relapse. Discharge planning/preparation groups are an ideal way of doing this and an area where occupational therapists can contribute advantageously.

# In what way does the role of occupational therapy fit with early intervention?

As an emerging role, there is currently little peer reviewed published literature on the role of occupational therapy in this area. Therefore, this section is based on a limited number of studies, and interviews with occupational therapists working in this field.

## Psychosis, development and occupation

Those working in the field of early intervention for psychosis have suggested that recovery from psychosis should be considered from a developmental context. This is to avoid individuals missing out on normal developmental steps (Brown 2011). With this in mind, the fact that psychosis usually occurs during a critical transition period of social and physiological development is vitally important, as the individual is transitioning from childhood to adult roles (Brown 2011).

From a neuroscience perspective, there is growing evidence of physiological, biological and behavioural changes associated with continuing brain development through adolescence and late adolescence (Spear 2010).

Using a social perspective, Erikson (1995) described the ages 14 to 20 years as about 'identity', where the individual is forming an integrated self-concept, and a coherent set of values and beliefs. The stage after identity is referred to as 'intimacy', occurring between 20 and 35 years of age. This stage is about establishing close intimate relationships. More recent theories of adolescence suggest that the transition to adulthood is a dynamic and changing process, subject to its cultural context, where individuals must function effectively in order to prepare them for adult roles and responsibilities (Coleman 2011). Illness during this stage of development can have a detrimental impact.

In practice you will commonly find that individuals presenting with first episode psychosis were just starting the first year of university, starting to develop a trade or working in their first jobs. They are at a stage where their career and future work is a significant concern for them. Unruh (2004) similarly concluded that this stage is about constructing an occupational identity based on achieving meaningful work. At the younger end of the spectrum it is common to see individuals who are working towards completing their GCSEs or A-levels. There is a strong awareness of their peer groups and wanting to be engaged in age-appropriate activities.

During the acute phases of psychosis, individuals are often struggling with distressing and unpleasant symptoms that make it difficult or impossible to engage in normal and familiar occupations. In later stages when symptoms are in remission, individuals may feel disorientated and confused by their experience. In more recent years there has been increasing recognition that the experience of becoming psychotic itself can be very traumatic and difficult for individuals to come to terms with (NICE 2014). Often they struggle to understand the experiences that they have been through and may be concerned about how they will be regarded by others, because of having suffered a mental health problem (Makdisi et al. 2013). Some individuals may be very apprehensive about returning to previous activities, especially if they are associated with becoming unwell, for example, when they are experiencing high levels of stress at school or work. In addition, the negative symptoms of psychosis also impact on occupation and recovery in general.

## Psychosis and occupation from the individual's perspective

To understand the role for occupational therapists in first episode psychosis we must first understand the impact on occupation from the individual's perspective. Research into the experience of psychosis and occupation from the occupational therapist's point of view is very limited. Roy et al. (2009) argued that understanding how occupation is affected by the onset of psychosis is vital for occupational therapists.

The limited number of studies exploring individuals' perspectives and experience of psychosis suggest a complex picture of multiple interacting factors. First there is a general recognition that psychosis is an assault on an individual's identity (Makdisi *et al.* 2013), and is a crisis (Kupra *et al.* 2010) that significantly affects everyday life (Brown 2011). Secondly there are a large number of things that can be helpful or unhelpful when trying to regain occupation after the initial onset of psychosis (Cook & Chambers 2009). Consequently, a tailored and individualised approach is required (Hitch *et al.* 2013), that recognises and accurately assesses the impact of specific internal and external factors on the individual's occupation.

External factors include relationships, current and past activity, finance, medication, physical environment (Cook & Chambers 2009). In contrast, internal factors include resilience, experience of trauma, spirituality, fear, physical health difficulties and personal coping skills (Cook & Chambers 2009). A recent meta-synthesis of relevant qualitative research summarises these various factors into four themes: emotions, identity, health and wellbeing, and relationships (Hitch *et al.* 2013).

The author's master's research study (Parsonage 2012) found three key phases to regaining meaningful occupation after the initial onset of psychosis. Transition from one phase to another was impacted by the individual's internal and external worlds. The three phases were named the 'unknown self' or crisis phase, 'locating the self' or adapting phase and finally the 'new self' or regeneration phase. In each of these phases the personal meaning of occupation underwent change as part of the process to recovery. There was a clear difference in what individuals needed at each stage of the recovery process to regain occupation.

The findings of these studies provide a clear idea of the role occupational therapy can have in supporting occupational recovery. These findings could be summarised as:

**1.** Adopt a developmental framework when planning to address occupational needs (Brown 2011).

**2.** Remember to adopt a client-centred approach which gives specific attention to support around difficult occupational transitions (Brown 2011). Ensure that current capabilities are appropriately matched to the specific demands of the activity; therefore appropriate goal setting and planning is required (Kupra *et al.* 2010) as is attention to energy levels (Roy *et al.* 2009).

**3.** Support individuals' efforts to engage in productive roles (Brown 2011). Career-related activity is highly significant for this population. Academic rehabilitations as well as the more well known vocational rehabilitations should be offered. This can include support to return to educational settings such as university, liaising with educational institutions, teaching study skills or encouraging buddying (Roy *et al.* 2009).

**4.** Recognise the importance and complexity of relationships in recovery of occupation. Aim to create a good therapeutic relationship and provide interventions that support positive social interaction. This can take the form of support around issues of disclosure, dealing with stigma, teaching self-advocacy, and providing social skills training (Kupra *et al.* 2010, Roy *et al.* 2009). It might also involve anxiety management, peer support or social-based groups to regain confidence and reduce isolation in the early stages after the onset of psychosis (Bryant *et al.* 2012).

**5.** Promoting and teaching the principles of lifestyle balance (Kupra *et al.* 2010). Specific emphasis should be given to support an individual to make their own interpretation of what lifestyle balance means for them in the different phases of their recovery.

**6.** Psychoeducation can help individuals process their emotional experience related to psychosis and increase an individual's sense of self-advocacy and self-management (Hitch *et al.* 2013, Kupra *et al.* 2010). This can include education about psychosis itself, stress management, how to cope with voices, and information about medication etc. Occupational therapists do not have exclusivity in this area and it is important to recognise when to involve the multi-disciplinary team.

**7.** Establish appropriate partnerships in the community, e.g. with local universities or services.

**8.** Assessment of the physical environment including functional Activities of Daily Living (ADL) assessments (Roy *et al.* 2009).

## Juggling the role of care coordinator and the role of occupational therapist

The role of occupational therapists in this field frequently, but not exclusively, involves generic tasks associated with care coordination. The philosophy underpinning the practice of occupational therapy can easily be adapted to the role of care coordinator with some success. Levels of specific occupational therapy assessment and intervention will depend on local contract agreements for the post. In some cases there may be a defined split between care coordination and occupational therapy. It is best to establish this early when joining a team as it can be more challenging to change the role once expectations are established.

## Using models in early intervention services

Generally speaking, any model that is recognised for use in a mental health setting is appropriate. So the Canadian Occupational Performance Measure (COPM) (Law *et al.* 2014), Kawa River Model (Iwama 2006), the Model of Creative Ability (MOCA) (Du Toit 2009), and the Model of Human Occupation (MOHO) (Kielhofner 2002) are appropriate to use.

The author's own experience is largely with the model of human occupation. The Model of Human Occupation Screening Tool (MOHOST) (Parkinson *et al.* 2006), the Worker Role Interview tool (WRI) (Braveman *et al.* 2005) and the Occupational Self-Assessment tool (OSA) (Baron *et al.* 2006) have seemed most useful. The MOHOST is an overall assessment tool that supports the occupational therapist to assess and identify the strengths and weaknesses an individual has in various areas that impact on engagement in occupation (Kielhofner 2002). Vocational issues are particularly relevant to this group of service users, making the worker role interview a useful tool when supporting individuals to return to the working environment. An important limitation experienced with this tool is that the questions are not as relevant to those who have not worked before. In contrast, the occupational self-assessment tool is particularly useful for supporting a collaborative approach to goal planning.

The model of creative ability is well known and frequently used in mental health services in South Africa, and recognition is growing in the UK. Application of this model in a community-based early intervention service is currently limited, as the levels within the model itself are not sufficiently sensitive. The exception to this is where learning disabilities and psychosis are experienced by the individual. In such cases the model can be very useful in informing intervention planning and appropriate activity analysis. The remaining two models have not been used by the author in the context of early intervention.

## Other skills the job requires

**Patience**: occupational therapists will need to exercise patience. Each individual will take time to adjust and adapt to the experience of becoming psychotic and may be reluctant to engage with planned interventions. Identifying the need does not necessarily mean the individual is ready to deal with the issue presented or indeed that it is a priority for them. They will need patient coaching and support to address personal challenges.

**Advanced communication skills**: psychosis is known to distort an individual's sense of reality. Individuals can experience intense beliefs and hallucinations during the acute phases and these can feel very real and frightening. Effective communication skills are required to reassure and to engage the service user in his/her own recovery, for example: effective communication with an individual in the acute phases of illness can mean the difference between the person's agreement to go to hospital informally rather than through use of the Mental Health Act (1983/2007).

**Flexibility**: occupational therapists should be able to adapt, as the needs of this client group are often unpredictable. You need to be able to respond in times of crisis or need.

**Perseverance**: first episode psychosis can be a challenging area. Individuals may be in denial about their illness, and not take on board advice given, and inevitably relapse. It is vitally important that staff remain supportive in spite of opposition and help service users to learn to manage their illness. Additionally, many early intervention teams have numerous systems and processes that consume work time.

**Ability to engage with families**: occupational therapists need to be able to engage quickly and effectively with members of the families of those suffering psychosis. They should be honest about what can be offered, taking care not to raise expectations that cannot be delivered. Information giving should be timely and delivered with care to avoid overloading families. Family interventions should be led by the nature of the family, e.g. some families may prefer a more humorous approach, others may require a more serious factual approach and still others may require a more listening approach with only occasional information and advice given. Be cautious with families who are experiencing exhaustion with services after a long struggle trying to get help for their child. Be mindful that some families may have experienced intense disruption from the illness and from emergency services, such as home treatment teams, prior to your involvement. Be alert to the fact that you may be labelled and receive anger from family members as they come to terms with the trauma they and their loved one have just been through. It is common that people look for other people to blame for the onset of psychosis or indeed to deny that a person was ever psychotic. It is often helpful to persevere with families, offering shorter visits to start with and longer visits later. Make every effort to build trust and adapt communication style to one that works for the family. Carer assessments should be completed and in some cases the use of a family therapist or family behaviour skills may be appropriate.

**Self-management**: is vital to performing well in this area and to reduce stress associated with working in this field. Ensuring you take an organised approach, such as keeping lists, and identifying daily priorities, will help to manage stress and keep on top of increasing workloads. Regular supervision is important to review caseload and manage workload. Support can also be found informally from the multi-disciplinary team.

# Case studies

Several case studies (Boxes 14.6, 14.7, 14.8, 14.9) are provided to illustrate the way in which occupational therapists in early intervention services may provide interventions to promote occupational recovery in and alongside their care coordinator role.

## Box 14.6: Case study 2

**Background**: Alice is a 17-year-old girl, who became psychotic a year after leaving school. She was badly bullied at school and left without any qualifications. She was referred to the occupational therapist on the team for anxiety management and to improve independence and add structure to her daily routine.

At the time of referral Alice was compliant with taking 1000mg divalproex sodium (Depakote) BD and 500mg quetiapine (Seroquel) OD and was cyclothymic. Alice had no friends and was too anxious to initiate relationships with others her own age. Functionally she relied heavily on her mother and was unwilling to leave the house without her mother. Her one activity outside the house was a volunteering role, which her mother drove her to and from once a week.

### Occupational therapy intervention:

● Anxiety management therapy and practical sessions, looking at thoughts, emotions and behaviours. Providing education, distraction techniques, relaxation and breathing techniques, thought records, recognising negative thinking, how to risk assess accurately, developing positive thinking and behavioural experiments.

## Graded exposure

- Family work – exploring roles within the home
- Looking at age-appropriate behaviour
- Role playing scenarios
- Functional assessments – looking at her ability to identify risk and act accordingly
- Independent travel
- Extra qualifications.

**Outcomes**: Alice started to work part-time and volunteered twice a week. She is now able to organise her own weekly timetable, gets herself up and organises her own meals. She is able to utilise public transport independently and develop positive friendships with people of the same age, including finding a boyfriend. Alice now cooks for herself and administers her own medication. She is also involved in a mentor scheme and looking at gaining qualifications.

## Box 14.7: Case study 3

**Background**: Alexandreina was a 23-year-old Romanian woman. She had been in the UK for a number of years but was not entitled to benefits. Prior to becoming unwell with psychosis she had been made redundant from the food industry and it became evident during assessment that her work life balance had been poor. Losing her work role was particularly difficult for her as she valued the work role highly, needed to help pay the rent and also supported family back in Romania. She carried a strong sense of responsibility for her alcoholic mother, her father and the two children her sister had abandoned. Recently married, Alexandreina was also experiencing marital conflict at the time of her psychosis and was also very isolated from other social support. There was also a history of psychosis in the family.

Alexandreina became psychotic very quickly and did not experience a period of noticeable decline in functioning prior to acute symptoms. She experienced terrifying visual and auditory hallucinations. She described her experience as like that of living in a horror film. She stated that the house looked as if it had been burned down around her; consequently she felt anxious when she returned home. Her husband was very supportive after her admission but at times struggled with the caring role as he was also struggling with personal issues. She was care coordinated by an occupational therapist and it was clear, following the assessment, that she wanted to return to work.

### Generic interventions:

**1.** Psychoeducation – Alexandreina was supported to develop an understanding of psychosis and how stress had contributed to the onset of psychosis. Focus was given to developing her personal relapse signature and prevention plan.

**2.** Opportunities to talk through experiences provided openings to deal with the trauma of her psychotic experiences.

**3.** A carer assessment was completed with the husband and, as a result, supportive counselling was introduced.

**4.** Family therapy was offered.

### Occupational therapy interventions:

**1.** Stress management education

**2.** Teaching relaxation and distraction techniques to help her manage anxiety to feel safe in her home

**3.** Support to build up readiness to return to work. This included goal planning and support with developing career aspirations

**4.** Discussed occupational balance – to help her adopt a better work/life balance and avoid relapse

**5.** Assertiveness training was also incorporated to help her avoid saying yes when leaned on to do extra work

**6.** Supported the development and acquisition of new hobbies and interests, including gardening and craft work, to help her reduce stress

**7.** Discussed options where she could meet other Romanian women and other social activities to combat isolation.

**Outcomes**: Alexandreina was able to explore her future career and completed an NVQ as a teaching assistant, and volunteered as a leader for after-school activities clubs. She got a job in a school kitchen and later was promoted. She eventually decided that although she enjoyed helping with the after-school clubs she would rather work in catering. She was also able to gain confidence in saying no when people took advantage of her willingness to help others. This enabled her to establish more personally helpful boundaries and keep her stress levels manageable. She also linked into a new church with a good understanding of mental illness and felt more connected to her local community. Additionally she developed new hobbies and interests that she looked forward to when she came home, including painting and working on an allotment.

## Box 14.8: Case study 4

**Background**: Mark is a 19-year-old man who became unwell during his first year at university. He suffered significantly through hearing voices and even with medication he continued to experience distressing voices that criticised him and told him he was worthless. He frequently self-harmed in response to the voices. At times he also thought about suicide. Over time Mark became aware that his voices were worst when he felt low in mood or particularly stressed. Mark was referred to occupational therapy to support him with his exam resit.

### Occupational therapy intervention:
Took a history of his preparation for his exams and how he coped with stress. Helped him to plan his revision strategy that compensated for poor concentration levels and incorporate protective behaviours to avoid his becoming over-tired and low in mood. Supported him to develop hobbies and other interests to improve lifestyle balance. Education around mood management. Supported him to develop a Recovery and wellbeing plan to enable him to decide how he would manage his mood and how he would be able to cope with the voices when he returned to college full-time.

**Outcome**: Mark reported that he felt calmer when he took his resit exam. He also reported that his friends had noticed that he seemed more relaxed and happy since making his lifestyle changes. He felt more confident about how he would manage his illness following his return to university.

## Box 14.9: Case study 5

**Background**: John is a 17-year-old living at home with his alcoholic mother. He is estranged from his father. John experiences the relationship with his mother as highly critical and regularly gets into arguments with her. At times when he is acutely psychotic these arguments have become highly confrontational and the police have been called on several occasions by the neighbours.

He became psychotic shortly after finishing school with poor grades, and has never worked. He regularly went to the gym with his friends and was on job seekers allowance. John had a long history of drug and alcohol misuse and when he became psychotic he heard voices telling him to harm his mother. He wanted to live away from home as he found it difficult to live with his mother and his voices were worse when he was at home. Consequently, he spent little time at home and wandered the street for long periods during the day.

**Occupational therapy intervention:**

1. Occupational functional assessment – to identify what level of supported accommodation would be most appropriate
2. Education on healthy living and lifestyle balance, e.g. alcohol and drug misuse, focus on encouraging leisure interest and encouraging exploration of work aspirations
3. Support around disclosure to friends.

**Generic intervention:**

1. Completion of supported housing application, and submission to housing panel
2. Support with practicalities of moving in and leasing, with support services
3. Offered referral to drug and alcohol services
4. Family therapy interventions
5. Carers assessment.

**Outcomes**: John was settled in appropriate accommodation that helped him to develop skills for independent living. He hopes to go on and have a flat of his own. John has reduced his drug and alcohol consumption: he continues to use at times but is aware of his warning signs and personal limits, and he recognises the need to take medication to minimise the risk of relapse. His relationship with family has improved but remains difficult. John has renewed contact with friends. He goes out regularly and attends the gym. He is considering part-time work of a manual nature such as construction or removals.

# Other essential information

## Managing risk

The management of risk is a vitally important aspect of working in mental health. It should be considered at all times when planning and working with individuals with mental health difficulties. While the reality is that most clients are more likely to be a threat to themselves than anyone else, there is a small group who present a risk to others. The nature of psychosis is that for those suffering, their reality and comprehension of the world is altered. To look at it a different way, if we believed that the people we saw around us were trying to kill us, we would react to protect ourselves in whatever way we could. In the experience of psychosis, when trusted senses inform one's world view and tell you there is a threat, you will react to protect yourself.

This is why an understanding of the nature of the delusions and hallucinations is important information to gather from a service user. It is one of the best ways of understanding the risk a client may present. It is also an effective way of understanding the barriers which may affect the individual when engaging in specific occupations, and indeed his/her engagement with you as a therapist.

When considering risk, it is important to think about fixed risk factors and fluid risk factors. Fixed factors relate to an individual's history and unchangeable facts such as gender, diagnosis, previous risk events. In early intervention for psychosis, young men have the highest risk of suicide. Fluid factors are factors which vary from time to time such as mental state, feelings of hopelessness or periods of increased stress.

First episode psychosis is challenging as the risks are unknown and there is no history to help assess risk. Therefore, lone workers should give careful consideration to risk management when planning to meet people in the community.

# The legal side

An occupational therapist's main concern lies within occupation but an awareness of the legal aspects that influence care is essential when working in early intervention and indeed any mental health setting. It is essential to understand the key components of the Mental Health Act (Ministry of Justice 1983/2007), the Mental Capacity Act (Ministry of Justice 2005), and the Deprivation of Liberty Safeguards (Ministry of Justice 2008).

## Mental Capacity Act (2005)

When devising a treatment, it is vital to assess the individual's capacity to consent (Mental Capacity Act 2005). The Mental Capacity Act (2005) is clear that for each decision made, a separate capacity assessment is required. This is because an individual may have the capacity to make decisions in some areas of their life but find it more difficult in others. Decisions being capacity assessed are also time-specific as capacity can fluctuate. The assumption is that someone has capacity unless proved otherwise. The key parts of an assessment are:

1. Do they have an impairment of a nature that may affect capacity?

2. Can they take on board information?

3. Can they retain information?

4. Can they weigh up the pros and cons of the decision?

5. Can they communicate their decision?

If they are deemed not to have capacity then treatment is decided by the multi-disciplinary team taking a best interest decision.

In some cases where a person lacks capacity and is treated for psychosis under best interest on a ward, a Mental Health Act (1983/2007) assessment may be sought. Where a person lacks capacity but is prevented from leaving a specific care home or unit (and they are not subject to detention under the Mental Health Act 1983/2007) then a Deprivation of Liberty Safeguards' Best Interests Assessment should be requested, having made an urgent authorisation to detain them under the Mental Capacity Act (2005). Failure to do so is a breach of human rights and is unlawful.

## Mental Health Act (1983/2007)

The Mental Health Act (1983/2007) enables people to be detained against their will for their protection or the protection of the public. It takes into account the nature and degree of their presentation. The most commonly used parts of the act are: Section 2 which gives 28 days for assessment, and Section 3 which is for treatment for up to six months with annual reviews thereafter. Occupational therapists acting as care coordinators will be required to write social circumstances reports for tribunals and hospital manager hearings; they may also be called on to provide a 'second opinion'.

## How to communicate with individuals about their delusions and experience of being psychotic

First and most importantly, don't be afraid of talking to people who have psychosis. People experiencing psychosis mostly want to be listened to just as much as any other individual does. They also want and need to be understood and be shown empathy. Good communication skills are the basis of developing a good rapport with people who have psychosis.

It is worth remembering that those who are acutely psychotic for the first time are undergoing an experience as traumatic and as potentially life changing as a car crash. One lady once described her experience of being psychotic as like 'living in a horror movie'. The experience of being detained under the Mental Health Act (1983/2007), or admitted to hospital, can be equally distressing and traumatic especially if you are feeling confused, disorientated or that your life is threatened.

It is important to remember that when something happens to us that we have never experienced we want to understand what has happened. We do this by trying to put together the evidence as we see it and draw conclusions as a result. If you listen to or read narratives from those with psychosis you will frequently come across the desire to understand their experiences and be understood. Many of those experiencing psychosis want to understand what is happening even when they are still acutely psychotic. This is why working with individuals as soon as possible following the psychotic episode is important. Helping an individual to understand what is happening can reduce anxiety and aid recovery. In the author's experience, once a delusion has been established for some time, it can be harder to challenge the conclusions drawn.

One woman who had experienced psychosis shared how difficult it is to know whether you can trust the reality you are experiencing. What she meant was that she understood, now that she was well, that she had been psychotic; but during the period of psychosis all her senses and ways of understanding the world had felt just as real to her. She sought reassurance as to what was actually real. It is important to remember that delusions and hallucinations feel real to those experiencing them, and equally important to validate the subjective experience of the individual but not to collude with it because that is what they are experiencing. For example, see Box 14.10.

## Box 14.10: Case study 6

Ruby believed that she was a victim of some conspiracy, that she had been arrested by the police wrongfully and victimised. She strongly believed that she did not have a mental illness and did not believe that she should be in hospital. What was evident from listening to her explain what had happened to her was that she had been very frightened by the whole episode and found it traumatic. The trauma of her experience was acknowledged and this helped to establish rapport. We agreed to talk about her experience in terms of a trauma and its impact on her life, rather than as a mental illness. This opened the door for a later explanation about psychosis and how that alters perception. It also prevented unnecessary barriers which might block engagement, by enabling communication which validated her experience.

## Planned approach

The approach to someone with any mental illness can have a significant impact on the outcome of that meeting. The first approach can be improved by clear introductions, explaining the purpose of the meeting and asking for permission from the service user to continue with the meeting. The Motivational Interviewing (MI) approach emphasises the importance of asking for permission. This means the individual is empowered to say no if they do not want to talk about something or are not ready to meet. Being sensitive about the timing of the meeting can also be important; also, where possible, giving the individual some choice over the time and venue of meetings.

## Warnings

Caution is required when individuals are acutely unwell. It is important to be mindful of how long it is appropriate to stay talking with someone when they are unwell, as talking can be stimulating and tiring for them. Being asked lots of questions, especially if you have already been asked them by three other people that morning, can also be frustrating and tiring. One should be cautious when addressing areas that may be particularly sensitive, especially if you do not feel confident about handling information that may be difficult.

It is also important to be aware that for some people the experience of becoming psychotic is a positive one. Some people describe gaining comfort from the voices they hear, especially if they feel lonely; others enjoy the energy levels and feelings of power associated with mania, and may find coming down from a 'high' very difficult indeed. There are also those who describe being psychotic as like being on a drug trip. This is why it is so important to grasp the individual's own narrative and the specific effects of their own psychosis.

# Useful resources

- Centre for Mental Health: an independent national mental health charity aiming to inspire hope, opportunity and a fair chance in life for people of all ages living with or at risk of mental ill health: http://www.centreformentalhealth.org.uk.

- IRIS: A national website which provides knowledge of resources about early intervention in psychosis, in particular to front line services: http://www.iris-initiative.org.uk/

- Mental Health Matters: A mental health charity offering services, plus support and information about local services, organisations, news and resources: http://www.mentalhealthmatters.com

- Mind: A mental health charity with many useful resources: http://www.mind.org.uk

- Orygen: The national centre for excellence in youth mental health: http://orygen.org.au

- Rethink Mental Illness: A charity that supports those with mental health concerns and seeks to challenge stigma: http://www.rethink.org

# References

Baron, K., Kielhofner, G., Iyenger, A., Goldhammer, V. & Wolenski, J. (2006). *Occupational Self Assessment (OSA), Version 2.2.* Chicago: University of Illinois.

Bertolote, J. & McGorry, P. (2005). Early intervention and recovery for young people with early psychosis: consensus statement (on behalf of the World Health Organization and the International Early Psychosis Association). *British Journal of Psychiatry* 187 (Suppl 48) 116–119.

Bond, G. (2004). Supported employment: evidence for an evidence-based practice. *Psychiatric Rehabilitation Journal*, 27 (4), 345–359.

Braveman, B., Robson, M., Velozo, C., Kielhofner, G., FIsher, G., Forsyth, K. & Kerschbaum, J. (2005). *Worker Role Interview (WRI), Version 10.0.* Chicago: University of Illinois.

Brown, J. (2011). Talking about life after early psychosis: the impact on occupational performance. *Canadian Journal of Occupational Therapy,* 78 (3), 156–163.

Brown, M., McGowan, S., Powell, R. & Johnson, K. (2003). *A Window of Opportunity: a Practical Guide for Developing Early Intervention in Psychosis Services.* London: The Sainsbury Centre for Mental Health.

Brunet, K. & Birchwood, M. (2010). 'Duration of untreated psychosis and pathways to care' in *Promoting recovery in early psychosis*, eds. P. French, J. Smith, D. Shiers, M. Reed and M. Rayne. UK: Wiley-Blackwell.

Bryant, W., Fieldhouse, J. & Bannigan, K. (eds) (2014). *Creek's Occupational Therapy and Mental Health*, 5th edn. London: Churchill Livingstone Elsevier.

Bryant, W., Parsonage, J., Tibbs, A., Andrews, C., Clark, J. & Franco, L. (2012). Meeting in the mist: key considerations in a collaborative research partnership with people with menal health issues. *The Work Journal of Prevention, Assessment & Rehabilitation*, 43 (1), 23–31.

Cardinal, R. & Bullmore, E. (2011). *The Diagnosis of Psychosis.* Cambridge: Cambridge University Press.

Chudleigh, C., Naismith, S., Blaszczynski, A., Hermens, D., Redoblado-Hodge, A. & Hickie, I. (2011). How does social functioning in the early stages of psychosis relate to depression and social anxiety? *Early Intervention in Psychiatry* 5 (3), 224–232.

Coleman, J. (2011). *The Nature of Adolescence,* 4th edn. London: Routledge.

College of Occupational Therapists (2006). *Recovering Ordinary Lives: the Strategy for Occupational Therapy in Mental Health Services 2007–2017.* London: COT.

Cook, S. & Chambers, E. (2009). What hinders people with psychotic conditions doing what they want in their daily lives. *British Journal of Occupational Therapy* 72 (6), 238–248.

Department of Health (2001). *The Mental Health Policy Implementation Guide.* DoH: TSO.

Dodgson, G. & McGowan, S. (2010). 'Early intervention service models' in *Promoting Recovery in Early Psychosis,* eds. P. French, J. Smith, D. Shiers, M. Reed and M. Rayne. UK: Wiley-Blackwell.

Du Toit, V. (2009). *Patient Volition and Action in Occupational Therapy* 4th edn. Pretoria: Vona & Marie Du Toit Foundation.

Erikson, E. (1995). *Childhood and Society,* 2nd edn. London: Vintage Books.

Harrop, C. & Trower, P. (2001). Why does schizophrenia develop at late adolescence? *Clinical Psychology Review* **21** (2), 241–265.

Hitch, D., Genevieve, P. & Stagnitti, K. (2013). Engagement in activities and occupations by people who have experienced psychosis: a metasynthesis of lived experience. *British Journal of Occupational Therapy* **76** (2), 77–85.

Iwama, M.K. (2006). T*he Kawa Model: Culturally Relevant Occupational Therapy.* London: Churchill Livingstone, Elsevier.

Kielhofner, G. (2002). *Model of Human Occupation: Theory and Application*, 3rd edn. Baltimore, USA: Lippincott Williams and Young.

Kupra, T., Woodside, H. & Pocock, K. (2010). Activity and social participation in the period following first episode psychosis and implications for occupational therapy. *British Journal of Occupational Therapy* **73** (1), 13–20.

Law, M., Baptiste, S., Carswell, A., McColl, M.A., Polatajko, H. & Pollock, N. (2014). *Canadian Occupational Performance Measure,* 5th edn. Ottawa: CAOT.

Lloyd, C., Waghorn, G., Lee-Williams, P., Harris, M. & Capra, C. (2008). Early psychosis: treatment issues and the role of occupational therapy. *British Journal of Occupational Therapy* **71** (7), 297–304.

Mackrell, L. & Lavender, T. (2004). Peer relationships in adolescents experiencing a first episode of psychosis. *Journal of Mental Health* **13** (5), 467–480.

Makdisi, L., Blank, A., Bryant, W., Andrews, C., Franco, L. & Parsonage, J. (2013). Facilitators and barriers to living with psychosis: an exploratory collaborative study of the perspectives of mental health service users. *British Journal of Occupational Therapy* **76** (9), 418–426.

Marshal, M. & Rathbone, J. (2011). 'Early intervention for psychosis' (Cochrane Review). *The Cochrane Library,* **6**.

Ministry of Justice (1983/2007). *Mental Health Act 2007: Code of Practice.* London: TSO.

Ministry of Justice (2005). *Mental Capacity Act 2005: Code of Practice.* London: TSO.

Ministry of Justice (2008). *Mental Capacity Act 2005: Deprivation of Liberty Safeguards: Code of Practice to supplement the main Mental Capacity Act 2005 Code of Practice.* London: TSO.

National Institute for Health and Clinical Excellence (2014). *Psychosis and Schizophrenia in adults: Prevention and Management.* NICE Guideline (CG178).

Oxford University Press (1997). *New Shorter Oxford English Dictionary.* Oxford: Oxford University Press

Parkinson, S., Forsyth, K. & Kielhofner, G. (2006). *The Model of Occupation Screening Tool (MOHOST),* Version 2.0. Chicago: University of Illinois.

Parsonage, J. (2012). *Gaining 'meaningful occupation' following first episode psychosis: a service user perspective.* Unpublished Thesis (MResCP), St George's University, London.

Roy, L., Rousseau, J., Fortier, P. & Mottard, J. (2009). Perception of community functioning in young adults with recent-onset psychosis: implications for practice. *British Journal of Occupational Therapy* **72** (10), 424–433.

Spear, L. (2010). *The Behavioural Neuroscience of Adolescence.* New York: W.W. Norton.

Unruh, A. (2004). 'So ... What do you do?' Occupation and construction of identity. *Canadian Journal of Occupational Therapy* **71** (5), 290–295.

Wunderink, L., Sytema, S., Nienhuis, F. & Wiersma, D. (2009). Clinical recovery in first epsiode psychosis. *Schizophrenia Bulletin* **35** (2), 362–369.

# Chapter 15

# Working with people with personality disorder

## Keir Harding

## Introduction

This chapter describes the author's journey to working in the field of personality disorder services, highlights some ideas about useful ways of thinking about personality disorder and considers some of the challenges that working with personality disorder can entail. I'll finish up with some suggestions for interventions which, while by no means exclusive, might help answer the question 'but how can I help?'

## Key points

- Working with people with personality disorder can be highly challenging.
- The work involves a considerable degree of 'therapeutic use of self' in that the nature of the interactions between therapist and service user is key; the 'therapy' takes place largely through this relationship.
- Be wary of falling into the 'rescue trap'.

## Preparation?

It might be useful to think about the journey that I took before I became a specialist practitioner in a personality disorder service. Personality disorder was never mentioned in my graduate training. My first job was in a special security hospital and when I started work there in around 2000, one of the patients had just been released after he had successfully convinced the court that, as he was diagnosed with personality disorder, an untreatable condition, it was unlawful that he should be detained in a hospital. After his success it felt like everyone in the place with a similar diagnosis was arguing the same and refusing intervention of any kind. The court's later decision, that the nursing environment constituted treatment, was not received well by the residents, but what I'm trying to illustrate is an environment where people with personality disorder were deemed to be 'untreatable'.

I moved from this job to an acute ward in London where I have a clear memory of a lead nurse pointing out someone with a diagnosis of personality disorder and explaining how, because of this, nothing could be done to help him. My 'education' continued in this vein and I grew into a clinician who saw people with personality disorder as difficult, dangerous, and people to be avoided at all costs. Despite this, while working in a community mental health team, I started to get feedback that I was good at working with people with a personality disorder diagnosis. I'm not sure what 'good' meant but I seemed able to maintain a relationship with those that others struggled to, and to help them to reduce some of the behaviours that most damaged their relationships with services. As a result of this I was asked if I wanted to work in a day Therapeutic Community (TC) for people with personality disorder. It would mean working with a group of them all day on a Monday for at least a year. I refused at once: why on earth would I want to do that? After thinking about it some more I became curious about a new way of working and managed to get myself seconded into the service for a year. That year was career changing for me as I grew to see the members of the TC as human and not a diagnosis. I saw them falling apart and holding each other together. I saw them caring for each other while holding each other to high standards. That year in the TC had a seismic effect on my career and, after successfully fighting for my secondment to continue, when it eventually had to stop, I knew that this was the area I wanted to work in.

What follows is some of the knowledge that I've gained throughout my work in this field, but it's important that I'm not held up as some kind of exemplar of perfect practice. I have had all the urges to reject, punish, break boundaries and rescue that are typical in this line of work and I've acted on those urges plenty of times. This chapter is aimed less at being brilliant and more at helping us to be 'good enough'.

## What is this thing called 'personality disorder'?

Whenever I'm running training courses on personality disorder, the first questions people generally ask are 'what are the different types?' and 'what are the signs and symptoms?' Generally, knowledge of these doesn't help people with their work and I think these requests represent an attempt to understand what is going on for people with a personality disorder diagnosis so as to feel more knowledgeable and competent around them. The National Offender Management Service have produced a book which contains a detailed account of personality disorder classification and those facts are there if you want them (DoH 2011). With Borderline Personality Disorder (BPD), in the DSM-5 there are nine diagnostic criteria of which you need to display five to get a diagnosis (American Psychiatric Association 2013). In reality this means that two people can have a diagnosis of BPD while only sharing one characteristic. Bearing in mind that it is rare for people to have their personality difficulties in one defined cluster, and the majority have difficulties in other personality types, trying to force a complex presentation into an easily definable box seems less than helpful.

The oversimplified way that helps me to best think about people with personality disorder is as 'having difficulties containing strong emotions, difficulties managing relationships and using ways of coping that are self-destructive'. A more articulate definition might read like this:

> … an enduring pattern of inner experience and behaviour that deviates markedly from the expectations of the individual's culture, is pervasive and inflexible, has an onset in adolescence or early adulthood, is stable over time and leads to distress or impairment …
>
> (summary from information in the DSM-V 2013)

What is useful about this is that it helps us see difficulties as fixed (as opposed to relapsing/remitting) and unusual for the social environment. The difficulties occur across a range of situations and they cause distress. In other words the difficulties are persistent, pervasive and problematic. If you have little concern for the feelings of others and will do anything to achieve your goals you might well thrive on the frontline in battle or as the head of a Wall Street bank. In public life in general these traits are likely to bring you to the attention of the police. It's useful as occupational therapists to think about how the environment defines whether personality is disordered or not, and it's also useful to think about how the environment shapes personality.

The use of the term 'personality disorder' is often contentious, loaded as it is with all the stigma that years of unsuccessful treatment can bring. It's often seen as a judgement, that someone is broken or contaminated in some way. In services it can often be used as a way of dismissing people from care. I've worked with people who have loved having their problems labelled as it has made them feel that they were not as 'freakishly different' from the rest of the world as they had suspected. It's let them know that what they've experienced is a recognised problem for which there are theories and treatments. Others have railed against the diagnosis and fought for some different label other than the one they've seen given to the least popular clients in services (NIMHE 2003).

# Prevalence

With this label of personality disorder, which may or may not be useful and is certainly a shorthand way of describing a very complex presentation, let's have a think about how likely we are to come across it. Figures for how prevalent all personality disorder is in the population as a whole can vary substantially from 5 to 13 per cent (Coid *et al.* 2006). Everyone agrees that this number increases as you move into services with higher levels of security and structure with up to 30 per cent in primary care, up to 50 per cent in secondary care, up to 70 per cent in drug and alcohol and eating disorder services and up to 78 per cent in prison (Moran 2003). I've met a lot of people who claim that they don't work with clients with personality disorder; however, looking at those figures you realise that if they are working in mental health then they must be.

# Developmental theory

Frustratingly there is no one theory that can categorically explain how personality disorder evolves. From the extremes of it being something people are born with to the idea that it is solely shaped by the environment to the lazy search for one traumatic event in someone's life to pin all their problems on, theories are varied. As ever in life, the truth is likely to lie somewhere in the middle and using a bio/psycho/social model is often quite useful in making sense of a person's presentation (Bateman & Krawitz 2013). Here the 'bio' refers to what we leave the womb with – inherited traits, neurochemistry, IQ and physical abilities. 'Psycho' describes thinking, attitudes, self-esteem and ways of coping, while 'social' refers to our experiences of school, family and culture. While I can intellectually accept the influence biological factors have on the development of our personality, my occupational therapy background leads me towards placing an emphasis on our actions, how the environment responds, and how we interpret it to make further actions. The frequency with which I see clients who have difficulty managing their emotions, whose parents had difficulty managing their emotions, and whose grandparents were the same, somehow pushes me away from inherited traits and towards people learning to manage as best they can, given the teaching and examples that they have received. Some psychoanalytic theory can be useful to back this up. This would say that the newborn baby gets attached to its primary care giver and through their attention and feedback it learns about itself and the world. In scenarios where this doesn't happen, where the care giver vanishes or is inconsistent or is actively malevolent, the baby develops ideas about its worth, the behaviour of others and how to get its needs met (Danquah & Berry 2013). Whatever difficulties someone with personality disorder presents with, it is rare that their past experiences don't manifest in the difficulties they encounter now.

# Occupational therapy and personality disorder

Given that the process of assessing what someone wants to do, needs to do, and has the capacity to do within the environment around them, is individual to everyone, I'm not going to spend much time talking about how to do occupational therapy with people with personality disorder; instead I'll talk more about what the challenges to effective work might be.

## Stigma

My experience of a patient being pointed out and identified as 'unworkable' is by no means unique. This happened to me over ten years ago but students will happily share similar experiences with me today. In training, attendees will frequently describe people with personality disorder as 'difficult, frightening, dangerous, a waste of time' and use many more equally noxious labels. It's worth considering what our motivation to work with someone we thought of as the above might be when their referral lands on our desk. If I carried the above views I would be more likely to try to avoid the person, try to keep them out of the service and look for reasons to make their problems someone else's business. If I was the service user who walked through the door of a place that was supposed to help me and met someone with these attitudes, I wonder how motivated I would be to work with them? I wonder whether I would feel safe enough to be honest with them and whether their preconceptions might lead me to respond in a way that confirmed all the prejudices that they held.

The impact and reality of stigma is evident in services and recent research (e.g. Lam *et al.* 2015) showed how a label can hugely affect the effectiveness of practitioners. It is useful to be aware of how we think about personality disorder so that we can ensure our preconceived ideas don't influence what we do in our work.

## Relationships

What someone with a diagnosis of personality disorder is likely to bring to a relationship is a long history of struggling with interactions. The factors that influence this are infinite; however, we might expect them to come from a background where the people who were supposed to care for them might have neglected, abandoned or hurt them. When we step into the role of 'someone who is supposed to help', it would be odd if our client's previous experiences did not show up in our relationship. We might feel that a look at the clock is a way of keeping on top of the timing of the sessions, while our client might see this as confirmation we are not interested. Our missed session due to sickness might seem to be confirmation that we would abandon them as others have. Our defensive reply to being accused of being vindictive, uncaring or uninterested might be confirmation that we will tell them how they are wrong like everyone else has. If we don't expect and understand the difficulties our clients have had in their previous relationships, we are highly likely to repeat them, then go home, cursing ourselves for being bad therapists and hating our clients for 'making' us feel that way. In many ways, 'being able to maintain a therapeutic relationship' can be a useful goal with the difficulties that emerge, informing further intervention.

## Risk

Despite self-harm being only one of the criteria for borderline personality disorder, it is one of the most common associations clinicians have when personality disorder is mentioned. People with personality disorder often use self-harm for a variety of reasons (Motz 2009). The most common reason is that it works for whatever means they use it for. People might self-harm to get a release from tension, to punish themselves, to communicate their distress, to distract themselves, to give them a reason to care themselves or a different reason or a mix of any and all the above. Very often self-harm is a bigger problem for the clinician than the client themselves. For the client, it is the way of coping that they have used effectively for years. For the clinician it is a symptom that must be cured – how can anyone be a good therapist while their client is carving lines in their arms? Aside from our urge to stop self-damaging behaviour we need to also consider the socio-political environment we operate in. We have a 'duty of care' to our clients and a responsibility to 'help'.

It can be highly distressing to have clients on your caseload who manage life in a way which means they might die. The thought of sitting in a court while a barrister berates you for not saving your client is chilling. An effective (for the clinician) way of managing this distress is to shift the duty of care to someone else, perhaps a different colleague or a service who can do more – a crisis team, an acute unit or specialist out of area placement where the responsibility for the client's safety can be held by others. Another effective way is to discharge them from the service. Both of these do our clients a terrible disservice and my experience (which I am certain does not encompass all occupational therapy services) is that in general, clients who are high risk are not seen as an occupational therapist's business. Rethinking the duty of care to frame things like keeping the client as autonomous as possible, working towards long-term goals and not doing things that make the situation worse can be hard to hold in mind while we worry for our professional registration, but it is vital to focus on how effective care rarely involves taking control away from the client. By all means we should target occupations that are life threatening, but to have any success doing this, reducing self-harm has to be the client's goal as well as ours. Sometimes we need to accept that we can help someone improve their functioning while they maintain dangerous ways of coping in their lives.

## Motivation

The best clients, the ones that make us feel like good occupational therapists, are the ones who listen to our opinion, do what we agree together and get better. Alas the majority of our clients with a personality disorder diagnosis will turn up to our meetings feeling worthless, useless, having little locus of control to change their situation and feeling that a professional somewhere has the answer. These will all get in the way of an intervention working and our impulse is likely to be to cry 'no motivation' and 'get them out of our service'. I've worked in services where a low score on the Occupational Circumstances Assessment Interview and Rating Scale (OCAIRS) 'readiness for change' section was reason for exclusion rather than something to be curious about. Something tends to stop us trying to understand why a client didn't turn up for their appointment in the same way we would break down why a client dropped their plate in the kitchen. It's as if the idea that a lack of belief in yourself and others is a reason to keep someone out of a service rather than a skill deficit to be addressed.

## Helplessness

'But what do I do with them?' is a question I'm frequently asked when working with clinicians. It's as if clinicians with years of mental health experience have nothing to offer people with relationship and emotional difficulties who put themselves at risk. It is all too comforting to think (like the clients) that the answers lie with someone else rather than consider how to be effective within our own role. Despite the multiple treatments for personality disorder that are out there, the biggest factor in making effective change is not the particular mode of therapy that is used; it is not the specific profession nor the experience of the clinician; it is the quality of the therapeutic alliance (Martin *et al.* 2000). A huge oversimplification of this term might break it down as the quality of the relationship the client and clinician have incorporating a joint understanding of the problem, a rationale for overcoming it, a belief that the clinician is interested and an ability to repair breaches in the relationship. It's essential to hold these in mind whether you are cooking, weaving, teaching, boxing, talking, psychoanalysing or dissecting schemas. The value is in not what you do, but the way that you do it.

# Some thoughtful ways of working

## Working with (or not) the diagnosis

Some clients will embrace the diagnosis, feeling that it describes and explains the difficulties they have experienced over the years. They felt freakish, an outsider and they didn't fit. They are reassured that their difficulties are so common that there is a name in a book to describe them. Other clients will rail against it. They feel it labels them as broken, flawed and less worthy than others. I have yet to have any success arguing with someone who doesn't accept their diagnosis that they are wrong and I'd suggest it isn't worth doing. It's been useful for me to get alongside clients and forget about diagnosis while trying to come to an understanding with them of their problems, how they impact on their lives and what the two of you can do improve things. As occupational therapy is concerned with function rather than diagnosis, this is entirely consistent with our holistic approach and accepting that diagnosis (or identification with the diagnosis) doesn't really matter can be a big step in helping clients and clinicians progress.

## Assessment/formulation/understanding

Perhaps the greatest asset you and your client can create in your work together is a shared understanding of the difficulties that they bring. This is likely to involve a lengthy and ongoing period of assessment and won't come from an hour ticking boxes on a questionnaire. While working with clients with personality disorder we do all the things that we would usually do in our assessments, while paying special attention to what has led our clients to where they are now. For the client to understand themselves and for the clinician to maintain empathy, it is essential to develop a clear idea about why the issues of today make sense, based on the issues of the past. Someone taking a non-lethal overdose is stressful for the clinician. We can think of them as selfish, manipulative or 'a time waster'. If we have taken the time to explore how the only time they received care as a child was when they were hurt, how their parents would beat them for being upset, how they only had the example of acting on emotional pain rather than talking about it and how treatment in hospital was the only time they felt truly cared for, it is difficult to maintain the mental picture of 'a vindictive, manipulative time waster'. Whatever the problem/behaviour/issue we are faced with, we will hold far greater capacity to be effective clinicians if we can be curious about and try to make sense of it as opposed to assuming we know. The Dialectical Behaviour Therapy (DBT) maxim that the client is trying their best, given the skills and experience that they have, is useful to keep in mind (Linehan

1993). While doing my assessments I try to be especially mindful of the client's early environment, their experience of having people who cared for them, whether they saw useful role models of effective interpersonal skills, whether they were taught appropriate ways of managing frustration and distress and what has brought them to a place where they are now meeting with a therapist.

I've often heard people explaining a client's behaviour as 'bad' because they assume the client knows that it is morally wrong. An example might be a client who assaults people when they refuse to meet their needs. Most of us come from a background of 'good enough' early life experiences and will have been taught that hurting people is wrong. To keep our empathy for the client we need to be able to think about how we would tell right from wrong if our father had fought anyone who looked at him the wrong way, if we had been beaten when we annoyed our parents too much or if mum had encouraged us to fight the children who wouldn't play with us. It's imperative that we don't interpret our client's behaviour through the lens of our own experience. Instead, we need to understand their way of seeing the world and help them to understand how their current ways of managing might cause them problems.

## Goals

Once our initial assessment has been completed we should have an idea of what the client wants to get out of our relationship. It's useful to turn broad goals into specific objectives so that you both agree what is going to be done and how it's going to be achieved. Very often I come across clinicians who have worked with a client for years with little idea about what the purpose of their contact is. This is frequently a deeply uncomfortable relationship for all concerned, especially as it's impossible to tell if it's working.

With clients who have little experience of being able to change their circumstances, who are reliant on others to get their needs met or who have no confidence that things may be different, we might be tempted to *suggest* changes that we think could improve their lives. This is an understandable and laudable option; however, it comes with the danger of the therapist providing all the motivation and responsibility for things changing. Having been there I can assure you that this is a miserable situation to find yourself in, particularly as the buzz you get from being helpful fades very quickly when you feel that you are the only one invested in the relationship. Sometimes a client's goals will be 'to feel better' or 'to feel normal' and it's essential to break these down into occupations or activities that can be achieved. Once that is done (even if the goal is to spend time to get a greater understanding of the client's difficulties) we can then tell the client what we can offer that will help them achieve this goal. Sometimes the goals will be outside our expertise or belong in a different service – we need to be clear about what we can and can't do.

Once we have a goal and a plan for how to get there, we need to think about what might get in the way. The client's experiences with carers in the past will affect their relationship with you as a carer so it's useful to think of the pitfalls and how you will both respond. With some clients, if they miss a session, it might be useful to chase them up showing that you are interested in their absence and eager to think about how to help them get there next time. With other clients you might want to reduce their passivity and consciously wait for them to make contact. Either way it's useful to try to agree some of these responses *before* they are needed so that you and the client are jointly responsible for how things proceed.

Finally, it is useful to think about what would have to happen for your services to stop being offered. This might be a certain number of Did Not Attends (DNAs), reoccurrence of particular behaviours or anything else that really affects your motivation or makes successful therapy impossible. When these things do occur it's an opportunity to explore with the client what is getting in the way and to give them the chance to do something different. Work might also end because you have achieved the things you set out to. While this is often cause for celebration we should be mindful that for people who have been frequently abandoned, the end of a positive relationship is a poor reward for achieving your goals so the difficulties around endings will need a lot of thinking about.

Having a joint plan for what you are doing together and when it will end are critical for ensuring that you're goal-focused and working on what you have agreed to be helpful. I've found this is a much more rewarding experience than muddling along with people and wading through recurring crises.

## Keeping it real

If our clients have difficulties with their relationships one of the most useful things we can do is use our relationship as a 'lab' where the process of being with someone can be scrutinised. I've lost count of the number of clinicians who have told me that they are so angry, fed up, frightened or baffled by their clients but who never voice it in their hearing. There's often a sense that it might be unprofessional, uncaring or inappropriate to do this but the alternative is often that relationships end suddenly, which is a lot more of all the above.

It can be useful for the therapist to professionally vent what they are feeling in a thoughtful way: 'when you say/do this I feel x and then I want to y' gives clients clear feedback as to what is happening in your relationship in that moment and gives them an opportunity to do something different. Letting a client know recently that her turning up to sessions after not eating for three days resulted in me feeling like a rubbish therapist, unable to help someone change, wondering if there was any value to the work we were sitting down to do, was a major factor in her redoubling her commitment to care for herself. Not because it was important to her to look after herself, but because she wanted to preserve our relationship. Being respectfully honest with our clients is much more ethical than letting them think the issues that significantly affect us are of no consequence. Again, 'putting it out there' in a way the client can hear means that solving the issue is a problem for both of you, and not something the therapist has to swallow alone.

## Supervision/reflection

The experience of working with people who have high levels of risk and relationship difficulties can be challenging. One of the most valuable things I've had in my career is a space to be able to share my thoughts and feelings about the work and have these accepted. I remember a time when the mantra of 'unconditional positive regard' would be repeated in the service. It was as if having strong negative reactions to clients was 'wrong' and that a better therapist would think differently. Good supervision gives us a place to air our feelings about our work and feel justified in what we feel. While I have often had this and felt its benefits, there is a danger in getting too much validation. My most valuable supervisors have been those who have accepted how I feel but also challenged me to examine the basis of my feelings. When I have wanted to flee they have helped me to explore what it might be like to stay. When I have wanted to hold on I've been encouraged to think of the benefits of letting go. When I have been sure that the client has singled me out for ill treatment purely for the pleasure they will get from knowing I suffer, I've been offered another hypothesis explaining why their actions make sense in the context of their past experience.

The experience of having another mind to think about difficulties is invaluable in this line of work. Where it isn't available, using peers to help us validate how we feel can help us to keep motivated. In the absence of a critical friend to challenge us it's vital to spend time reflecting on the work and what drives our urges to act. Much of our work in this area involves helping our clients to decrease the gap between thoughts and action and it's useful to try to do this for ourselves.

## Some things to try

Often when assessing the environment around a client we will find things that inhibit adaptive functioning or reinforce occupational behaviour that destroys relationships. A fictional amalgam of a couple of my ex-clients is given in Box 15.1 to illustrate this.

## Box 15.1: Case study – John

John was admitted to hospital due to having strong suicidal urges. In the community John had gained some relief from his distress by carefully cutting with a Stanley knife that he kept clean in a box with dressings to clean himself up afterwards. On the ward John had his knife taken away from him. Unable to relieve his distress in the usual way John began to cut whenever people weren't looking, with broken cups, torn drink cans, with his nails. The hospital was unable to tolerate this and removed everything he could cut with. John began locking himself in the toilet and wrapping ligatures around his neck, throwing himself down the stairs and smashing his head against the wall. The number of staff allocated to John increased and his freedom and privacy vanished. It was forgotten that John's admission had been to briefly manage his suicidality and instead it became a mission to free him of self-harm, something he didn't want, something that had not been a factor in his admission but was the sole reason for him being detained on the ward.

John remained on the ward for over a year, becoming increasingly unpopular with staff who felt that managing this behaviour wasn't their job. He was eventually sent to an expensive private unit. In the private unit his restrictions and levels of security were increased further. John's self-harm had become a huge problem for other people and he wasn't going to be let out until he made everyone feel better about it.

My work with John mostly involved going through his old notes, building a case that John was significantly less risk to himself when he was looking after himself in the community. His behaviours were controlled and his methods of coping significantly less lethal. I highlighted the proportional link between the levels of restriction around him and the lethality of his ways of coping. My brief individual contact with John involved meeting John in the unit, agreeing his priorities (to get out), agreeing with his view on the relationship between security and risk, and getting his informed consent to push for discharge to the community. Interestingly, everyone was convinced by the argument that the level of restriction was a direct contributor to John's risk behaviour but this did little to change ways of working with John or reassure people that he would be safer with less help. Even though it was clear that our help was hurting John, we couldn't tolerate not helping in the hope it would make him safer. It was only through sharing this view with clinicians on every level and managers with greater and greater authority that change came about, admittedly with some clinicians convinced John would kill himself the moment he was released and ruing the madness of letting him go. Eventually John did transfer to a house with support but no restriction. He showed some of the same behaviours that he had shown prior to his admission but nothing compared with what happened when we worked hardest to keep him safe.

As occupational therapists are more interested in the nature of the problem, rather than what name it has in a textbook, we are in a unique position to be able to objectively assess the difficulty and the effect of the environment around it. Interventions like the one above are contentious but likely to be popular with clients who despise being incarcerated and services that pay hundreds of thousands of pounds a year for interventions that might do more harm than good.

## Less direction – more empowerment

Over the years I have fallen in love with working with people using the principles of a therapeutic community. In the past, therapeutic communities tended to be institutions people would move into and immerse themselves in an environment where they took on the responsibility for their progress. Doctors were not in charge and patients made decisions. Despite the proven success and cost-effectiveness of TCs their popularity has waned; however, the spirit of the TC lives on in the Enabling Environment project and in the Day Therapeutic communities that can be found around

**247**

the country, particularly in the North. I can talk for hours about the clinical and ethical values of the TC – shared decision making, shared responsibility for the service, having people who have lived through similar experiences supporting those who are going through them now, helping people to learn what works rather than giving them theoretical answers ... instead, I'll try to make the day TC or enabling environment relevant to occupational therapists.

The group is not run by staff. Therefore, the members have to take on the roles that allow the group to function. This involves members stepping into unfamiliar circumstances and getting clear feedback from their peers around their performance. The roles can be anything but there is obviously a grading between the person who writes the attendance list and the one who chairs the meeting. The rules of the group are made by the members who can constantly refine their ways of doing things so that there is both flexibility and consistency. In reality this means that the group is responsible for its success but also learns from its experiences. The role of staff is not to rescue the group but to help them break down and understand what has happened in order to adjust their actions next time. The TC becomes like a laboratory for people to display what goes on that causes difficulties in their life outside. They receive feedback from staff and peers around what it is like to be around them. Their peers might suggest techniques or strategies that they have benefited from themselves. The service user is encouraged to question, challenge or object to any aspect of the day. All the above give the service user ongoing experience of putting their difficulties into words so that they do not have to act them out. I feel that the process of attending and contributing to the group, taking on different roles and responding to feedback is one of the purest examples of people healing through activity in mental health.

I've been lucky enough to work in a couple of day TCs; however, the principles of the TC or enabling environment can be used in shorter groups. I think the idea of handing responsibility to clients with personality disorder can be uncomfortable for staff and service users; however I'll suggest that this way of working can fundamentally change the dynamic of the relationship with people who have not responded to what we normally provide. Certainly it is better than continuing to do what doesn't seem to work and more ethically sound than offering nothing or discharging people who don't fit with what we like to provide.

I think that with the TC focus on empowerment, independence, use of activity, all within a non-diagnostic framework, occupational therapists are particularly suited to work in this way.

# Dialectical Behaviour Therapy skills

Dialectical Behaviour Therapy (DBT) is a therapy designed by Marsha Linehan who has a diagnosis of personality disorder herself (Linehan 1993). While DBT is a comprehensive therapy in its own right, there are elements that occupational therapists can make use of in their work. It takes the view that personality disorder (particularly BPD) is a problem of emotional regulation. Strong feelings lead people to act in ways that take them away from their long-term goals by harming themselves and their relationships.

Once we have assessed our clients and identified what occupations they want and need to do, we come to the skills that they need in order to do them. Dialectical behaviour therapy provides a number of teachable skills in the fields of mindfulness, distress tolerance (things to do to avoid self-harm), emotional regulation and interpersonal effectiveness (assertiveness). I'm sure Linehan would agree that these skills are not particularly original, but what she has done is collected skills that we might have seen in interventions such as assertiveness, anxiety management, healthy living and living skills and applied them to personality disorder (Linehan 1993). Obviously, the answer to working with clients with personality disorder isn't to just do DBT skills with them; however, if our assessment indicates that skill deficits are interfering with our clients' functioning, *and* they agree that the skills could be useful, then practising these skills with them would be a valid intervention.

## Conclusion

While this chapter was supposed to discuss a new role for occupational therapists, I've tried to give the impression that if you're working in mental health, you are working with personality disorder anyway. The process of occupational therapy remains the same regardless of our client group. What I'd like occupational therapists to take from this chapter is a belief in process, and an understanding of how the risk and relationship difficulties associated with personality disorder can knock that process off track. Occupational therapists have the potential to make huge differences to this client group. It's time we recognised the contribution we can make and started to lead.

# Useful resources

- Try to get on a 3 day KUF (Knowledge and Understanding Framework) Awareness course. These run around the country and are often free if run within your organisation.

- http://apt.rcpsych.org/content/7/5/365 – this gives information on therapeutic communities.

- http://www.enablingenvironments.com/ – this gives information on and standards for an enabling environment if you wanted to build a service/group based on those principles.

- http://www.emergenceplus.org.uk/images/Documents/meeting-the-challenge-making-a-difference-practitioner-guide.pdf – this is a guide for working with personality disorder written by people with personality disorder. I would highly recommend this.

- Hirons, A., Rose, R. & Burke, K. (2010). The journey day service: an occupational groupwork programme for people with personality disorder. *Mental Health Review Journal* **15** (4), 51–57. This describes an occupational therapy-specific intervention in a specialist personality disorder service.

- https://www.justice.gov.uk/downloads/offenders/mentally-disordered-offenders/working-with-personality-disordered-offenders.pdf – this has lots of information on types of personality disorder and suggestions of useful ways of working.

- Main, T. (1957) 'The Ailment' (Main 1957) is one of the best papers I have read for describing the difficulties of personality disorder without ever mentioning it.

# References

American Psychiatric Association (2013). *Diagnostic and Statistical Manual of Mental Disorders: DSM-V,* 5th edn. Washington, D.C: American Psychiatric Association.

Bateman, A.W. & Krawitz, R. (2013). *Borderline Personality Disorder: An Evidence-based Guide for Generalist Mental Health Professionals.* Oxford: Oxford University Press.

Coid, J., Yang, M., Tyrer, P., Roberts, A. & Ullrich, S. (2006). Prevalence and correlates of personality disorder in Great Britain. *British Journal of Psychiatry* **188** (5), 423–431.

Danquah, A.N. & Berry, K. (eds) (2013). *Attachment Theory in Adult Mental Health.* Oxford: Routledge.

Department of Health (2011). *Working with Personality Disordered Offenders: A Practitioners Guide.* London: TSO.

Lam, D.C.K., Salkovskis, P.M. & Hogg, L.I. (2015). Judging a book by its cover: an experimental study of the negative impact of a diagnosis of borderline personality disorder on clinicians' judgements of uncomplicated panic disorder. *British Journal of Clinical Psychology* DOI: 10.1111/bjc.12093.

Linehan, M.M. (1993). *Cognitive-behavioural Treatment of Borderline Personality Disorder.* New York: The Guilford Press.

Main, T.F. (1957). The ailment. *British Journal of Medical Psychology* **30** (3), 129–145.

Martin, D.J., Garske, J.P. & Davis, M.K. (2000). Relation of the therapeutic alliance with outcome and other variables: a meta-analytic review. *Journal of Consulting and Clinical Psychology* **68** (3), 438–450.

Moran, P. (2003). *The Epidemiology of Personality Disorders.* http://www.dh.gov.uk (last accessed: 5.2.2016).

Motz, A. (2009) 'Self-harm as a sign of hope' in *Managing Self-harm, Psychological Perspectives,* ed. A. Motz. Oxford: Routledge.

National Institute for Mental Health for England (2003). *Personality Disorder: no Longer a Diagnosis of Exclusion. Policy Implementation Guidance for the Development of Services for People with Personality Disorder, Gateway Reference 1055.* London: NIMH(E).

# Chapter 16

# Working with people with eating disorders

## Clare O'Reilly with Lucy Johnson

## Introduction

This chapter will identify the functional implications of eating disorders, highlight the opportunities for therapists to work in a variety of settings and describe common interventions used with this client group. It aims to explore the scope for working in the field, including using core occupational therapy skills and expanding to developing areas such as Dialectical Behaviour Therapy (DBT). It will focus largely on the interventions used with those with moderate to severe difficulties. Although these represent the minority of individuals with eating disorders they are more likely to receive occupational therapy than those with a milder presentation.

## Key points

- Eating disorders have a significant impact on the daily lives of those who experience them.
- Occupational performance in all key areas can be severely affected due to the impact of physical and psychological consequences of eating disorders.
- Individuals with long-term eating disorders can struggle to fulfil their potential in many occupational areas including realising career goals and having romantic relationships.
- Those with eating disorders, particularly anorexia nervosa, are often ambivalent about change and the occupational therapist can be effective at motivating people through focusing on functional goals and outcomes.
- The occupational therapist has a key role in supporting the individual to shop for, prepare and eat foods that they have been avoiding due to their eating disorder.
- Occupational therapists can enable an individual to develop competence in other areas of occupational performance such as progressing with their career or expanding leisure

interests and participation. This serves to reduce the focus and importance a person places on their shape and weight.

● Therapists can further enhance a person's recovery through facilitating development and use of skills such as those delivered using Dialectical Behaviour Therapy (DBT) as an alternative to using eating disorder behaviours as a means of managing distress.

# Eating disorders – the background

It is widely acknowledged that eating disorders are complex conditions that impact on many aspects of health and wellbeing (NICE 2004, PwC 2015). The potential global impact on occupational performance is equally recognised, including 'social isolation, compromise of educational and employment plans and occupation in the areas of self-care, daily living and productivity of employment and/or education' (NICE 2004, p. 14).

With almost 725,000 people in the UK experiencing an eating disorder at present (PwC 2015), these conditions affect a significant proportion of the population. Recent studies indicate that the incidence of eating disorders is increasing (Micali et al. 2013). It is also known that eating disorders often occur alongside other mental health problems such as depression, anxiety and substance disorders (Braun et al. 1994) and a range of personality disorders (Reas et al. 2013). Clinical experience echoes these empirical findings and suggests that individuals are presenting with more severe and complex problems. The majority of those presenting with eating disorders for the first time are young females (PwC 2015). Equally, eating disorders are being experienced more widely by men and within a variety of cultural groups and contexts (Pike et al. 2014).

Eating disorders are somewhat unique in their effect on both an individual's physical and mental health. Occupational therapists are well equipped to work in this area due to their ability to consider the impact of a variety of physical, psychological, social and environmental factors on an individual's occupational performance (Townsend & Polatajko 2007). Additionally, their focus on functional outcomes serves to engage and motivate this client group who are widely acknowledged to be ambivalent about change and recovery (Geller & Drab 1999, Vansteenkiste et al. 2005). Clark and Nayar (2012) detailed the key role for occupational therapists in supporting individuals to recover from eating disorders.

# Eating disorders' features and presentation

People with eating disorders are characteristically preoccupied with their shape and weight. They place excessive emphasis on their bodies as an expression of their worth and value (Fairburn 2008). This difficulty is compounded by an individual's distortion of their body image, often believing themselves to be overweight or to have an undesirable shape when they are in fact normal or average weight or indeed extremely thin or emaciated (American Psychiatric Association 2013). The focus on this aspect of one's life results in disordered eating patterns, including dietary restraint (excluding things from the diet) and restriction (eating too little), rigid adherence to food rules and engagement in compensatory behaviours such as vomiting, taking laxatives and compulsive exercise. Individuals use these behaviours in an attempt to reduce their weight and control their body shape. The particular pattern of weight control behaviours, and the effect of these on an individual's weight, determines which specific eating disorder diagnosis they receive.

In addition to its role in attempting to control weight and shape, an eating disorder often functions to affect a person's emotions (Corstorphine 2006). For example, starvation and dietary restriction can result in blunting of emotions (Keys *et al.* 1950). Similarly, vomiting and laxative use can relieve emotional distress and alleviate guilt caused by eating 'forbidden foods' and bingeing can be used as a strategy to cope with and avoid unwanted feelings. Furthermore, focusing attention on one's eating, weight and shape can serve to distract from problematic thoughts, disturbing memories or distressing life situations.

The most common eating disorders are Anorexia Nervosa (anorexia), Bulimia Nervosa (bulimia) and Binge Eating Disorder (BED). The term 'Other Specified Feeding and Eating Disorders' (OSFED) is used to describe eating disorders that may present similarly to anorexia or bulimia but do not meet all criteria. It can additionally refer to conditions in which the individual has disordered eating unrelated to their weight or shape including Avoidant/Restrictive Food Intake Disorder (ARFID), pica (the consumption of non-food items such as paper) or rumination disorder (persistent regurgitation of food) (American Psychiatric Association 2013). Such difficulties are more commonly experienced by children than adults.

Eating disorders may present in a number of ways depending on individuals' experiences. Some people demonstrate a range of impulsive behaviours to manage their emotions including eating behaviours, self-harm and substance use. Others exhibit more controlled and perfectionist approaches to their eating and many people can experience high anxiety, low mood and poor self-esteem. Practitioners need to be mindful, therefore, not just of the person's diagnosis but of their individual difficulties. An occupational therapist can play a valuable role in observing a person's behaviour in the context of their environment, identifying the function of behaviours and choosing appropriate interventions to ameliorate difficulties based on the understanding developed. Thus an informed occupational formulation based on knowledge of both eating disorders and an occupational framework is highly valuable. Box 16.1 (below) summarises the main subjects/topics which the occupational therapist needs to be knowledgeable in when working with people with eating disorders.

## Anorexia nervosa

People with anorexia nervosa demonstrate an intense fear of fatness and a relentless pursuit of thinness above other goals (Crisp 2006), including preservation of life in severe cases (Tan *et al.* 2003a). A person may experience extreme distress at eating particular foods that are considered threatening. Similarly, any experience of weight gain or shape change can be terrifying. Through dietary restriction and use of compensatory behaviours a person can reach an extremely low body weight. In order to receive the diagnosis, an individual's body mass index (BMI) is less than 17.5Kg/m². As a healthy BMI range for adults is between 20 and 25, sufferers are significantly suppressing their weight to very unhealthy levels. Thus, the medical consequences of anorexia are often severe and have both short- and long-term effects on health. Indeed, clinicians are acutely aware that the illness can be fatal and that anorexia has the highest mortality of any mental health problem (Birmingham et al. 2005, Hoang et al. 2014). Reversible medical complications include low immunity, reduced heart rate, liver dysfunction and anaemia (Miller et al. 2005). Osteoporosis and reduced fertility can further affect a person's health and quality of life over a prolonged period.

# Bulimia nervosa

Many of the features of bulimia nervosa are similar to those of anorexia, particularly the central importance of shape and weight and the presence of weight control behaviours. Individuals living with bulimia engage in binge eating followed by compensatory strategies including vomiting and laxative use. Binge eating is frequently preceded by severe dietary restriction and many hours fasting, resulting in great hunger and cravings for foods that have been forbidden. Bingeing involves eating excessive quantities of food at one time. People can experience a sense of losing control when overeating during these periods and often report distress following binge episodes (Fairburn 2013). As a consequence of binge eating, those with bulimia nervosa are often within the healthy weight range. Many will experience the effects of starvation, due to going long periods without eating, although the effects will generally be fewer and less severe than in those with anorexia.

# Binge eating disorder

Individuals with binge eating disorder will engage in recurrent binges in a similar manner to those with bulimia, without the subsequent compensatory behaviours. These behaviours can result in physical pain, embarrassment and emotional distress (American Psychiatric Association 2013). Due to the large amount of food consumed, obesity is a common effect of binge eating.

**Box 16.1: Eating disorders: knowledge base**

**Topics specific to eating disorders:**

- Knowledge of eating disorder symptoms and behaviours
- Effects of starvation
- Importance of regular eating
- Effects of vomiting and laxatives on food absorption and potential harmful physical effects of these behaviours

- Starvation and restriction binge cycle
- Harmful physical effects of eating disorders, including basic knowledge of the necessity and type of physical monitoring required
- Principles of healthy and unhealthy (compulsive) exercise
- Motivation and the cycle of change.

**General topics relevant to the area:**

- Effects of anxiety; anxiety management including use of exposure strategies
- Self-esteem and perfectionism
- Emotional dysregulation.

# Occupational formulation

Obtaining nutrition is essential for all living creatures. Although this is very basic biological information it is something that clients with eating disorders often have great difficulty accepting. Many people have told me that they wish they didn't have to eat or that they have just decided they will not eat again or that they will totally exclude entire food groups from their diets. As humans we need to eat at regular intervals, up to six times every day, in order to function effectively in daily life and to meet our potential. Activities associated with eating pervade our daily lives, from planning meals, shopping, preparing food and eating at home or in the workplace to socialising with friends or colleagues in restaurants. While healthy individuals take our human digestive and metabolic physiology for granted, these associated daily activities can cause enormous anxiety and distress for people with eating difficulties. It is understandable therefore that occupational therapy authors identified difficulties in all occupational performance areas as a consequence of eating disorders (Costa 2009, Orchard 2003, Singlehurst *et al.* 2007). In addition to the effects of eating habits, Gogarty and Brangan (2004) elicited the significant impact of body image distress on an individual's ability to engage in activities including shopping for clothes, pursuing leisure activities and being physically intimate. While the effects on eating-related activities will be most pronounced, difficulties within educational, work and leisure domains persist (Gogarty & Brangan 2004, Lock & Pépin 2011).

The symptoms of the conditions are exacerbated by the physical, cognitive, emotional and behavioural effects of starvation. These effects were first documented by Keys *et al.* (1950) who found that previously healthy men who had been starved displayed a myriad of symptoms including extreme weight loss, fatigue, weakness, sensitivity to the cold, preoccupation with food, low mood, irritability and lack of sexual interest. In individuals with eating disorders, particularly anorexia, the characteristic cognitive rigidity can become increasingly entrenched as the person restricts their diet or loses further weight. Consequently, it can be progressively more challenging for a person to

**255**

respond to the challenges faced in their environment as their physical strength and cognitive abilities deteriorate. It is similarly increasingly difficult for clients to engage in and benefit from treatment as they become more starved.

The disorders present a challenge in conceptualising an individual's occupational performance and eliciting true values. For example, understanding a person's volition to act is complex as actions can be motivated exclusively because of their effect on weight rather than directed towards functional outcomes. Kielhofner (2008) argued that in such cases an individual is acting on avoidance motivations rather than approaching desired goals. This is particularly pertinent with regard to exercise as individuals may feel compelled to be active, as in the case of 'activity anorexia', a physiologically driven urge to be active when starved (Pierce et al. 1994). Psychologically, a person may compulsively exercise in order to avoid the unwanted emotional consequences of a failure to exercise such as guilt (Meyer et al. 2011). Additionally, one may choose not to engage in valued occupations, including social events and enjoyable leisure activities, due to the presence of food or inability to be sufficiently active. I am frequently surprised that those who I work with experience dread at going to the cinema or taking a long train journey. Often, when an individual has experienced an eating disorder for an extended period of time, they may find it difficult to distinguish between actions motivated by the eating disorder and those indicating a personal preference or real choice. The therapist can use strategies such as Socratic questioning (Padesky 1993) to engage in meaningful discussions regarding these dilemmas. Occupational therapy assessments including the Occupational Performance History Interview (OPHI) (Kielhofner et al. 2004) and Occupational Circumstances Assessment and Interview Rating Scale (OCAIRS) (Forsyth et al. 2005) can also be used to facilitate reflection on individuals' motives and goals.

Understandably, the dominance of the eating disorder thoughts and motives has a significant impact on a person's habits such that days can be consumed by rituals regarding food, body checking and compensatory behaviours. A person may also be engaged in complex behaviours to maintain the secrecy of the disorder including avoiding meals with others, hiding binge foods and leaving evidence to convince others they have eaten. In the long term the accumulation of these habits leads to disturbance in occupational performance. These factors can be particularly pertinent as eating disorders often first present during adolescence (PwC 2015), a period of significant global development. They can result in compromising physical and psychological development and can interrupt the achievement of important milestones including achievement of academic goals, development of meaningful relationships and establishment of independence. For example, a person may spend much of their late adolescence and early adulthood in hospital and may find it difficult to reintegrate into social groups with their peers. Quiles-Cestari and Ribeiro (2012) found that the majority of individuals with anorexia nervosa in their study were not in romantic relationships. They additionally stated that participants experienced loss of major roles including worker, friend and hobbyist.

**256**

In some contrast to the described presentation, individuals with severe eating disorders can, at times, present as extremely competent. For example, a person may achieve very high academic grades or work full-time in a challenging role immediately prior to being admitted to hospital severely underweight and at risk of physical harm. This can be conceptualised in one way by the principle of 'apparent competence' (Linehan 1993). In these instances, people can, understandably, be very reluctant to relinquish any part of their vocational role despite the fact that continuing to pursue it can put them at risk (e.g. working long hours without breaks). In my experience such people will demonstrate marginalisation of other occupational areas, most notably in self-care and social leisure activities. Box 16.2 gives a case study illustrating an occupational approach to a formulation.

## Box 16.2: Case study – occupational disruption

Cristina is a 27-year-old lady with a long history of anorexia which was diagnosed in her early teens. She is a very kind, thoughtful and caring person who enjoys keeping in touch with friends through writing letters and making cards. Cristina enjoys writing articles for a local magazine and blogs about her experiences frequently. She also likes cross-stitch and knitting and has established groups for people who enjoy these activities. She has also engaged in volunteer roles related to these activities. Cristina is extremely resourceful. She has developed relationships with magazines and retailers to secure donations of materials to support her projects and to boost the self-esteem of others who have eating disorders. Cristina has also used her hobbies of writing and stitching to raise awareness of mental health problems, including anorexia, and to reduce the stigma associated with these conditions. In the long term Cristina would dearly love to be married and to start a family. She also has a dream of becoming an occupational therapist. Cristina will often be seen scouring charity shops to find shoes to add to her large collection or sorting through her mountain of craft materials to choose items for a new project!

Cristina's anorexia follows a relapsing and remitting pattern. It has been difficult for her to establish a healthy daily routine and to develop independent living skills as much of her adult life has been peppered with recurrent admissions to specialist eating disorders units to enable weight restoration. Cristina finds it difficult to trust her own perception of the adequacy of her diet, the amount of exercise she requires and the pattern of her weight.

She eats a very limited diet and leaves long hours between meals, often eating her breakfast very early in the morning and not eating again until very late in the evening. When Cristina is unwell she will only allow herself to eat a small range of foods. One of the most limiting factors is Cristina's intense need to be constantly physically active, resulting in her walking throughout the day. She often chooses to prioritise her walking over other valued activities such as spending time with friends. This aspect of her eating disorder has a prominent impact on all occupational performance areas and her need to be on the move can dominate the habits and routines of her day. Cristina starts every day with a very early morning walk as she will not allow herself to stay in bed.

## Occupational performance components

### Physical

When she is particularly unwell and underweight, Cristina can feel extremely cold, resulting in her wearing many layered clothes even in hot weather. She can experience pain in her feet from walking long distances. Cristina can feel dizzy and weak, making it difficult to carry heavy objects or climb stairs. She often feels tired through lack of sleep and weary from her long walks. When she is feeling particularly anxious and at a low weight, Cristina can experience pain in her chest which is frightening and upsetting for her.

### Cognitive

Many of Cristina's thoughts are dominated by food, shape and weight. This can result in difficulty concentrating on tasks. Her assessment of her weight can often be inaccurate and her overall appraisal of her health becomes less reliable as her weight decreases. Cristina demonstrates inflexible thinking patterns and finds it more difficult to think rationally as her difficulties progress.

### Affective

Cristina can experience great distress, particularly when her walking habits are disturbed. She can demonstrate great anxiety with any fluctuations in her weight; either fearing that she is gaining weight or feeling hopeless at times with repeated relapses or exacerbations of her difficulties. Cristina commonly becomes increasingly irritable when her weight is particularly low. She can find it extremely difficult to tolerate distress and can act impulsively to relieve distress. This can result in her being unable to continue with plans that are established with her such as continuing with a planned treatment programme or challenging herself to achieve a goal that she has established.

### Self-care

Cristina has worked hard to develop her independent living skills in recent years. She has managed to live alone and in shared accommodation and to support herself financially through jobs she enjoyed. Cristina has great difficulty maintaining a regular pattern of eating. She has limited experience of preparing balanced meals and of trying novel foods. Cristina is aware of healthy food portion sizes. She is able to use her knowledge and experience to prepare meals with support while in a hospital environment but finds it difficult to complete these tasks independently in the community. Cristina enjoys wearing pretty clothes and shoes. When she becomes more unwell she loses interest in her appearance and dresses in a drab fashion.

### Productivity

Cristina has worked in a number of jobs, including in the care and service industries. She can find it difficult to maintain a job over a long period of time as her health is often unstable and can require frequent lengthy hospital admissions. At times of ill-health, her low energy and poor strength can make it difficult to fulfil all aspects of her role such as carrying heavy objects and supporting patients with mobility problems. Within care positions Cristina has found it very challenging to support her clients with eating tasks. In addition to the above difficulties, Cristina further evaluates her job role based on the impact it will have on her eating disorder rituals, in particular her ability to engage in long walks throughout the day. Cristina's difficulty in sustaining a regular work routine can lead to financial challenges, thus compromising her independent living. She has worked to find a compromise between jobs she finds satisfying and helpful and those that have a negative impact on her health.

### Leisure

Cristina has a wide range of leisure interests as outlined above. The primary area that is affected by her difficulties is her social leisure. Due to her prolonged involvement in specialist treatment settings, Cristina's main peer group are also those with eating disorders. Due to her caring nature she can be very concerned for individuals who she has known through treatment and it can be difficult for her to stabilise her own health when her peers are deteriorating. Cristina has found that her relationships, both friendly and romantic, can be interrupted by her anxiety about eating with others, having meals out and engaging in activities perceived as too restful such as having a lie in or going to the cinema.

Cristina continues to learn from her experiences and over time is practising prioritising her life goals over her desire to maintain a low weight despite her anxieties about this.

# Role of occupational therapists in different settings

Interventions for individuals with eating disorders are often provided via a stepped model of care, increasing in intensity and speciality depending on the severity of the disorder and the level of risk to health (e.g. Nicholls 2013, Welsh Assembly Government 2009). Distribution of clients across services is pyramidal, with the majority of individuals receiving intervention at primary care level and fewer requiring intensive multi-disciplinary input. Palmer (2000) identified that although the majority of sufferers can be effectively treated as outpatients, individuals with severe anorexia nervosa require extensive service input over a prolonged period including hospitalisation in some cases.

The NICE guidelines (2004) similarly advocate community-based treatment while simultaneously acknowledging the potential need for inpatient admission to remedy physical health problems and provide a supportive structure to restore weight and regulate eating. Intensive community day treatment is also available in certain areas, enabling individuals to receive concentrated intervention while maintaining their personal social support systems. Inpatient treatment may be provided in a general medical setting, an acute psychiatric ward or a specialist eating disorder facility depending on individual need. Long-term psychiatric rehabilitation services are also increasingly being utilised to provide opportunities for clients with chronic difficulties to sustain changes in eating behaviour and increase occupational participation to improve their quality of life.

For those individuals with complex difficulties it will be necessary for staff across services to work collaboratively to ensure smooth transitions for clients. For example, health professionals in a community mental health team (CMHT) may need to liaise with specialist eating disorder services or staff on a medical ward. Seymour (2015) highlighted the complementary role and responsibilities of the therapists in secondary mental health services in comparison with those in specialist teams. Occupational therapists provide a useful bridge between services, identifying the specific skills the person needs to maintain their health throughout and beyond treatment. They can reduce barriers to engagement through addressing the impact of the illness on individuals' function rather than exclusively focusing on weight or symptoms.

Occupational therapists may intervene with clients in any of the above services and will provide different treatment depending on the person's stage of illness and treatment. The occupational therapist in a general psychiatric ward may support the client during a short admission to choose food items from a ward trolley or to identify activities to engage in to manage distress after meal times. In a specialist inpatient service, the therapist can provide the individual with an opportunity to develop an extensive menu and practise shopping for and preparing foods to sustain their health. The occupational therapist is likely to play a key role in the team, structuring the environment to enable individuals to become increasingly independent in the setting and scheduling activities to grade food-related challenges. Within a specialist setting the therapist and client are often afforded the luxury of working together for a significant period of time to develop skills and improve confidence in preparation for discharge. Similarly, specialist community therapists can continue to build on the progress made in inpatient settings and enable clients to adapt to the reduction in structure and support that was present in hospital.

## Engagement and therapeutic relationship

As previously outlined, the majority of people with eating disorders are ambivalent about recovery from the illness. Individuals strive to achieve and maintain low weight and value their control over food. Consequently, the illness can be deemed by many to be 'egosyntonic', a term indicating that the behaviours of the eating disorder are consistent with the individual's own personal values (Vitousek et al. 1998). It may additionally be serving a purpose, including regulating emotions, providing comfort or it can represent familiarity and safety. Thus, a person may have great difficulty committing to making changes in eating-related behaviours. Additionally, health staff may recognise that their goals of supporting a person are in conflict with the individual's goals to lose weight (Wright & Hacking 2012). These factors can make it difficult for a person to engage in active treatment and to build a relationship with health staff. Therefore, an individual's motivation for recovery and the therapeutic relationship need careful attention during the interactions and interventions.

In considering a person's motivation for change, Prochaska and DiClemente's transtheoretical model (1984) forms a useful foundation for discussing how an individual evaluates their own motivation. It enables the person to identify what 'stage' of change they are at and how ready they feel to implement changes. This can help to normalise and verbalise ambivalence and enables both parties to commit to engaging in a collaborative therapeutic relationship. Addressing motivation is often an integral part of active treatments such as Cognitive Behavioural Therapy (CBT) (Fairburn 2008). Equally, interventions focusing on motivation without expecting or discussing change can be used when individuals are unable to make progress with active treatment. In following a motivational approach it can be particularly challenging for the therapist to maintain a 'neutral stance' regarding an individual's intention to change. As those with eating disorders are often keen to please others, they can often verbally agree to change or embark on a treatment programme without truly intending to alter their behaviour. Waller (2012) highlighted that the evidence for the use of such motivation based interventions is limited. However, Jakubowska *et al.* (2013) identified that over 40 per cent of those who engaged in 'contemplation' groups subsequently undertook change-oriented interventions. In my experience such programmes have been helpful in enabling clients to reflect on pertinent issues such as the role of the eating disorder and its effect on relationships, future goals and values. Such reflections can assist the individual and team to make decisions about the most effective pathway of care. These topics are additionally highly relevant to the occupational therapy process and can facilitate exploration and identification of goals for treatment.

The issues of engagement and motivation are complex when working with individuals with eating disorders. For example, Waller (2015) outlined that therapists can often be scared to use treatment strategies that patients report disliking, e.g. weighing, body image work, supporting a client to eat challenging foods. As an occupational therapist with an embedded client-centred philosophy, this was one of the things I found challenging in working with this client group. I reflected that it was my role to support the part of the person that wished to be healthy rather than the unhealthy part. My experience was that in the short term this occasionally caused difficulties in therapeutic relationships, for example, if I was sticking to boundaries to ensure an individual used adequate food portion sizes during meal preparation or if I highlighted eating disorder behaviours at the table. However, in the longer term I considered that clients would trust that I would maintain consistency and would not collude with their eating disorder. Further challenges regarding engagement are presented when an individual lacks capacity to make healthy decisions as a consequence of their eating disorder (Tan *et al.* 2003b). As a consequence, individuals in inpatient treatment programmes who are particularly ill need to assume responsibility for their own food intake in a very gradual

**261**

manner. The occupational therapist can be invaluable in structuring the inpatient programme to support successful graded self-management. For example, the occupational therapist may initially identify that a person is ready to participate in some group food preparation and to eat snacks out in the community. Later they may progress to serve their own portions with supervision and ultimately may be able to eat unsupervised.

# Occupational therapy assessment

The assessment of an individual is very dependent on the timing and context of the assessment. In certain settings, the occupational therapist may be one of the first mental health professionals to meet with the individual. If this is the case, the therapist will wish to form the foundation of a collaborative relationship with the person and to assess the nature and severity of the eating disorder to manage risk and inform treatment decisions (Fairburn 2008, Palmer 2000).

The approach to assessment will also vary throughout the illness. For example, if the person's health is stable the therapist may wish to conduct a broad top-down assessment such as the Occupational Circumstances Assessment and Interview Rating Scale (OCAIRS) (Forsyth et al. 2005), spending time understanding the person's current roles, habits and hopes for the future. In contrast, if the individual is deteriorating, relapsing or recently discharged from a specialist treatment programme it may be beneficial to focus particularly on eating and meal preparation skills. In the case of individuals recently discharged from hospital, the therapist will wish to capitalise on the momentum gained in treatment as people often deteriorate on return to the less structured home environment.

In an inpatient setting the occupational therapist will have many opportunities to assess the individual. The assessment will be guided by a person's physical health, progress with weight restoration and proximity to discharge. The therapist may conduct a holistic assessment or focus on specific skills and goals, particularly food preparation, in order to make the best use of the limited time available. Further assessments may be conducted to determine if a client is suitable for a particular group or aspect of the treatment programme.

Occupational therapy assessment can be a particularly valuable process in engaging and motivating clients with eating disorders. The therapist is in a privileged position to be able to address functional goals, particularly when other clinicians may be focusing on physical parameters, risk and dietary intake. In my clinical practice I have used occupational therapy assessments as engagement tools and outcome measures when commencing generic interventions such as CBT. Clients have reported finding it beneficial to consider the ways in which their eating disorder impacts on their daily lives and to identify the goals they wish to achieve through treatment. In a similar manner the therapist can use the assessment process to explore with the client not only their ability to engage in a chosen activity but additionally their motivation for doing so (Abeydeera et al. 2006). This can be particularly prudent when considering physically exerting activities as decisions to engage can often be driven by a person's eating disorder. In this manner the assessment can enable the client and therapist to formulate the individual's occupational participation based on an understanding of personal preferences and eating disorder patterns.

In assessing an individual's food preparation ability, a therapist can use a combination of interview, formal assessment and observation. In a hospital setting there are many occasions to observe a person eating and handling food. It can be useful for the occupational therapist to observe meal times on a regular basis, such as one meal and one snack per week. It is often effective to engage an individual in food preparation at a reasonably early stage in treatment, providing an opportunity to assess their ability to choose food, select adequate portions and manage food appropriately, for example spreading butter on bread. This can be a useful overall assessment of how well an individual is progressing and can provide effective information for the whole clinical team. Collaborative goal setting can be achieved through discussion to identify the type of food an individual needs and wishes to prepare. It can be particularly useful to enquire about an individual's 'goal meal' – one that they previously enjoyed but which contains a number of foods that are feared or forbidden. The therapist can subsequently grade preparation, gradually introducing elements of the goal meal into successive cooking sessions. A formal assessment, such as the Eating and Meal Preparation Skills Assessment (EMPSA) (Lock *et al.* 2012), identifies the particular aspects of meal preparation that a person finds challenging and additionally measures their motivation for performing the required skill. In a similar way a therapist can assess further food-related tasks including food shopping and social eating. The combined approaches to assessment enable collaborative goal setting and outcome measurement.

## Box 16.3: Case study by Lucy Johnson – 'Charlotte'

### General history

Charlotte is a 20-year-old female with a longstanding history of anorexia nervosa and several inpatient admissions to both adult and Child and Adolescent Mental Health Services (CAMHS) units. She has a history of self-harm, and professionals are questioning whether she has borderline personality disorder. She has been studying for her A-Levels for four years as a result of frequent inpatient admissions which have interrupted her studies. When Charlotte has been ill, her family have attended her CPA meetings and engaged in family therapy sessions. She is, however, wanting to go to university to study medicine. On admission to the inpatient unit her BMI was 12.

### Formulation

Maintaining factors:

- No responsibility when ill – hasn't moved out of home or finished A-levels.
- Feels safe in hospital, as this is more familiar or 'known' than being in the outside world where she feels out of her comfort zone and anxious.
- Co-dependence with mum – illness keeps them both together?

Predisposing factors:

- Long history of eating disorder.
- Parents' divorce when young – lots of arguments, loss of nuclear family base.
- Mum's own mental health problems and how this impacts on Charlotte – Charlotte caring for mum and siblings when mum was ill but mum caring for her when she became ill with eating disorder.

Precipitating factors:

- Having to think about the future – applying for university, finishing college, achieving grades, leaving mum, moving out, etc.
- Pressure around exams – has already had to re-sit, and younger sister is now applying for university too – feelings of failure for not already being at university.

## Occupational therapy process

Upon admission, an occupational therapy assessment based on the Model of Human Occupation (MOHO) (Kielhofner 2008) was completed. This is because the MOHO has a practical approach and focuses on behaviour, which is an integral part of an eating disorder. In Charlotte's case it was particularly suitable and useful around the work that was done regarding her overcoming ingrained behaviours around food. This looks at skills, environment (home and location), motivation for daily occupations, her mood and the impact it has on her functioning, and at future hopes/aspirations.

The Occupational Self-Assessment (OSA) (Baron et al. 2002) was completed around admission to establish a baseline of level of functioning. The OSA is a self-rating assessment that looks at values and competence in terms of a wide range of occupations. It covers self-care ('taking care of myself'), productivity ('getting done what I need to do') and leisure ('relaxing and enjoying myself'). Areas for change are then identified and then therapy goals are completed based on these, which forms the basis of the occupational therapy interventions. The OSA is particularly helpful as it is client-centred and allows collaborative working. These features are of particular importance when working in eating disorders as the OSA facilitates 'doing with' the client rather than 'doing to' the client.

Goals were also formulated with Charlotte on what she would like to change. Intervention was designed, which was based on the goals, in the form of one to one occupational therapy. Charlotte chose 'expressing self to others', 'doing what I like', 'relaxing and enjoying myself', and 'having a satisfying routine' as the goals to address as a priority.

The Eating and Meal Preparation Skills Assessment (EMPSA) (Lock et al. 2012) was chosen to assess Charlotte's abilities to prepare a meal. She prepared a sandwich for herself and the EMPSA highlighted difficulties around (a) using the correct amounts as outlined in the dietitian-approved recipe; and (b) making a decision regards what to make.

With these skill deficits identified, the occupational therapist worked with Charlotte to formulate new goals to address/challenge these difficulties. The nursing staff were able to assist in carrying out some of the intervention objectives/tasks with Charlotte: graded meal preparation at the hospital followed by her beginning to prepare meals for her family using recipes from the hospital.

Charlotte began a ten-week occupational therapy-led meals out-patient programme focusing on meal preparation, and on eating in the community setting. The first snack in the community was assessed by the occupational therapist, and Charlotte struggled to have a hot chocolate. The assessment was an observational assessment created by the occupational therapist for that particular unit; it used elements of activity analysis, e.g. rating Charlotte's ability to look at the menu options, make a decision, complete the snack, manage emotions/feelings in relation to being in public/away from the safety of the unit, engage in conversation, etc. The assessment has a rating scale which is helpful in determining the amount of support a person needs and also provides numeric data which demonstrates progress from initial assessment to re-assessment (thus an outcome measurement is given).

This was reviewed by Charlotte and the occupational therapist and new goals/objectives were set where Charlotte would challenge herself to have something to eat. The goal was graded by looking at what Charlotte used to enjoy eating and starting with those foods. The ongoing assessment highlighted difficulties around decision making and being able to eat without having prompting/reassurance from staff. Several sessions later, the occupational therapist noted that Charlotte was able to choose a cookie but appeared very anxious about this, trying to use her phone to calculate the calories, and breaking the cookie into tiny pieces before eating it. Also, she asked to leave as soon as she had finished despite the occupational therapist still having half a cup of tea left.

The occupational therapist continued to work with Charlotte by making regular reviews of progress with her, allowing Charlotte to have control of the pace of progress. In time, Charlotte becomes more confident in decision making, is able to eat a cookie in a more appropriate manner, and is able to sit at the table having completed the snack to chat. Further progress is then made on decision making and challenging herself to eat foods which she particularly fears ('fear foods') such as pasta.

Charlotte also practises buying a snack on her own and bringing it back to the unit, where the 'safety net' of staff checking her snack is suitable allows her to practise taking responsibility. She eventually progresses to having a snack out on her own and is able to practise this when she has to get a train to go on home leave.

Alongside the food-related goals, the occupational therapist works with Charlotte on assertiveness and social skills so that she is able to communicate her needs more effectively, rather than using her eating disorder to express her distress at different situations, i.e. her parents' divorce, the stress of exams, and her feelings of uncertainty about her future.

Regarding self-harm, the occupational therapist and Charlotte worked together on seeking alternative methods of managing emotions. This became particularly relevant when a discharge date was mentioned at a CPA, following which Charlotte's mood and weight declined. She began restricting her food intake and hiding food when at the table. She eventually admitted that she had been having doubts about studying medicine but felt unsure about how to broach this with her parents. The occupational therapist explored her options with Charlotte who concluded that she didn't want to study medicine as this was her parents' expectation rather than her own. The occupational therapist supported Charlotte in deciding on and pursuing the application process for a biology degree instead. Once Charlotte had informed her parents of her decision, she appeared more settled in mood, with a reduction in self-harming and eating disordered behaviours being noted. This allowed her to re-engage with the therapeutic programme and to work towards a discharge date.

The discharge planning included the use of a Wellness Recovery Action Plan (WRAP) (Copeland 2016) which helped Charlotte to anticipate what would keep her well. In addition, it helped her to identify what her triggers were and plan how she would manage these.

At this stage, an Interests Checklist (Heaseman & Salhotra 2008) is carried out to establish what Charlotte's interests are and a Leisure Motivation Scale (Beard & Ragheb 1983) to look at what motivates her in terms of leisure occupations. Both assessments are useful in that they can be completed by the client with the therapist present, allowing them to take ownership of this. The Interest Checklist is useful because it provides a wide range of activities, but also looks at participation in past, present or future, which allows the therapist to establish a history of the changes in Charlotte's participation and what the reasons for these were.

From this, Charlotte is encouraged to re-connect with previous leisure occupations (painting) and try new activities (crochet and yoga). Occupational balance is considered in anticipation of the forthcoming demands of college/job along with self-care and leisure in Charlotte's life. Prior to discharge, Charlotte and the occupational therapist formulate a timetable for her to follow which incorporates all these elements.

A discharge OSA is completed and compared with the admission OSA. When used in this way, with a 'before' and an 'after' assessment, a tool such as the OSA can measure clinical outcomes. The OSA lends itself to this because it is quantifiable. Charlotte was able to acknowledge in the face of the OSA giving her concrete evidence that she had made a lot of progress, and she also acknowledged there was still room for further changes.

Charlotte was discharged after nine months with a BMI of 18.

Case study written by Lucy Johnson

# Treatment and intervention

Within my posts in both community and specialist inpatient eating disorders services I have provided interventions specific to occupational therapy and also treatments that can be delivered by a variety of health professionals. In the following sections I will discuss specific occupational therapy interventions and also generic evidence-based eating disorder treatments. I will highlight the aspects of generic treatments which render them particularly suitable to the skills of an occupational therapist.

# Specific occupational therapy interventions

The principle of using meaningful occupation to support recovery from an eating disorder is explored by Clark and Nayar (2012). The authors identify that the mechanism of recovery includes improving individuals' self-esteem through facilitating successful engagement in chosen activities. Through progressive development of skills and competence, individuals can improve their ability to care for themselves and to work towards meaningful life goals. Additionally, achievement of goals such as employment can often serve as both a motivator for individuals to improve or maintain their physical health and as a focus to reduce the importance of weight and shape (Abeydeera et al. 2006).

Occupational therapy interventions can address occupational performance directly, through engaging in specific activities such as cooking or indirectly through improving performance components, for example, cognitive and behavioural skills to manage anxiety. Furthermore, therapeutic activity can be used as a means to improve performance components. Depending on the setting and the needs of the client group, including their stage of treatment and recovery, a therapist may provide treatment in either a group or individual setting. For example, social eating or food preparation may be conducted on a one-to-one basis initially and graded to become a group activity.

Direct interventions include addressing food-related occupations, personal care activities related to body image, vocational, leisure and creative activities (Seymour 2015). Box 16.4 provides a sample of interventions that can be provided.

Box 16.4: Sample community occupational therapy interventions in key occupational performance areas

### 1. Self-care

Centred around supporting people to be able to eat at home alone or with their families, and in the community. It also has included helping people to manage their body image difficulties when clothes shopping. It has involved:

- Enabling people to plan healthy meals, shop for food, cook meals in their own homes and then be able to eat them
- Working with carers and families in the home environment to eat together

**267**

- Supporting people to eat in community facilities
- Budgeting skills
- Clothes shopping/sizing
- Facilitation identification of appropriate accommodation
- Liaising with support workers in supported housing services.

## 2. Productivity

Helping people to make decisions about their future and take the necessary steps towards employment or education and includes:

- Supporting people to attend open evenings at colleges
- Referrals to career advisers
- CV writing
- Support in accessing voluntary work
- Liaising with employers and providing support in returning to work
- Problem-solving regarding work issues.

## 3. Leisure

- Supporting people to access community resources, discover hobbies, interests and reduce social isolation
- Exploring past interests and potential new ones
- Accompanying people to sports venues
- Supporting people to enrol on courses.

## Food preparation interventions

Lock et al. (2012) described a group meal preparation intervention in which participants planned and prepared a selection of individualised, affordable and culturally appropriate meals over a minimum of ten sessions. The data from the study concluded that the intervention was effective in improving individuals' ability and motivation in the skills required for meal preparation. Personal experience reflects similar outcomes as a result of food preparation interventions. The authors of the study describe how group members were supported to follow healthy boundaries, including incorporating adequate food portions and completing food in an allotted period of time (Lock et al. 2012). Strategies such as challenging distorted cognitions were utilised to manage individuals' difficulties.

Personal experience in clinical work has shown that by providing information and guidance, including food portion guidelines and direction regarding cooking skills, a therapist can act as a role model to clients during food preparation and social eating. This can involve freely measuring rather than weighing food items, adding foodstuffs high in calories or fat, eating at a normal pace and ordering foods they enjoy in social settings. As with any other therapeutic activity, the client is encouraged to become more independent over time and to use available resources to support their decisions. A clear example of this can be when the person is repeatedly asking for information and reassurance regarding portion sizes. The therapist can facilitate the client to use the portion guidelines to guide these decisions, rather than relying on the therapist. In my experience it can be enjoyable to enable a person to prepare a meal that they have previously enjoyed and to eat it with them while engaging in normal, casual conversation. Such collaboration can also provide the person with experience dividing and portioning food and eating in front of others.

Social eating interventions provide individuals with an opportunity to eat in public, spend money on food, order items from a menu or counter and socialise with peers. It can often be helpful to reduce the focus on eating by incorporating other goals. For example, a craft group can be held in a coffee shop, enabling individuals to work on craft activities while consuming a snack.

## Creative activity

Abeydeera *et al.* (2006) describe using creative groups to enable participants to express themselves, socialise with others, solve problems and develop communication skills. Creative activity can also be used to support individuals to manage common traits that interfere with fulfilment of goals, for example perfectionism. Creating products that can be sold can improve individuals' self-esteem and engaging in projects (such as marketing goods or establishing a temporary shop for products) can develop complex skills.

# Occupational therapists delivering generic treatments

In addition to specific occupationally focused interventions, the therapist may collaborate with other professionals to deliver education and skills training such as communication and assertiveness, anxiety management including relaxation and interventions to manage body image distress within the therapeutic group programme.

Occupational therapists may also have an opportunity to provide formal evidence-based interventions. Within this section I will outline the main approaches to treatment that I have experience of and will highlight the ways in which they are aligned with core occupational therapy skills and approaches.

## Motivational interventions

Motivational Interviewing (MI) was initially developed for working with people with difficult to change behaviours (Treasure 2010). The use of motivational interviewing can be particularly useful with people with anorexia nervosa as these patients can be uncertain about change (Blake *et al.*

1997). Feld *et al.* (2001) found that through motivational interviewing, patients with eating disorders reported fewer depressive symptoms and increased self-esteem. In using this approach the therapist facilitates the client engaging in 'change talk' to discuss and consider the possibility of change. Treasure (2010) emphasised that this can lead to the person taking personal responsibility and experiencing mastery. Motivational interviewing techniques would include asking open ended questions, e.g. 'what will that achieve?', listening reflectively, or summarising what the person has said and affirming, finding something positive to say. It is particularly important that the therapist does not attempt to 'push' change on the person and has no expectations that they will decide to change but rather maintains a neutral stance and enables the individual to reach their own decisions.

People with anorexia may present as shy and inhibited and might therefore find the concept of motivational interviewing quite difficult so conversation may be somewhat slow (Treasure & Schmidt 2007). This means that the therapist needs to be flexible in their approach and consider other avenues of motivational interviewing. It is worth noting that motivational interviewing alone will not be effective in treating the eating disorder and other interventions such as CBT need to be used alongside this (Treasure & Schmidt 2007).

## Groupwork

In some ways, groupwork in eating disorders is similar to that of other mental health groups – for example, use of psycho-education groups. However, what makes these types of groups different is that there needs to be consideration of content and whether it is appropriate to discuss in an eating disorder setting, for example, being mindful when discussing food, weight, exercise or appearance and ensuring you are enabling the person rather than their eating disorder. Similarities to other mental health settings would be the need for ground rules, lack of motivation within the group and potentially sabotaging behaviours, e.g. sleeping, not engaging, etc.

Groups can be offered in different ways, with some specialist units offering a therapeutic programme at which attendance is compulsory, and with other units having a stepped programme with patients requiring assessment for suitability for particular groups or a 'sign up' process in place. The difficulty of compulsory attendance, based on the author's experience, is managing mixed stages of recovery within the group, which can be challenging with relapse prevention groups, for example. This can cause dynamics which are unhelpful to other members of the group and raises the question of whether compulsory attendance is of benefit for some people.

Groups to consider would include: relapse prevention, anxiety management, mindfulness, creative/art groups, body image, etc.

## Food- and eating-related interventions

As outlined earlier in the assessments section, there is a great deal of scope for occupational therapy input regarding eating and food related difficulties. As humans, being able to feed oneself and prepare meals is integral to survival, and when a person is unable to do this, whether this be due to a physical or cognitive impairment, it can cause a range of issues.

**270**

# Cognitive behavioural therapy for eating disorders

Enhanced Cognitive Behaviour Therapy for eating disorders – CBT-E (Fairburn 2008) (see Box 16.5) is the most evidence-based treatment for eating disorders (NICE 2004). Equally it has been used largely with those with bulimia rather than anorexia. While people with bulimia represent the majority of individuals with eating disorders, those who are likely to present to secondary and tertiary care services will be more likely to have a diagnosis of anorexia.

## Box 16.5: CBT-E main stages and principles

Enhanced cognitive behaviour therapy for eating disorders follows these main stages and principles:

- Initial engagement and formulation including motivational elements and therapeutic weighing
- Establishment of a regular eating routine
- Elimination of compensatory behaviours
- Increase in quantity of food eaten to restore weight (for those who are underweight). Individuals work towards a goal of restoring 0.5Kg per week
- Review of treatment after six sessions
- Following reasonable weight restoration, focus on body image tasks and goals.

Occupational therapy skills and therapeutic techniques are very well suited to many of the tasks of CBT-E. The therapist's skill in collaborating with the client to solve practical problems regarding eating regularly is particularly useful. Additionally, a main task of the treatment is to facilitate the client in expanding occupational roles and developing interests to reduce the focus on their shape and weight. In my experience supporting people to build a life can be key to progress and recovery. Further goals include inclusion of feared foods and the principle of grading can be beneficial. In contrast to other professionals the occupational therapist may practically support a client to include these foods and develop their skills in preparing and serving appropriate portions in collaboration with dietetic colleagues. In the advanced stages of treatment an occupational therapist can support a person to address body image difficulties (Seymour 2015). Again, it is most effective to work with an individual to set functional goals in relation to body image such as wearing particular clothes or using communal changing rooms.

# Dialectical Behaviour Therapy

Dialectical behaviour therapy is an intensive year-long treatment that was developed for individuals with severe difficulty regulating emotions who engaged in self-harming and suicidal behaviour (Linehan 1993). The principles of intervention involve replacing harmful ways of coping with more skilful approaches. Participants attend weekly groups to learn the skills and engage in individual sessions aimed at solving the problems that lead to harmful behaviours and urges. The therapist works with the client to identify which skills will be most effective in each individual situation. Thus, when working with individuals with eating disorders, behaviours including vomiting, laxative use, over-exercise and dietary restriction are monitored and alternative solutions to difficulties are generated. The pragmatic, problem-solving approach of an occupational therapist is particularly valuable in delivering this treatment. Lynch *et al.* (2013) described a 'radically open' DBT inpatient treatment approach for those with anorexia nervosa. This treatment encompassed many elements of core DBT and additional aspects to enable those who exhibit excessive control of their emotions to use more effective mechanisms of engaging and communicating with others.

## Acceptance and Commitment Therapy

Pronounced like the word 'act', Acceptance and Commitment Therapy (ACT) treatment is highly compatible with occupational therapy practice and philosophy. It utilises mindfulness strategies and facilitates achievement of valued goals. The treatment aims 'to create a rich, full and meaningful life while accepting the pain that inevitably goes with it' (Harris 2009, p. 7). In contrast to cognitive behavioural models the intervention does not seek to challenge or change thoughts or feelings. Instead it cultivates strategies to manage thoughts and feelings that arise and encourages individuals to commit to actions that are in line with values-driven goals. Psychologically, the therapist aims to increase the client's flexibility of thought and most importantly of behaviour. The emphasis therefore is not on the content of an unhelpful thought but rather on the extent to which the client is fused or attached to the thought. Heffner and Eifert (2004) developed a self-help workbook to enable individuals with anorexia nervosa to identify values and work towards goals through applying skills. Within my clinical practice I have found the ACT strategies to be helpful in enabling individuals to manage the distress associated with weight restoration and to continually recommit to engaging in healthy behaviours. Certain aspects of the intervention appear particularly acceptable to clients, including the frequent use of metaphors, the novel aspects of some of the skills and ideas and the straightforward nature of the approaches. For example, one suggestion to manage distressing thoughts is to sing them to a simple tune such as 'twinkle twinkle little star'. Such approaches provide amusement and can dissipate intense emotions experienced alongside distressing thoughts. Although this approach to working with individuals with eating disorders is relatively new, I have found it to be effective in engaging clients in treatment.

## Specialised supportive clinical management

It is recognised that anorexia is associated with frequent relapses (Strober *et al.* 1997) and that, in complex presentations, it can persist as a chronic illness (Wentz *et al.* 2009). Authors have identified that a proportion of sufferers develop a Severe and Enduring Eating Disorder (SEED) (Robinson 2009). Touyz and Hay (2015) advocate a staged model of the illness, highlighting that individuals be treated according to the duration and severity of the condition as well as their initial diagnosis. The authors further argue that clinicians should focus more on improving quality of life for individuals with Severe and Enduring Anorexia Nervosa (SE-AN) rather than exclusively aiming to alleviate symptoms. Interventions such as specialised supportive clinical management (SSCM) have been developed to work with this client population. Specialised supportive clinical management provides a structure to set goals in valued life domains alongside improving symptoms (McIntosh *et al.* 2010). Occupational therapists, being highly skilled at collaborative goal setting, are well suited to deliver such interventions. In my experience this principle of focusing on both a person's eating difficulties and their life goals alongside one another has been a helpful one to use with clients to maintain hope of recovery and support ongoing change.

# Reflection and final considerations

In my experience it has been extremely rewarding to work in this clinical area. It has equally been challenging at times, requiring patience, understanding and knowledge of each individual and of eating disorder features and presentations. Such challenges have provided an opportunity for extensive professional and personal development and enabled me to acquire a wide variety of skills, strategies and approaches to engage and motivate individuals and support them to overcome their difficulties and achieve their goals. Equally, when working with clients with eating disorders their progress can often be slow and limited and frequent relapses may be observed. This can impact on a therapist's confidence in their own professional ability. As with any clinical area it is vital to utilise clinical supervision to enable the therapist to reflect on interactions with clients, identify any personal or professional difficulties and work towards providing best practice. I have found it beneficial to utilise clinical supervision within the specialist field and also within occupational therapy structures. Collaboration and consultation with other occupational therapists working with individuals with eating disorders can be invaluable and enable sharing of innovative practice, development of new ideas and validation of progress and struggles. Occupational therapy special interest groups in eating disorders have been an extremely valuable resource to receive such support and have included local groups (Seymour 2015) and national eating disorders special interest study days (via the College of Occupational Therapists' Specialist Section in Mental Health – see www.cot.co.uk/cotss-mental-health/eating-disorders-forum).

# Useful resources

- BEAT-UK eating disorder charity. This has lots of useful information for professionals, families and people with eating disorders. https://b-eat.co.uk. *European Eating Disorders Review*, which is the professional journal of BEAT. Lots of up to date research on eating disorders. BEAT also runs a conference for professionals usually in March each year. Details can be found on the BEAT website.

- COT special interest group for eating disorders. Visit the COT website and Specialist Section Mental Health pages for more details. https://www.cot.co.uk/mental-health/mental-health

- http://www.hungertorecover.com – Useful American website with lots of helpful resources for people with eating disorders, family/friends and professionals. Includes blogs, poetry, recovery stories, ideas that can be used in groups and useful links.

- http://joyproject.org – Non-profit, grassroots project in America. Lots of helpful resources and ideas for groups with templates for worksheets, meal plans and tools for recovery.

- http://www.seedeatingdisorders.org.uk – UK-based charity set up by the parents of Gemma Oaten (former Emmerdale Actress) who is now the patron. Gemma suffered from an eating disorder for 13 years. The website has lots of resources ranging from drop-in sessions, information on nutrition, online workshops and blogs/inspirational stories. They are based in Hull.

- Pinterest: lots of helpful ideas for eating disorder recovery including group ideas, art projects, therapy and inspirational quotes. https://uk.pinterest.com/

- The internet is a very useful resource with a wealth of information available but networking with other professionals working in eating disorders, not just occupational therapists, is also highly beneficial.

# References

Abeydeera, K., Williams, S. & Forsyth K. (2006). Occupation focused assessment and intervention for clients with anorexia. *International Journal of Therapy and Rehabilitation* **13** (7), 296.

American Psychiatric Association (2013). *Diagnostic and Statistical Manual of Mental Disorders*, 5th edn. Washington DC: The APA.

Baron, K., Kielhofner, G., Iyenger, A., Goldhammer, V. & Wolenski, J. (2002). *The Occupational Self Assessment (OSA),* Version 2.0. Chicago: University of Illinois.

Beard, J.G. & Ragheb, M.G. (1983). Measuring leisure motivation. *Journal of Leisure Research* **15** (3), 219–228.

Birmingham, C., Su, J., Hlynsky, J., Goldner, E. & Gao, M. (2005). The mortality rate from anorexia nervosa. *International Journal of Eating Disorders* **38** (2), 143–146.

Blake, W., Turnbull, S. & Treasure, J.L. (1997). Stages and processes of change in eating disorders: implications for therapy. *Clinical Psychology & Psychotherapy* **4** (3), 186–191.

Braun, D.L., Sunday, S.R. & Halmi, K.A. (1994). Psychiatric comorbidity in patients with eating disorders. *Psychological Medicine* **24** (4), 859–867.

Clark, M. & Nayar, S. (2012). Recovery from eating disorders: a role for occupational therapy. *New Zealand Journal of Occupational Therapy* **59** (1), 13–17.

Copeland, M.E. (2016). *The Wellness Recovery Action Plan*. http://mentalhealthrecovery.com (last accessed: 11.2.2016).

Corstorphine, E. (2006). Cognitive-emotional-behavioural therapy for the eating disorders: working with beliefs about emotions. *European Eating Disorders Review* **14** (6), 448–461.

Costa, D.M. (2009). Eating disorders: occupational therapy's role. *OT Practice* **14** (11), 13–14.

Crisp, A. (2006). In defence of the concept of phobically driven avoidance of adult body weight/shape/function as the final common pathway to anorexia nervosa. *European Eating Disorders Review* **14** (3), 189–202.

Fairburn, C.G. (2008). *Cognitive Behaviour Therapy and Eating Disorders*. London: The Guilford Press.

Fairburn, C.G. (2013). *Overcoming Binge Eating,* 2nd edn. New York: The Guilford Press.

Feld, R., Woodside, R.D., Kaplan, A.S., Olmsted, M.P. & Carter, J.C. (2001). Pretreatment motivational enhancement therapy for eating disorders: a pilot study. *International Journal of Eating Disorders* **29** (4), 393–400.

Forsyth, K., Deshpande, S., Kielhofner, G., Henriksson, C., Haglund, L., Olson, L., Skinner, S. & Kulkarni S. (2005). *The Occupational Circumstances Assessment, Interview and Rating Scale (OCAIRS).* Chicago: Model of Human Occupation Clearing House, Department of Occupational Therapy, College of Applied Health Sciences, University of Illinois.

Geller, J., Drab, D.L. (1999). The Readiness and Motivation Interview: a symptom-specific measure of readiness to change in the eating disorders. *European Eating Disorders Review* **7** (4), 259–278.

Gogarty, O. & Brangan, J. (2004). The lived body experience of women with eating disorders: phenomenological study of the perceived impact of body image disturbance on occupational performance. *The Irish Journal of Occupational Therapy* **33** (2), 11–19.

Harris, R. (2009). *ACT made simple*. California: New Harbinger Publications.

Heaseman, D. & Salhotra, G. (2008). *Interest Checklist*. http://www.cade.uic.edu (last accessed: 9.2.2016).

Heffner, M. & Eifert, G.H. (2004). *The Anorexia Workbook: How to Accept Yourself, Heal Your Suffering, and Reclaim Your Life.* New Harbinger Publications: California.

Hoang, U., Goldacre, M.M. & James, A. (2014). Mortality following hospital discharge with a diagnosis of eating disorder: National Record Linkage Study, England, 2001–2009. *International Journal of Eating Disorders* **47** (5), 507–515.

Jakubowska, A., Woolgar, M., Haselton, P.A. & Jones, A. (2013). Review of staff and client experiences of a motivational group intervention: meeting the needs of contemplators. *Eating Disorders* **21** (1), 16–25.

Keys, A., Brožek, J., Henschel, A., Mickelsen, O. & Taylor, H. L. (1950). *The Biology of Human Starvation.* Minnesota: University of Minnesota Press.

Kielhofner, G. (2008). *Model of Human Occupation: Theory and Application,* 4th edn. Philadelphia: Lippincott, Williams and Wilkins.

Kielhofner, G., Mallinson, T., Crawford, C., Nowak, M., Rigby, M., Henry, A. & Walens, D. (2004). *The Occupational Performance History Interview-II (OPHI-II), Version 2.1.* Chicago: Model of Human Occupation Clearing House, Department of Occupational Therapy, College of Applied Health Sciences, University of Illinois.

Linehan, M.M. (1993). *Cognitive Behavioural Treatment of Borderline Personality Disorder.* New York: The Guilford Press.

Lock, L., Williams, H., Bamford, B. & Lacey, J.H. (2012). The St. George's eating disorders service meal preparation group for inpatients and day patients pursuing full recovery: a pilot study. *European Eating Disorders Review* **20** (3), 218–224.

Lock, L.C. & Pépin, G. (2011). 'Eating disorders' in: *Occupational Therapy in Mental Health; A Vision for Participation,* eds. C. Brown and V.C. Stoffel. Philadelphia: F.A. Davies.

Lynch, T.R., Gray, K.L.H., Hempel, R.J., Titley, M., Chen, E.Y. & O'Mahen, H.A. (2013). Radically open-dialectical behavior therapy for adult anorexia nervosa: feasibility and outcomes from an inpatient program. *BMC Psychiatry* **13**, 293.

McIntosh, V.V.W., Jordan, J. & Bulik, C.M. (2010). 'Specialist supportive clinical management for anorexia nervosa' in *The Treatment of Eating Disorders; A Clinical Handbook*, eds. C.M. Grilo and J.E. Mitchell. New York: Guilford.

Meyer, C., Taranis, L., Goodwin, H. & Haycraft, E. (2011). Compulsive exercise and eating disorders. *European Eating Disorders Review* **19** (3), 174–189.

Micali, N., Hagberg, K.W., Petersen, I. & Treasure, J.L. (2013). The incidence of eating disorders in the UK in 2000–2009: findings from the General Practice Research Database. *British Medical Journal: Open* **3** (5), doi: 10.1136/bmjopen-2013-002646.

Miller, K.K., Grinspoon, S.K., Ciampa, J., Hier, J., Herzog, D. & Klibanski, A. (2005). Medical findings in outpatients with anorexia nervosa. *Archives of International Medicine* **165** (5), 561–566.

National Institute for Clinical Excellence (2004). *Eating Disorders: Core Interventions in the Treatment and Management of Anorexia Nervosa, Bulimia Nervosa and Related Eating Disorders.* London: NICE.

Nicholls, D. (2013). *Towards a Stepped-Care Approach for Child and Adolescent Eating Disorders: The role of Early Intervention.* Dublin: European Society of Child & Adolescent Psychiatry.

Orchard, R. (2003). With you, not against you: applying motivational interviewing to occupational therapy in anorexia nervosa. *British Journal of Occupational Therapy* **66** (7), 325–327.

Padesky, C. (1993). *Socratic Questioning: Changing Minds or Guided Discovery?* Keynote address delivered at the European Congress of Behavioural and Cognitive Therapies.

Palmer, B. (2000). *Helping People with Eating Disorders: A Clinical Guide to Assessment and Treatment.* West Sussex: Wiley & Sons.

Pierce, W.D., Epling, W.F., Dews, P.B., Estes, W.K., Morse, W.H., Van-Orman, W. & Herrnstein, R.J. (1994). Activity anorexia: an interplay between basic and applied behavior analysis. *The Behavior Analyst* **17** (1), 7–23.

Pike, K.M., Hoek, H.W. & Dunne, P.E. (2014). Cultural trends and eating disorders. *Current Opinion in Psychiatry* **27** (6), 436–442.

Prochaska, J.O. & DiClemente, C.C. (1984). *The Transtheoretical Approach: Towards a Systematic Eclectic Framework.* Homewood, IL, USA: Dow Jones Irwin.

PwC (2015). *The Costs of Eating Disorders: Social, Health and Economic Impact.* London: BEAT.

Quiles-Cestari, L.M. & Ribeiro, R.P.P. (2012). The occupational roles of women with anorexia nervosa. *Latin American Journal of Nursing* **20** (2), 235–242.

Reas, D.L., Rø, Ø., Karterud, S., Hummelen, B. & Pedersen, G. (2013). Eating disorders in a large clinical sample of men and women with personality disorders. *International Journal of Eating Disorders* **46** (8), 801–809.

Robinson, P. (2009). *Severe and Enduring Eating Disorder (SEED): Management of Complex Presentations of Anorexia and Bulimia Nervosa.* Sussex: John Wiley and Sons.

Seymour, A. (2015). Integrated eating disorders services in Wales. *OT News* **23** (12), 38–39.

Singlehurst, H., Corr, S., Griffiths, S. & Beaulieu, K. (2007). The impact of binge eating disorder on occupation: a pilot study. *British Journal of Occupational Therapy* **70** (11), 493–501.

Strober, M., Freeman, R. & Morrell, W. (1997). The long-term course of severe anorexia nervosa in adolescents: survival analysis of recovery, relapse, and outcome predictors over 10–15 years in a prospective study. *International Journal of Eating Disorders* **22** (4), 339–360.

Tan, J., Hope, T. & Stewart, A. (2003a). Competence to refuse treatment in anorexia nervosa. *International Journal of Law and Psychiatry* **26** (6), 697–707.

Tan, J.O.A., Hope, T., Stewart, A. & Fitzpatrick, R. (2003b) Control and compulsory treatment in anorexia nervosa: the views of patients and parents. *International Journal of Law and Psychiatry* **26** (6), 627–645.

Touyz, S. & Hay, P. (2015). Severe and enduring anorexia nervosa (SE-AN): in search of a new paradigm. *Journal of Eating Disorders* **3**, 26 doi: 10.1186/s40337-015-0065-z

Townsend, E.A., & Polatajko, H.J. (2007). *Enabling Occupation II: Advancing an Occupational Therapy Vision for Health, Wellbeing, and Justice Through Occupation.* Ottawa, ON: CAOT Publications ACE.

Treasure, J. (2010). 'Understanding models of health behaviours and the processes used to facilitate change' in *The Clinician's Guide to Collaborative Caring in Eating Disorders*, eds. J. Treasure, U. Schmidt and P. Macdonald. London: Routledge UK.

Treasure. J, & Schmidt, U. (2007). 'Motivational interviewing in the management of eating disorders' in *Motivational Interviewing in the Treatment of Psychological Problems*, eds. H. Arkowitz, H.A. Westra, W.R. Miller, and S. Rollnick. London: The Guilford Press.

Vansteenkiste, M., Soenens, B. & Vandereycken, W. (2005). Motivation to change in eating disorder patients: a conceptual clarification on the basis of self-determination theory. *International Journal of Eating Disorders* **37** (3), 207–219.

Vitousek, K., Watson, S. & Wilson, G.T. (1998). Enhancing motivation for change in treatment-resistant eating disorders. *Clinical Psychology Review* **18** (4), 391–420.

Waller, G. (2012). The myths of motivation: time for a fresh look at some received wisdom in the eating disorders? *International Journal of Eating Disorders* **45** (1), 1–16.

Waller, G. (2015). *Exposure-based Treatment for Eating Disorders: Terrified Patients and Scared Clinicians,* 12th London International Eating Disorders Conference. London, 18th– 20th March 2015, Workshop Presentation.

Welsh Assembly Government (2009). *Eating Disorders – A Framework for Wales.* Cardiff: Welsh Assembly Government.

Wentz, E., Gillberg, I.C., Anckarsäter, H., Gillberg, C. & Råstam, M. (2009). Adolescent-onset anorexia nervosa: 18-year outcome. *British Journal of Psychiatry* **194** (2), 168–174.

Wright, K.M. & Hacking, S. (2012). An angel on my shoulder: a study of relationships between women with anorexia and healthcare professionals. *Journal of Psychiatric and Mental Health Nursing* **19** (2), 107–115.

# Chapter 17

# Occupational therapists as cognitive behaviour therapists

## Nick Dutton and Jane Clewes

### Introduction

This chapter offers the reader an insight into one way in which an occupational therapist can undertake a role using Cognitive Behaviour Therapy (CBT). It is not prescriptive; the use of CBT as a therapy or part of therapy can be delivered in various ways (such as within a skills training programme or as an underpinning approach by a team/ward). In this instance, Nick has become a cognitive behaviour therapist and lost the title of occupational therapist, though he uses transferable skills from his occupational therapy background.

## Key points

- Occupational therapists' unique skills in activity analysis bring this particularly useful expertise to the practice of CBT, such as when devising desensitisation hierarchies.
- Occupational therapists naturally ensure that the 'B' in 'CBT', the behavioural aspect, is considered, realising that it is key to the clinical outcomes.
- Those considering undertaking such a role might be wise to consider the political landscape and the demands of the training prior to embarking on a CBT role.

## Cognitive Behavioural Therapy

Occupational therapists understand the therapeutic power of 'doing'; they understand how this fits and interplays with 'being' and 'becoming' (Wilcock 1998). They are armed with a knowledge and appreciation of how habits and routines impact on a person's health and wellbeing, habits including, perhaps, the automatic habits of thinking patterns. Occupational therapists are well placed to use various techniques and tools (e.g. Platkin 2002) in their therapeutic practice towards enabling people to achieve change. It could be said that learning has occurred only when it can be demonstrated that a change has taken place. As shown in *Hartrampf's Vocabularies* (1935), 'change' is synonymous with:

'alter'; 'modify'; 'transform'; 'metamorphose'; 'shift'; and 'supersede'. This focus on activity, which occupational therapists utilise, equips them well for practising cognitive behavioural approaches, especially with those people who respond better to the 'B' in CBT (Cognitive Behavioural Therapy) than to the 'C'. Activity analysis skills enhance goal setting through assisting a clear understanding of the what (components) and why (purpose) of that goal, so that when the service user undertakes (does) the goal it is likely to be more 'near the target' (see Paley *et al.* 2006).

With this in mind, occupational therapists can put these strengths forward when seeking to take up opportunities such as a post as a cognitive behavioural therapist or a therapist working in an Improvinging Access to Psychological Therapies (IAPT) service (see Chapter 18). It is noted that there are formalities around the terminology used when describing what a therapist is using in their practice, and that it may be prudent to beware of adopting a title or description of what you are doing as being CBT unless there is a suitable training course completed or qualification attained. Nevertheless, occupational therapists have been using ideas from cognitive and behavioural approaches and theories for decades albeit having been described with different wording.

## The Cognitive Behavioural Therapist

Nick Dutton is an occupational therapist who has gone on to become qualified in CBT and then moved into a specific cognitive behavioural therapist post in secondary mental healthcare. His post sits within the directorate for psychological services and his title is cognitive behavioural therapist. The post requires a mental health clinician with professional registration (a social worker; a clinical psychologist; a mental health nurse; a psychiatrist; or an occupational therapist). He mainly provides one-to-one therapy though could be called on to lead some groupwork or assist colleagues within the psychological service to deliver groupwork. Posts such as this, in other secondary healthcare organisations, are likely to be arranged within the hierarchical structure in various ways. For Nick's work, he receives referrals which have already been screened by a consultant psychologist who, through the screening process, has identified Nick as being the suitably skilled and suitable match of person for that service user. For example, Nick has a special interest in psychosis and has a background of having undertaken studies of and experience of clinical practice with psychosis. Also, he is male, has a practical and applied approach and is able to augment the core CBT work with bespoke interventions.

## What the work entails

Nick tends to work with an individual for up to 20 sessions (or for those where there are particular reasons, such as difficulty engaging, or who have symptoms such as from a psychosis causing distraction, up to 25). He has an initial meeting appointment with the person where he ascertains their readiness and motivation level for engaging with the CBT. If there is agreement to go ahead, then the sessions commence and a review date, such as at ten weeks into the therapy, is set. Depending on the findings from the initial appointment, an initial offer of, say, up to ten sessions might be made, and then at a review towards the end of that a further offer might be made for another period. Nick's referrals are people who are care clustered at four or above, and these groups of people are likely to require the longer courses (of approximately 20 sessions) than those who attend CBT services in primary care settings. The nature of CBT involves a range of specific thinking and questioning techniques and tools for change; therefore, once the person has learned the theory of it, they are then able to use the information themselves; 20 weeks should be more than enough to understand and use the information and so further sessions are not offered. It might be that at a later period, if the person is struggling, a 'refresher' or 'top up' might be offered (there is evidence that, particularly with psychosis, repeated episodes of therapy – even if per episode only moderately successful – can prime someone to benefit eventually).

As with many talking/psychological therapy services, there is a huge non-attendance ('did not attend', DNA) problem. Nick offers up to four appointments within one working day, and on average will have at least one of the four DNA or cancel. For those who repeatedly DNA, they are asked to return at a later date if and when they feel able to engage better; they might be told that their poor attendance is a sign that they are 'not ready'. Nick would not recommend CBT during times of crisis, but does recommend that soon after a time of crisis is a good opportunity to engage in CBT as the recall of the crisis is fresh and can enhance the undertaking of reflection on the material from the crisis to good effect.

## Box 17.1: Case study – Katherine

### Background

Katherine, aged 50, always considered herself to be a worrier but her level of worry became acute and excessive following an ear infection and associated balance problems. Psychological interventions were tried unsuccessfully and an admission to psychiatric hospital proved traumatic and compounded the problem. Already suffering with fibromyalgia, she felt she had no option but to leave her job in nursing.

Four years later, chronically anxious, low in mood, desperate to get better but sceptical about both medication and talking therapies, Katherine was referred for CBT. She had been assessed for CBT early in her illness but had not been ready to commit at that stage.

### Assessment

Katherine identified her main problem as being excessive worry over many issues, with key themes being health (physical and mental), work and relationships with other members of the family. A second problem was low mood associated with the negative conclusions reached from ruminating on problems (past and present) and predicting further, insoluble, problems in the future. After an initial education session on excessive worry and the CBT approach she consented to an intervention aimed at addressing the maintaining factors, to be followed by work on low mood.

## Intervention

In the first phase of the intervention Katherine and her therapist mapped out in some detail what happened when she worried. Katherine recognised that some level of worry is absolutely normal but that in her case it had got out of control and was dominating her life. The aim was to reduce her worry to a level that was normal and acceptable for her by working on her thinking and behaviour.

One of the things that stood out when Katherine's pattern of worrying was examined was her difficulty coping with any kind of uncertainty. She went to great lengths to try to control the outcome of all situations by taking excessive responsibility. For Katherine worry had the function of making things certain because of its quality of covering all possible outcomes (though mostly negative ones). In therapy Katherine made two important discoveries: first that it is never possible to be completely certain, no matter how hard we try, and secondly that inability to cope with uncertainty is the fuel which worry needs in order to get completely out of hand. From this she appreciated the need to learn to live with uncertainty via a series of 'uncertainty experiments'. Starting with modest tasks (such as going out for a meal without researching the menu in advance), she completed increasingly challenging ones over time (eventually being able to go away on holiday instead of insisting on never being away from home because of her belief that she could not sleep without having blackout curtains). At first she experienced a lot of internal anxiety but noticed that the more experiments she completed, the more natural she felt.

Whilst continuing and pushing uncertainty experiments, Katherine began to evaluate problem solving as an alternative to worry for 'here and now' concerns. Her skill level and confidence in this area had historically been good, if rather neglected during her illness. In the sessions Katherine's method of problem solving closely matched a 'textbook' version; in between-session homework she successfully applied this method to current issues and went on to combine problem solving and uncertainty experiments in other tasks.

For much of the time that Katherine was working on worry she also kept a 'positive data log' which regularly showed that some positive things were happening in her life but were previously overpowered by negative thinking and therefore discounted. Listing positive events made it far more difficult to discount them and provided robust evidence in the next phase of the work.

Over a period of weeks Katherine learned to identify when she was thinking negatively; then, instead of uncritically accepting the thoughts as true, to step back from them and scrutinise them. She often found that the evidence (including that from the positive data logs) not only failed to support the negative thoughts but also often undermined them. This allowed Katherine to create alternative 'balanced' thoughts which not only fitted the facts better but were also much more helpful for her. She was then able to take action to show which of the competing thoughts was nearer to the truth – for instance contacting her daughter, from whom she had heard nothing for a period of time, to test whether she had caused her daughter offence in some way or whether there was a less charged explanation, such as the daughter being busy, preoccupied, etc.

From this Katherine went on to challenge some longstanding negative beliefs about herself and the 'rules' she had formulated in an attempt to compensate for them. One key area she looked at was her drive to be a high achiever in her career in order to compensate for her belief that she was 'useless'. Once again, using robust evidence, she was able to form a more balanced and helpful view of herself and introduce some flexibility into her 'rules'.

Throughout the course of CBT Katherine had been setting herself increasingly complex goals (including resuming going to family gatherings and football matches and to resume driving) and by the end she was combining this with all the other major strands of her CBT work (tolerating uncertainty, challenging negative thoughts and having more flexible 'rules') to investigate the possibility of a return to some kind of caring role.

At the end of therapy Katherine produced a personalised staying well plan and attended three 'top-up' sessions before being discharged. Six months post-therapy she reported continued improvement despite having experienced negative life events such as bereavement.

Created by Nick Dutton (anonymised) 2015.

## The CBT training course

The opportunity to undertake the post-graduate diploma in CBT with complex conditions (PG-Dip) came when Nick's employing Trust had made a one-off arrangement with a local university to train a number of the Trust clinicians as the Trust wanted to improve and expand the CBT availability within the service. He had to attend an interview to be sent on to the training course. This selection process included his having to carry out a blind, time limited appraisal and answer written questions on a research study journal article; then he had a short interview and a role play where he had to play the therapist role.

The course lasted for 18 months and comprised three parts. There was formal teaching one day per week. One day a week there was role play around a specific technique or tool that was being learned; they used video playback to constructively criticise their performance. A small CBT caseload was required, and the supervision sessions which took place for this comprised part of the assessment towards the final pass. Throughout the course were a number of written assignments too; these were mainly case studies to be presented with a cognitive-behavioural explanation of the formulation, and to be underpinned with supporting evidence. Essays also included something on research techniques and adapting CBT to suit other cultures. Further assessment was through compiling tapes of sessions with people on the caseload, and being observed in set role plays. Both the practical and academic sides of the assessments had to be satisfactory before a pass was awarded. To embark on such a course should not, Nick says, be done without serious commitment as it is time and energy demanding; the heavy load of coursework takes over your weekends and evenings. However, such opportunities (to get funded training with at least *some* study time out) do not arise every day!

## Using occupational therapy skills in the role of cognitive behavioural therapist

Nick is of the opinion that the transferable skills which he uses are those core skills from occupational therapy, some of which are commensurate with those from other mental healthcare disciplines, such as being able to talk to people and having a thorough knowledge base. He finds the occupational therapy unique skill of activity analysis to be of great help with the devising of hierarchies. He finds that he is good at averting the avoidance mechanism of intellectualising; he focuses on the behavioural elements (such as the technique in CBT of devising and carrying out 'behavioural experiments'). The pragmatic approach of the occupational therapist ensures a realistic approach to writing a hierarchy which offers some achievable progress which in turn helps to motivate the person further to continue. Also, occupational therapists' problem solving expertise is usefully and frequently employed in the role, where the therapist gets the service user to undertake the problem solving themselves, rather than supply the solutions to them without the tool to seek answers themselves.

## Some advantages and disadvantages to consider

Nick is aware of some 'political' issues: for the non-psychologist practitioner, a post within a psychological services department as a cognitive behavioural therapist is viewed by managers who are clinical psychologists as 'uni-modal', considering the clinical psychologist as being 'multi-modal'. This can support the idea that practitioners in such posts as cognitive behavioural therapists, who are from disciplines other than clinical psychology, are not sufficiently skilled to be considered for advancement to higher graded posts. Systems such as having all referrals screened by someone other than oneself can also disempower a practitioner, and conversely might be given as reasons for supporting continued need for higher grades to carry out the screening, if presented convincingly. This is a strong example of a 'glass ceiling'.

Nick, however, is at a stage of his career where he prefers to focus on being a therapist with service users. When he first entered healthcare his intention was to help people with mental health problems through therapeutic interventions. Whilst his personal philosophy is very much that of an occupational therapist, his preferred role is one where he can provide the talking therapies. Having been a care coordinator before undertaking the CBT training, he appreciates the pressures of holding a massive caseload where less of the job is about delivering the actual interventions. Nick's prior roles have also included provision of a range of groupwork to acute mental health wards, and he has also trained in and delivered behavioural family therapy.

# Advice for those interested in CBT roles

It is advisable not begin a CBT diploma course without having first undertaken a good preparatory amount of study. Nick had done a number of short CBT courses as well as some self-directed study. He had already begun to specialise in CBT with psychosis even before starting the PG-Dip. This gave him a reasonable preparation as well as having a good idea of what the approach was. He suggests that experience such as his where he worked in acute psychiatry, leading groupwork and various therapies, built his skills in delivering therapies. There are a number of basic guides to CBT which offer a suitable overview to someone before they commit to going ahead with training. Within his initial cohort, Nick noted that about half of the intake had left or dropped out or failed the academic standard.

In addition, Nick urges other occupational therapists to be sure to consider their future career for steps available to them later on. It may be difficult to return to being an occupational therapist after a long time out being a cognitive behavioural therapist; although, having said that, the role of cognitive behavioural therapist in secondary care is undoubtedly different from that within primary care settings. The throughput in secondary services is slower and the cases are more complex, which offers the practitioner an opportunity to stray from the basic manual of CBT and augment the intervention with other similarly practical approaches borrowed from, for example, solution-focused therapy.

If you wish to register with the British Association for Behavioural and Cognitive Psychotherapies (BABCP), make sure that the CBT course you embark on is recognised by them as suitable for accepting you as a registrant.

# Useful resources

- http://www.babcp.com
- Practical guides to how to change habits and routines, e.g. Platkin, C.S. (2002). *Breaking the Pattern: The 5 Principles you need to Remodel your Life.* New York City: Red Mill Press.
- Resources from Dr Chris Williams such as workbooks (e.g. Williams, C. (2001). *Overcoming Depression – a Five Areas Approach.* New York: Hodder Arnold, Oxford University Press) and websites (e.g. http://www.live-lifewell. net/wp-content/uploads/2012/04/understanding-depression-workbook1.pdf;

# References

Hartrampf, G.A. (1935). *Hartrampf's Vocabularies: Synonyms, Antonyms, Relatives,* 6th British edn. Manchester: Psychology Publishing Company.

Paley, J., Eva, G. & Duncan, E.A.S. (2006). In-order-to analysis: an alternative to classifying different levels of occupational activity. *British Journal of Occupational Therapy* **69** (4), 161–168.

Platkin, C.S. (2002). *Breaking the Pattern: the 5 Principles you need to Remodel your Life.* New York City: Red Mill Press.

Wilcock, A.A. (1998). *An Occupational Perspective on Health.* Thorofare, NJ: Slack.

# Chapter 18

# Improving access to psychological therapies

Annoula Raptis

## Introduction

This chapter provides an overview of the work of the Psychological Mental Health Practitioner (PMHP) within an Improving Access to Psychological Therapies (IAPT) service. Personal experience is used to give the reader insights into the work and the challenges of the role.

## Key points

- The IAPT services provide part of the stepped model for mental health care, often providing short courses of brief therapies in a primary care setting.
- The role is usually as a generic therapist using a CBT approach, and can be quite prescribed with limited time slots and target-driven.
- The occupational therapist brings many core skills which are easily transferable to the role.

## Improving Access to Psychological Therapies services

The white paper *Our Health, Our Care, Our Say* (DoH 2006), a government led initiative, set out to achieve four main goals: provide better prevention services with earlier intervention; provide more choice and a louder voice; to do more on tackling inequalities and improving access to community services; and offer more support for people with long-term needs. Lord Layard's report (London School of Economics 2006) argued for the provision of psychological therapies to be made easily accessible to everyone in Britain, with the aim of this feeding back into the economy as people return to work. Improving Access to Psychological Therapies (IAPT) took precedence, with the objective of reducing the impact that mental illness has on the economy. Marzillier and Hall (2009b) challenged the Layard initiative, highlighting his economic analysis as flawed and problematic. They discuss the importance of stepping away from a 'simplistic illness model', acknowledging how anxiety and depression are part of the human condition that is exacerbated by social and economic factors, not necessarily a pathological illness or a fault in the individual that needs to be 'cured' with psychological therapies (Marzillier & Hall 2009b).

In the early stages of the IAPT service development, two demonstration sites were set up to collate evidence in order to establish its effectiveness and lead the way forward for the expansion of further IAPT services to be developed nationally. The IAPT 3-year report, *The First Million Patients* (DoH 2012) provided evidence of the successes and achievement of the IAPT service to date and the objectives and progression for the future vision of IAPT.

The IAPT service is a stepped-care model approach (NIMH 2006); it was set up to provide evidence-based psychological therapies as approved by the National Institute for Health and Care Excellence (NICE) guidelines for people with depression and anxiety disorders (Clark *et al.* 2009, London School of Economics 2006). There has been a greater emphasis on Cognitive Behavioural Therapy (CBT) providing the core treatment intervention with evidence indicating that it is as effective as medication and better at preventing relapse (Butler *et al.* 2006). The dominance of the CBT paradigm within the IAPT service has provoked much debate on the delivery of evidence-based treatments (Casement 2009, Rizq 2012). Rizq (2013) describes how the IAPT system has adopted a language of healthcare driven by the 'evidence-based regime' that can be likened to an Orwellian scientific 'Newspeak'. It has been recognised that in order to meet the needs of patients accessing this service and provide patient choice, an eclectic treatment approach and consideration of implementing alternative ways of working is paramount (Marzillier & Hall 2009a). Treatments within IAPT services vary, provision of other treatment approaches may include: Interpersonal Therapy (IPT), Dynamic Interpersonal Therapy (DIT), Acceptance and Commitment Therapy (ACT) and Mindfulness-Based Cognitive Therapy (MBCT). There may be other approaches that haven't been discussed in this chapter; this depends on individual IAPT service specifications and what they have been commissioned to provide. Improving Access to Psychological Therapies services have been running pilots for Severe Mental Illness (IAPT for SMI). This project aims to increase public access to a range of NICE approved psychological therapies for psychosis, bipolar disorder and personality disorders (DoH 2011a, Jolley *et al.* 2015).

There are seven Key Performance Indicators (KPIs). These are 'Datasets' (quantifiable measures) collected quarterly to establish if IAPT services are meeting the objectives set out by commissioners which enable them to monitor and measure the service progress (DoH 2011b). The KPIs outline that IAPT services need to be providing timely access (locally agreed waiting times) for patients entering and beginning treatment, this is to increase by 15 per cent per annum; 3.2 million people will access IAPT, receiving either advice (guided self-help) or a course of therapy. The aim is for 50 per cent of those completing treatment to move to 'recovery' and meaningful improvement in their condition. Recovery is measured through Patient Reported Outcome Measures (PROMs), the main ones being the PHQ-9 (Kroenke *et al.* 2001) and GAD-7 (Spitzer *et al.* 2006). Each time a contact is made with a patient the measures are collected and are recorded on IAPTus/PCMIS or other clinical record systems. The measures help determine if a patient is above or below 'caseness', meaning 'symptomatic of depression/anxiety': if a patient scores below 'caseness' this would indicate that they are moving towards recovery (DoH 2012, NIMH 2006). Other measures used in this service include: The Work and Social Adjustment Scale (W&SAS) (Mundt *et al.* 2002); Obsessive Compulsive Inventory (OCI) (Foa *et al.*1998); Penn State Worry questionnaire (PSW) (Behar *et al.* 2003); Social Phobia Inventory (SPIN) (Connor *et al.* 2000); Impact of Events Scale – Revised (IES-R) (Creamer *et al.* 2003); Panic Disorder Severity Scale (PDSS) (Shear *et al.* 2001) and the Health Anxiety Inventory (HAI) (Salkovskis *et al.* 2002).

More recently the IAPT service has been scrutinised for the efficacy of the analysis of outcome measures and the cost-effectiveness of the service. See Griffiths & Steen (2013a, 2013b), who found that the analysis suggested 'a cost per IAPT session of £102.38 for low intensity therapy, and £173.88 for high intensity therapy, compared to DoH impact assessment estimates of £32.50 and £55.20 respectively' (Griffiths & Steen 2013b, pp. 151–152). Their analysis led them to conclude that '[t]he evidence base claimed for recovery rates for IAPT is flawed' (Griffiths & Steen 2013a, p. 139).

# What to expect working in an IAPT service: an occupational therapist's perspective

Volition, habituation, performance capacity and environmental conditions always resonate together, creating conditions out of which our thoughts, feelings and behaviour emerge (Kramer *et al.* 2003, p. 58).

Having qualified as an occupational therapist, I work as a Psychological Mental Health Practitioner (PMHP) in primary care mental healthcare (Myles & Rushforth 2007). The position was advertised at a band 5 level and open to mental health nurses (RMN), social workers (SW) and occupational therapists (OT). As a newly qualified occupational therapist, I was keen to secure a band 5 position that would enable me to consolidate my core skills (Creek & Lougher 2011, Turner 2002) and learn some new ones along the way. Despite knowing that embarking on a generic mental health role would be challenging for a first post, my interest in psychological therapies outweighed my anxieties about the role.

The role of PMHP was created with a view to resolving difficulties recruiting 'Psychological Wellbeing Practitioners' (PWP). Retention of PWPs had been problematic for IAPT services and highlighted the role demands (high caseloads) and limitations (training and career progression) (Bogart 2015, Moreea 2015, Shepherd & Rosairo 2008). The PMHP role requires additional training; I undertook a 5-day training course in evidence-based low intensity treatment for common mental health problems to enable me to deliver guided self-help in: behavioural activation; exposure and habituation; cognitive restructuring; panic management; problem solving; and sleep hygiene (Richards & Whyte 2011). The PMHP role is the same job description as the PWP role but the job titles are different due to the background training of the individual.

I work alongside a multi-disciplinary team (MDT) comprising professionals from different backgrounds who include: psychological wellbeing practitioners who deliver low intensity treatment (step 2) trainees; qualified psychological mental health practitioners (band 5s from one of the core professions (OT/RMN/SW)) who also deliver low intensity treatment (step 2); CBT therapists who deliver high intensity treatment (step 3) (trainee and qualified); Gateway workers; counsellors; psychotherapists; and clinical and counselling psychologists.

Referrals come from GPs, stepped-down from secondary services, or other external organisations, and go through a Single Point of Access (SPA). Many IAPT services have self-referral systems in place. This is to ensure that people from all ages/backgrounds/minorities are able to access the service. Self-referral, though, can result in inappropriate referrals which may have added complications around risk management which impacts on service delivery and efficiency, and as a consequence there are often changes and developments taking place to restructure and produce more effective systems (Brown et al. 2010, Richards et al. 2012).

# The role of the psychological mental health practitioner

The role requires the practitioner to assess and treat common mental health problems such as depression, panic disorder, Generalised Anxiety Disorder (GAD), Obsessive Compulsive Disorder (OCD), social anxiety, health anxiety. The emphasis is on a guided self-help approach (low intensity) using CBT-based interventions (step 2). The PMHPs/PWPs deliver a high volume (30 in some cases, less or more depending on the service). Sessions are conducted on a one-to-one basis in a timely manner, less than 20–30 minutes a session at 4–6 sessions. This is done face to face or over the phone.

Guided self-help techniques include: using workbooks; computerised CBT programmes (cCBT); health promotion through psycho-educational groups; bibliotherapy (books on prescription); and signposting to other services (such as Relate, voluntary and community sector, employment advisers, e.g. Onside and Remploy); and health trainers. Such services are ever changing; therefore it is necessary to keep up to date with signposting options.

# Assessment

Triage assessment is a screening that enables the PMHPs/PWPs to allocate patients to suitable treatment and is carried out either face to face or over the phone. During this process it is not uncommon to assess people with more enduring mental health difficulties or other healthcare needs who have 'fallen through the gaps'. Referrals to other services are sometimes necessary at this stage – for example, this could be to: eating disorders services; early intervention in psychosis services; older adult mental health services; Community Mental Health Teams (CMHTs) and social services.

The *Reach Out* guide outlines exactly how and what to gather at assessment. It gives you a structure for how to collate information, formulate a problem statement and implement interventions and is very prescriptive (Richards & Whyte 2011).

During assessment I have found myself formulating/conceptualising the patient's situation from two schools of thought: that of the PWP and that of the occupational therapist. Although I use the *Reach Out* guide to structure my assessment, I also draw from the Model of Human Occupation (MOHO) by formulating using the elements of volition, habituation, occupational performance capacity, looking at habits, routines, roles, values, interests, environment, attitudes, motivation, Activities of Daily Living (ADL), and family and relationships (Kielhofner 2002). The patient is held with a view that change is possible, focusing on the patient's strengths and towards recovery (Cara & MacRae 2005). Once understanding the patient's narrative and 'formulating a problem statement', I support the patient to establish SMART goals. Occupational therapists are well trained in devising collaborative therapeutic goals and supporting patients to act in accordance with their values. Their knowledge of task analysis, activity analysis and activity adaption (Creek & Lougher 2011, Duncan 2011) and the careful consideration of factors that influence a patient's engagement in activity, i.e. environment, performance skills (physical, cognitive, psychological, interpersonal), facilitates effective goal setting. Occupational therapists are careful with the language they use and frame goals positively with the emphasis on what the client will do/achieve rather than what they will not do. They support the patient to develop problem solving skills by getting them to generate solutions and consider tasks that can help them to meet their goals (Duncan 2011). The use of problem solving is recognised as a useful therapeutic skill and intervention that can be used with a wide range of patients and central to occupational therapy practice (Duncan 2011). This is also considered an intervention within the PMHP/PWP role.

# Treatment/interventions

Behavioural Activation (BA) (Veale 2008) is used for clients who are presenting with depression. When people experience depression they are more likely to avoid activity, experiencing limited positive reinforcement from their environment. The intervention encourages the patient to record and reflect on their current activity levels, noting impact on mood. A personalised activity schedule is developed in which the patient acts according to the schedule, not what they 'feel' like doing. The therapist will support the patient to change, adapt and problem solve any difficulties they encounter according to their needs. Activities are catagorised as routine, pleasurable or necessary. I reflect on this in terms of occupational participation, self-care, leisure and productivity (Kielhofner 2002).

Behavioural activation has been shown to be highly effective and there is a strong evidence base for the efficacy of this treatment approach (Bennett-Levy et al. 2010).

Behavioural activation reflects the essence of occupational therapy philosophy: supporting clients to achieve change through meaningful occupation and occupational engagement. When working with patients who are experiencing depression, factors that can influence engagement in activity include motivation, volition and autonomy (Creek & Lougher 2011). From my occupational therapy training I draw upon different theories/skills to address the above challenges. These include: task analysis theory (Duncan 2011), Motivational Interviewing (MI) (Miller & Rollnick 2012), the transtheoretical model (Prochaska & DiClemente 2005), and theory of planned behaviour (Ajzen & Manstead 2007).

I undertook some low intensity training (step 2) for working with people with long-term health conditions (LTHC) (e.g. chronic pain, diabetes, fibromyalgia, chronic obstructive pulmonary disease). The training demonstrated how, if a person is no longer able do an activity as a consequence of their LTHC, then the PWP/PMHP would find out what it was about that activity they valued and support the patient in considering other ways of meeting that value. If a patient can still carry out an activity, considering adaptations and Selection Optimisation with Compensation (SOC) (Freund & Baltes 1998) were proposed as ways of augmenting treatment. During this training I reflected on how this isn't vastly different from what an occupational therapist might traditionally do; it seemed the only difference was the use of language in which they describe their approach. There was clear emphasis on using Socratic method (Padesky 1993) to support the patient to identify alternative activities themselves. Within occupational therapy practice, a humanistic approach is often applied (Turner 2002), respecting autonomy and seeing the patient as a partner in therapy. Occupational therapists will discuss and generate options collaboratively to support patients to make informed choices without exerting control over their decisions (Turner 2002). The Socratic method lends itself well to this.

Exposure and habituation is an intervention that involves devising a hierarchy with the patient to enable them to habituate to certain situations/environments. It is typically used for people experiencing phobias/agoraphobia and panic. Occupational therapists are already skilled in this area with their knowledge of activity analysis and grading and adapting (Duncan 2011). Other interventions used within this role include: cognitive restructuring, worry management, behavioural experiments, exposure and response prevention, relapse and prevention plans, and health promotion through guidance on food and mood, sleep hygiene, and medication advice (Bennett-Levy et al. 2010, Richards & Whyte 2011).

# Groupwork

As part of under-graduate training, occupational therapists learn client-centred group skills (Creek & Lougher 2011). Within this role groupwork may take up a large proportion of a PMHP/PWP's time either facilitating or designing group interventions, evaluating and considering the effectiveness of group interventions through reviewing outcome measures/feedback. Group topics might include: anxiety and depression; confidence; stress; anger; worry; and long-term health conditions. Again, this depends on individual services. The style at this level tends to be more directive due to the psycho-educational approach being used. Despite this high level of structure, I have found that there will still be challenges in managing group dynamics (Cole 2005), even more so with self-referral systems in place. The PWPs/PMHPs often have to facilitate groups with more complex participants. I reflect on how further guidance and training for group skills could be considered for these roles and how protected time to evaluate and further develop group interventions is crucial.

## Supervision and clinical meetings

Case management and clinical skills supervision is given an hour a week. I have recently been introduced to a new model of supervision known as 'the seven-eyed model of supervision' (Hawkins *et al.* 2012). This enables discussion, exploration and reflection on the wider context of ethical, organisational, contractual, social and cultural aspects of the work. I have found that due to high demands of my role and many changes within the organisation, the peer supervision group has ceased. Similarly, for step 2, attending clinical decisions meetings has not been mandatory, although this provides opportunities for practitioners from the wider MDT to come together.

## Training and career progression

The PMHP training tends to be limited to low intensity interventions as this is what the role involves. This includes training for interventions on Cognitive Restructuring (CR), Behavioural Activation (BA), exposure and habituation, worry management for GAD, and Exposure Response Prevention (ERP) for OCD and health anxiety. Training opportunities for low intensity interventions are growing and recent areas of development for step 2 include social anxiety, perinatal care, working with older people, Post Traumatic Stress Disorder (PTSD) and long-term health conditions. I have had the opportunity to complete a 3-day experiential course in Acceptance and Commitment Therapy (ACT) which was made available to all practitioners within my service. I also take time out to undertake personal Continuing Professional Development (CPD) opportunities.

Many PWPs come from a psychology background in that they have completed an undergraduate degree in psychology. Scope for progression within the PMHP/PWP roles is limited. These posts have often been considered by many as a stepping stone into working in high intensity CBT or to provide experience to apply for clinical psychology posts (Moreea 2015). This has been recognised as problematic, and ways to make the role more attractive have been considered, with some services offering senior PWP posts (Richardson & Richards 2010).

# Advantages of the role for the occupational therapist

The PMHP role provides occupational therapists with experience of what it is like working for an IAPT service. This role has provided me with additional skills and experience that could enhance my occupational therapy practice in future. It has enabled me to develop resilience and improve my time management skills. The nature of the role enables the practice of motivational interviewing techniques and Socratic questioning, tools which occupational therapy graduates are familiar with. Developing a further understanding of the cognitive elements within psychological therapies is very useful and can provide good grounding for those who wish to progress to undertaking roles within high intensity CBT therapy provision.

# Limitations of the role

Occupational therapists have many skills and use many approaches, but could find themselves boundaried in what they can use due to how prescriptive this role is, given the service specifications. I consider that the limits on scope for creativity and autonomy could have further implications on practitioners' professional development and wellbeing.

Despite having opportunities to practice Socratic questioning and motivational interviewing, the time restriction and nature of the PMHP/PWP role (guided self-help) could limit the extent of development of these skills. I reflect that not being trained as a PWP has been a challenge to me, in particular in keeping to the allocated 30 minutes or less a session. The experience has been demanding due to the high volume caseload and administration requirements, giving a need to be efficient and resilient at all times.

# Challenges faced
## Professional identity

I have found that going into a generic post with such a specialised service straight after graduation meant that consolidating occupational therapy core skills was challenging. It requires commitment and time to stay updated and in touch with the occupational therapy world. I have done this through attending the OT Show at the NEC in Birmingham and networking through Facebook occupational therapy groups. I spend time reflecting and relating my practice back to occupational therapy theory to consolidate my skills. I take the opportunity to promote the occupational therapy role; however, people's lack of awareness of this role has been evident, i.e. being confused with occupational health or getting people back into employment. The PMHP's role has led to a level of ambiguity over my professional identity. Fortune (2000) explores the notion that occupational therapists could be perceived as filling in gaps; she discusses the importance of being able to ground practice in occupational therapy philosophies and reclaim the occupational therapy identity. I see the value in this but also recognise the importance of professionals not being perceived as implying superiority or exclusivity over their philosophical stance/approach; in practice this has apparently created barriers to collaborative practice.

## Collaborative practice

On previous placement experience I recall how the MDT members were brought together on a monthly basis as a mandatory exercise to share and present PowerPoints/discussions to each other which included topics about their role, interventions and models of practice. The organisational environment encouraged professionals to take an interest in each other's roles, to gain a better understanding of their theoretical background and develop a shared language.

Professional cultures can impact on inter-professional and collaborative working. Different professions have their own sets of beliefs, values, customs and behaviours (Hall 2005). Within the IAPT service there is a wide range of mental health professionals, all with different backgrounds, using different approaches. Some of the challenges of this are reflected in Davis' (2013) article 'We are all on the same side', where she discusses the criticisms she has received working in an IAPT service as a CBT practitioner. Equally from a different perspective Rizq (2012, 2013, 2014) expresses her frustrations regarding the IAPT service and the movement of evidence-based treatments. I reflect on how, coming from different schools of thought, professionals often present with varying clinical rationales which can lead to delays in the referral processes and throughput of patients. This can also create divisions between professional groups. Some of the challenges considered are the infrastructure, lack of resources and time constraints in people's working day placed by the service model; consequently in reality there is limited time for developing collaborative practices (Brown & Stoffel 2010, Jones & Delany 2014, Richards *et al.* 2012).

## Burnout and self-care

Every profession's Code of Ethics and Professional Conduct (e.g. COT 2010) will highlight the importance of looking after one's own wellbeing in order to provide the best care possible to others.

Burnout is considered to be a depletion of physical and mental resources (Steel *et al.* 2015). Therapists aren't immune to secondary trauma, compassion fatigue, emotional exhaustion, depersonalisation and burnout (Skovholt & Trotter-Mathison 2014). There have been limited publications about the experience and burnout of low intensity workers.

Ledingham (2015) conducted a qualitative study on mental health workers' perceptions and beliefs about burnout and found that participants struggled to disclose to others for fear of negative judgement and believed that they were weaker or less capable. Self-blame and self-stigmatisation meant that people would not address burnout and other perceptual biases led to them ignoring or minimising their symptoms. Thwaites *et al.* (2015) suggest that '[t]here are two main challenges to the role of the PWP, both of which are related to the high caseloads and throughput of the patient:

**295**

first it's finding time to reflect and learn from the wealth of the clinical experience in order to fine tune interventions; second is the prevention of practitioner burnout' (p. 311). Their study carried out a self-practice self-reflection programme for low intensity practitioners and found that it helped to enhance skills, maintain resilience and avoid burnout.

I acknowledge this field of work at times can feel lonely and isolating. There are times during my practice where I experience thoughts of being inadequate or feeling overwhelmed; I combat this by seeking support from my peers/colleagues friends and family, identifying training needs and making good use of supervision. I cultivate a sense of belonging that isn't just around my job but engaging in leisure activities out of work such as: art, music, running, and tending to my plants to enhance my experience of 'flow' (Csikszentmihalyi 2000) and wellbeing. I have realised since working in this post how important it is to consider scheduling in regular breaks/holidays to attend to my self-care needs. Working in this role has enabled me to further develop self-awareness (Creek & Lougher 2011), understand and better manage self-regulation (Brown & Stoffel 2010) and practise the art of balance.

# Ethical practice

Moral courage is needed (Murray 2010) for open discussions and deliberations regarding ethical dilemmas in practice. I pride myself on being an honest client-centred practitioner and not letting the target-driven culture impact on my treatment or the way I view patients. However, maintaining this moral viewpoint whilst working within an IAPT service could be challenging (as recognised by Bogart 2015, and Rizq 2012, 2013, 2014). In discussion with another colleague it was established that some PMHPs/PWPs in other IAPT services were expected to achieve/deliver 8–12 contacts a day whether this is done by phone, face to face, or with cCBT; I contemplate the implications of this and the impact on the patients, the service, the people trying to deliver this treatment, and society as a whole. I consider how helpful this could be for the patient journey: whether the patient felt they had a choice of intervention or how it was delivered, and how helpful their experience of that treatment was. Often in my practice I have worked with patients who have not been appropriate for low intensity treatment, and I am conscious of the fact I have to remain working with step 2 treatments that are unlikely to suffice in the longer term for my patients. I work within the realms of my remit for the role (PMHP) and seek support from my supervisor, but find it frustrating not being able to use other occupational therapy skills and knowledge to support my patients.

# Conclusion

Embracing a role like this provides the opportunity to be more reflective and inquisitive, comparing and contrasting differences which inadvertently leads to new learning and increased confidence in applying skills, theory and knowledge.

All services will be challenged by the ethical, organisational, contractual, social and cultural aspects of the work. I reflect on the usefulness of establishing whether your organisation's actions and views are consistent with your own personal values. This involves a level of exploration about the service and about yourself. If they aren't, there is a risk of experiencing dissatisfaction within the role, cognitive dissonance, and compromising your own morality and integrity. Reflecting can aid with this process and provide new understanding and insights. Bringing these difficulties to the forefront can assist in resolving or coming up with solutions, consideration of alternative ways of working, or challenging current ways of working. One of the main challenges for the PMHP/PWP role is the limited time for reflection, and the fact that any self-directed learning needs to be conducted in your own time.

People from different professional groups may use a different language, different outcome measures, different approaches, but ultimately it is about remaining client-centred and recognising what is 'best practice' for the patient; as Davies (2013) highlights, 'we are all on the same side'. Creek & Lougher (2011) present different frames of reference that highlight an occupational therapist's foundation in practice: these include, occupational performance (CAOT 1993), psychodynamic (Fidler & Fidler 1963), human developmental (Mosey 1968), cognitive behavioural (Beck 1976), rehabilitative (Deegan 1988), cognitive (Allen 1985), health promotion (Prochaska & DiClemente 1983) and occupational behaviour (Kielhofner & Burke 1980). Value is placed on drawing from a collection of ideas, theory and knowledge, to be able to holistically treat and meet the patient's needs. Appreciation, respect, and valuing the team's experience, knowledge and opinions, is fundamental to building positive professional relationships.

As an occupational therapist, I have been trained to view things holistically and do not hold a reductionist stance myself. The provision of psychological therapies services has come a long way. In order to further develop this, the inclusion of qualitative, participatory research and evaluations conducted in practice settings can aid in providing 'practice-based evidence' to build on 'evidence-based practice' (Green 2006, 2008, Williams 2015).

Williams (2015) states that 'the IAPT culture is arguably influenced by one research paradigm and such an influence can skew services only towards numerical outcome data as the only truth of "recovery". An interpretative paradigm could assist in shaping service-based cultures, alter how services are evaluated and improve the richness of CBT research' (p. 344). Green (2006) highlights that too much evidence comes from artificially controlled research that doesn't fit the realities of everyday practice.

# Useful resources

- Bennett-Levy, J. et al. (eds) (2010). *Oxford Guide to Low Intensity CBT Interventions*. Oxford: Oxford University Press.
- The CEDAR IAPT workbooks and resources from University of Exeter: http://cedar.exeter.ac.uk/iapt/iaptworkbooksandresources
- http://www.cci.health.wa.gov.au
- http://www.getselfhelp.co.uk/selfhelp.htm
- http://www.psychology.tools
- Westbrook, D., Kennerley, H. & Kirk, J. (2011). An Introduction to Cognitive Behaviour Therapy: *Skills and Application*, 2nd edn. London: Sage.

# References

Ajzen, I. & Manstead, A.S.R. (2007). 'Changing health-related behaviors: an approach based on the theory of planned behaviour' in *The Scope of Social Psychology: Theory and Applications*, eds. M. Hewstone, J.B.F. de Wit, K. van den Bos, H. Schut, & M. Stroebe. New York: Psychology Press.

Allen, C.K. (1985). *Occupational Therapy for Psychiatric Diseases: Measurement and Management of Cognitive Disabilities.* Boston: Little, Brown.

Beck, A.T. (1976). *Cognitive Therapy and the Emotional Disorders*. New York: International Universities Press.

Behar, E., Alcaine, O., Zuellig, A.R. & Borkovec, T.D. (2003). Screening for generalised anxiety disorder using the Penn State Worry Questionnaire: A receiver operating characteristic analysis. *Journal of Behaviour Therapy and Experimental Psychiatry* **34** (1), 25–43.

Bennett-Levy, J., Richards, D., Farrand, P., Christensen, H., Griffiths, K., Kavanagh, D. & Klein, B. (eds) (2010). *Oxford Guide to Low Intensity CBT Interventions.* Oxford: Open University Press.

Bogart, K. (2015). 'Sometimes, I feel that the psychological wellbeing practitioner role is undervalued'. *The Psychologist* 28, 236–239.

Brown, C. & Stoffel, V.C. (2010). *Occupational Therapy in Mental Health: A Vision for Participation.* Philadelphia, PA: FA Davis.

Brown, J.S., Boardman, J., Whittinger, N. & Ashworth, M. (2010). Can a self-referral system help improve access to psychological treatments? *British Journal of General Practice* **60** (574), 365–371.

Butler, A.C., Chapman, J.E., Forman, E.M. & Beck, A.T. (2006). The empirical status of cognitive-behavioural therapy: a review of meta-analyses. *Clinical Psychology Review* **26** (1), 17–31.

Canadian Association of Occupational Therapists (1993). *Occupational Therapy Guidelines for Client-centered Mental Health Practice.* Ottawa: CAOT.

Cara, E. & MacRae, A. (2005). *Psychosocial Occupational Therapy: A Clinical Practice.* UK: Cengage Learning.

Casement, P. (2009). Beyond words – the role of psychoanalysis. *The Psychologist* **22** (5), 404–405.

Clark, D.M., Layard, R., Smithies, R., Richards, D.A., Suckling, R. & Wright, B. (2009). Improving access to psychological therapy: initial evaluation of two UK demonstration sites. *Behaviour Research and Therapy* **47** (11), 910–920.

Cole, M.B. (2005). *Group Dynamics in Occupational Therapy: The Theoretical Basis and Practice Application of Group Intervention,* 4th edn. Thorofare, NJ: Slack.

College of Occupational Therapists (2010). *Code of Ethics and Professional Conduct.* London: COT.

Connor, K.M., Davidson, J.R., Churchill, L.E., Sherwood, A., Weisler, R.H. & Foa, E. (2000). Psychometric properties of the Social Phobia Inventory (SPIN) new self-rating scale. *British Journal of Psychiatry* **176** (4), 379–386.

Creamer, M., Bell, R. & Failla, S. (2003). Psychometric properties of the impact of event scale – revised. *Behaviour Research and Therapy* **41** (12), 1489–1496.

Creek, J. & Lougher, L. (2011). *Occupational Therapy and Mental Health.* Elsevier Health Sciences.

Csikszentmihalyi, M. (2000). *Beyond Boredom and Anxiety.* San Francisco: Jossey-Bass.

Davis, E. (2013) We are all on the same side. *Therapy Today* **24** (6), 15.

Deegan, P.E. (1988) Recovery: the lived experience of rehabilitation. *Psychosocial Rehabilitation Journal* **11** (4), 11–19.

Department of Health (2006). *Our Health, Our Care, Our Say.* London: TSO.

Department of Health (2011a). *Talking Therapies: Four Year Plan of Action.* London: TSO.

Department of Health (2011b). IAPT *Data Handbook, version 2.* http://www.iapt.nhs.uk (last accessed: 2.2.2016).

Department of Health (2012). *IAPT three-year report: The First Million Patients.* London: TSO.

Duncan, E.A. (2011). *Skills for Practice in Occupational Therapy.* New York: Elsevier Health Sciences.

Fidler, G.S. & Fidler, J.W. (1963) *Occupational Therapy: a Communication Process in Psychiatry.* New York: MacMillan.

Foa, E.B., Kozak, M.J., Salkovskis, P.M., Coles, M.E. & Amir, N. (1998). The validation of a new obsessive compulsive disorder scale: The Obsessive–Compulsive Inventory. *Psychological Assessment* **10** (3), 206.

Fortune, T. (2000). Occupational therapists: is our therapy truly occupational or are we merely filling gaps? *British Journal of Occupational Therapy* **63** (5), 225–230.

Freund, A.M. & Baltes, P.B. (1998). Selection, optimization, and compensation as strategies of life management: correlations with subjective indicators of successful aging. *Psychology and Aging* **13** (4), 531.

Green, L.W. (2006). Public health asks of systems science: to advance our evidence-based practice, can you help us get more practice-based evidence? *American Journal of Public Health* **96** (3), 406.

Green, L.W. (2008). Making research relevant: if it is an evidence-based practice, where's the practice-based evidence? *Family Practice* **25** (suppl 1), i20–i24.

Griffiths, S. & Steen, S. (2013a). Improving Access to Psychological Therapies (IAPT) Programme: setting key performance indicators in a more robust context: a new perspective. *Journal of Psychological Therapies in Primary Care* **2** (2), 133–141.

Griffiths, S. & Steen, S. (2013b). Improving Access to Psychological Therapies (IAPT) Programme: scrutinising IAPT cost estimates to support effective commissioning. *Journal of Psychological Therapies in Primary Care* **2** (2), 142–156.

Hall, P. (2005). Inter-professional teamwork: professional cultures as barriers. *Journal of Inter-professional Care* **19** (suppl 1), 188–196.

Hawkins, P., Shohet, R., Ryde, J. & Wilmot, J. (2012). *Supervision in the Helping Professions.* New York: McGraw-Hill Education.

Jolley, S., Garety, P., Peters, E., Fornells-Ambrojo, M., Onwumere, J., Harris, V., Brabban, A. & Johns, L. (2015). Opportunities and challenges in Improving Access to Psychological Therapies for people with Severe Mental Illness (IAPT-SMI): evaluating the first operational year of the South London and Maudsley (SLaM) demonstration site for psychosis. *Behaviour Research and Therapy* **64**, 24–30.

Jones, G.M. & Delany, T. (2014). What does collaborative practice mean within mental health care?: a qualitative study exploring understandings and proposing a definition. *Journal of Research in Inter-professional Practice and Education* **3** (3) 1–15.

Kielhofner, G. & Burke, J.P. (1980). A Model of Human Occupation, part 1: conceptual framework and content. *American Journal of Occupational Therapy* **34** (9), 572–581.

Kielhofner, G. (2002). *A Model of Human Occupation: Theory and Application*, 3rd edn. Philadelphia: Lippincott Williams & Wilkins.

Kramer, P., Hinojosa, J. & Royeen, C.B. (eds) (2003). *Perspectives in Human Occupation: Participation in Life.* Philadelphia: Lippincott Williams & Wilkins.

Kroenke, K., Spitzer, R.L. & Williams, J.B. (2001). The PHQ-9. *Journal of General Internal Medicine* **16** (9), 606–613.

Ledingham, M. (2015). *Beliefs and Perceptions about Burnout amongst Mental Health Professionals.* PhD thesis, Edith Cowan University, Australia.

London School of Economics and Political Science. Centre for Economic Performance. Mental Health Policy Group. (2006). *The Depression Report: a New Deal for Depression and Anxiety Disorders.* London: LSE Research.

Marzillier, J. & Hall, J. (2009a). Alternative ways of working. *The Psychologist* **22** (5), 406–407.

Marzillier, J. & Hall, J. (2009b). The challenge of the Layard Initiative. *The Psychologist* **22** (5), 396–399.

Miller, W.R. & Rollnick, S. (2012). *Motivational Interviewing: Helping People Change.* New York: Guilford press.

Moreea, O. (2015). *Northern IAPT Practice Research Network.* http://www.iaptprn.com (last accessed: 2.2.2016).

Mosey, A.C. (1968). Recapitulation of ontogenesis: a theory for the practice of occupational therapy. *American Journal of Occupational Therapy* **22** (5), 426–438.

Mundt, J.C., Marks, I.M., Shear, M.K. & Greist, J.M. (2002). The Work and Social Adjustment Scale: a simple measure of impairment in functioning. *British Journal of Psychiatry* **180** (5), 461–464.

Murray, J.S. (2010) Moral courage in healthcare: acting ethically even in the presence of risk. *Online Journal of Issues in Nursing* **15** (3), Manuscript 2.

Myles, P. & Rushforth, D. (2007). *A Complete Guide to Primary Care Mental Health.* London: Robinson.

National Institute for Mental Health (2006). *IAPT Outline Service Specification. Improving Access to Psychological Therapies Programme IAPT.* http://www.iapt.nhs.uk (last accessed: 5.10.2015).

Padesky, C.A. (1993, September). *Socratic Questioning: Changing Minds or Guiding Discovery.* Invited keynote address presented at the 1993 European Congress of Behaviour and Cognitive Therapies, London (Vol. 24), http:www.padesky.com (last accessed: 2.2.2016).

Prochaska, J.O. & DiClemente, C.C.(1983). Stages and processes of self change in smoking: towards an integrative model of change. *Journal of Consulting and Clinical Psychology* **51** (3), 390–395.

Prochaska, J.O. & DiClemente, C.C. (2005). 'The transtheoretical approach' in *Handbook of Psychotherapy Integration*, eds. J.C. Norcross & M.R. Goldfried, 2nd edn. New York: Oxford University Press.

Richards, D. & Whyte, M. (2011). *Reach Out: National Programme Student Materials to Support the Delivery of Training for Psychological Wellbeing Practitioners Delivering Low Intensity Interventions,* 3rd edn. London: Rethink Mental Illness.

Richards, D.A., Bower, P., Pagel, C., Weaver, A., Utley, M., Cape, J., Pilling, S., Lovell, K., Gilbody, S., Leibowitz, J. & Owens, L. (2012). Delivering stepped care: an analysis of implementation in routine practice. *Implementation Science* **7** (3), 1–11.

Richardson, G. & Richards, D. (2010). *Psychological Wellbeing Practitioners: Best Practice Guide.* http://www.iapt.nhs.uk (last accessed: 2.2.2016).

Rizq, R. (2012). The perversion of care: psychological therapies in a time of IAPT. *Psychodynamic Practice* **18** (1), 7–24.

Rizq, R. (2013). The language of healthcare. *Therapy Today,* http://www.therapytoday.net (last accessed: 2.2.2016).

Rizq, R. (2014). Perverting the course of therapy: the fetishisation of governance in public sector mental health services. Psychoanalytic Psychotherapy **28** (3), 249–266.

Salkovskis, P.M., Rimes, K.A., Warwick, H.M.C. & Clark, D.M. (2002). The Health Anxiety Inventory: development and validation of scales for the measurement of health anxiety and hypochondriasis. *Psychological Medicine* **32** (5), 843–853.

Shear, M.K., Rucci, P., Williams, J., Frank, E., Grochocinski, V., Vander-Bilt, J., Houck, P. & Wang, T. (2001). Reliability and validity of the Panic Disorder Severity Scale: replication and extension. *Journal of Psychiatric Research* **35** (5), 293–296.

Shepherd, M., & Rosairo, M. (2008). Low-intensity workers: Lessons learned from supervising primary care mental health workers and dilemmas associated with such roles. *Mental Health in Family Medicine* **5** (4), 237–245.

Skovholt, T.M. & Trotter-Mathison, M.J. (2014). *The Resilient Practitioner: Burnout Prevention and Self-care Strategies for Counsellors, Therapists, Teachers, and Health Professionals*. London: Routledge.

Spitzer, R.L., Kroenke, K., Williams, J.B. & Löwe, B. (2006). A brief measure for assessing generalised anxiety disorder: the GAD-7. *Archives of Internal Medicine* **166** (10), 1,092–1,097.

Steel, C., Macdonald, J., Schröder, T. & Mellor-Clark, J. (2015). Exhausted but not cynical: burnout in therapists working within Improving Access to Psychological Therapy services. *Journal of Mental Health* **24** (1), 33–37.

Thwaites, R., Cairns, L., Bennett-Levy, J., Johnston, L., Lowrie, R., Robinson, A., Turner, M., Haarhoff, B. & Perry, H. (2015). Developing metacompetence in low intensity cognitive behavioural therapy (CBT) interventions: evaluating a self-practice/self-reflection programme for experienced low intensity CBT practitioners. *Australian Psychologist* **50** (5), 311–321.

Turner, A. (2002). *Occupational Therapy and Physical Dysfunction: Principles, Skills, and Practice*, 6th edn. London: Elsevier.

Veale, D. (2008). Behavioural activation for depression. *Advances in Psychiatric Treatment* **14** (1), 29–36.

Williams, C.H.J. (2015). Improving Access to Psychological Therapies (IAPT) and treatment outcomes: epistemological assumptions and controversies. *Journal of Psychiatric and Mental Health Nursing* **22** (5), 344–351.

# Chapter 19

# The Approved Mental Health Professional role

## Gill Knott

---

### Introduction

This chapter is aimed at occupational therapists who would like to learn more about the role of the Approved Mental Health Professional (hereinafter referred to as 'AMHP'). The author has provided an overview of the purpose and main functions of the role, relevant legal frameworks, ethical dilemmas pertaining to the role, the approval procedure and an indication of occupational therapy skills and knowledge which may be transferrable to the role. There is a section discussing the independence and social perspective of the role, how this is applied in practice and the skills occupational therapists could bring to these aspects of the role. For occupational therapists who are uncertain whether to undertake training to become AMHPs, the author has provided information from personal experience of some of the situations that could be encountered in AMHP work; the aim here is to present a picture of what everyday life can be like for AMHPs. The author has also suggested a selection of activities that could be undertaken to give a clearer picture of what is involved in AMHP work and which may assist occupational therapists in deciding whether this is the right choice for them.

---

## Key points

This chapter:

- Provides information about what the AMHP role involves and why we need AMHPs
- Provides information on the knowledge and skills required to become an AMHP and the training required and the approval criteria
- Discusses ethical dilemmas for AMHPs
- Suggests activities to provide a broader perspective and deeper insight into AMHP work for those who are unsure whether it is the right career choice for them.

# Background

The Mental Health Act 2007 (UK Parliament 1983/2007), an amendment of the Mental Health Act 1983, governs compulsory assessment and treatment of people with mental disorders in England and Wales. In the UK, mental health law exists to balance the requirement to detain people compulsorily, to protect them from harm (i.e. suicide, self-neglect or other forms of self-harm), to protect others from harm, and to protect people's rights and autonomy. Mental health law safeguards against a person being inappropriately detained and treated without consent (Hall & Ali 2009, Mind 2011).

One major amendment to the Mental Health Act in 2007 was the broadening of professional groups eligible to undertake specific roles under the Act (see Box 19.1 for full details of amendments to Mental Health Act 1983). One of these roles was that of the approved mental health professional. For the previous 25 years, under the Mental Health Act 1983, this role had been known as approved social worker (ASW) and was carried out exclusively by social workers who had undertaken additional training to become 'approved' to perform statutory duties. The AMHP replaced the ASW and is now open to other mental health professionals, including chartered psychologists, mental health and learning disability nurses and occupational therapists. The new role was part of creating teams under the auspices of the *New Ways of Working* national workforce programme, which aimed to bring together mental health professionals to create a more flexible and adaptable workforce (DoH 2007a, DoH 2007b, DoH 2008, Hall & Ali 2009). The College of Occupational Therapists played a key role in the development of the amendments to the Mental Health Act and the creation of new roles for occupational therapists and embraced the changes as reinforcing the need for the profession to remain current and active in new modes of service delivery. Feedback was received that some occupational therapists felt this would be a positive direction to take with regards to their own professional development (COT 2006). It was also acknowledged that occupational therapists working as care coordinators, or within teams such as assertive outreach for example, who use a team-working approach when working with service users, were already regularly involved in discussion and decision-making processes about whether someone needed to be assessed under the Mental Health Act and frequently initiated the process. On this basis it was thought that occupational therapists possessed some of the required skills and were well-placed if wishing to train to become AMHPs, so inclusion of occupational therapists within the broadened groups eligible to undertake AMHP training was welcomed and regarded as a positive step. Not everyone, however, in the occupational therapy profession was in agreement with occupational therapists becoming eligible to become AMHPs – some saw the move as eroding professional philosophies and skills and losing the focus that occupational therapy brings to working with service users (McKay et al. 2008).

**Box 19.1: Summary of the main amendments to the 1983 Mental Health Act by the 2007 Mental Health Act**

- Introduction of single definition of mental disorder.
- Introduction of appropriate medical treatment test.
- Broadening of professional roles.
- Increased patient rights whereby patients can apply to have nearest relative under the Act removed by County Court.
- Widening of grounds for displacement of nearest relative.
- Civil partners to be included in the list of relatives.
- Earlier reference to Mental Health Act tribunal.
- Introduction of single tribunal for England alongside Welsh counterpart.
- Requirement that Hospital Managers must ensure that patients under the age of 18 are placed in age appropriate accommodation.
- Introduction of mental health advocacy service.
- Introduction of new patient safeguards in situations where electro-convulsive therapy is considered.

(based on Rapaport & Manthorpe 2008)

# What the AMHP role involves

## Mental Health Act assessments

One of the AMHP's main functions is to conduct Mental Health Act assessments of people deemed mentally disordered to determine whether they meet the criteria for detention (known as 'sectioning') and ensure that the law is applied correctly. When carrying out statutory duties AMHPs do so under the legal framework of the Mental Health Act. The *Mental Health Act Code of Practice* (2015a) and the *Mental Health Reference Guide* (2015b) explain how the law should be applied in practice. Approved mental health professionals are also expected to apply the 'five guiding principles' (see Box 19.2 and refer to *The Mental Health Act 1983: Code of Practice* (2015a), chapter 1 for further information) which is a framework of values and considerations which supports AMHPs in reasoning and decision-making processes in the unique and individual circumstances of each assessment (DoH 2015a, Knott & Bannigan 2013).

## Box 19.2: The five guiding principles of the Mental Health Act

**Least restrictive option and maximising independence**

Where it is possible to treat a patient safely and lawfully without detaining them under the Act, the patient should not be detained. Wherever possible, a patient's independence should be encouraged and supported with a focus on promoting recovery.

**Empowerment and involvement**

Patients should be fully involved in decisions about care, support and treatment. The views of families, carers and others, if appropriate, should be fully considered when taking decisions. Where decisions are taken which are contradictory to views expressed, professionals should explain the reasons for this.

**Respect and dignity**

Patients, their families and carers should be treated with respect and dignity and listened to by professionals.

**Purpose and effectiveness**

Decisions about care and treatment should be appropriate to the patient, with clear therapeutic aims, promote recovery and should be performed to current national guidelines and/or current, available best practice guidelines.

**Efficiency and equity**

Providers, commissioners and other relevant organisations should work together to ensure that the quality of commissioning and provision of mental healthcare services are of high quality and are given equal priority to physical health and social care services. All relevant services should work together to facilitate timely, safe and supportive discharge from detention.

A Mental Health Act assessment can take place in a number of different settings, including hospitals, care homes, police stations and in the community (i.e. the service user's home). There is no lower age limit so AMHPs can find themselves assessing children/teenagers. It is the AMHP's responsibility to organise and coordinate the assessment, which can involve a large amount of inter-agency working with other agencies, i.e. police and ambulance services, GP, consultant, bed management service, and any other professionals who have been working with the service user. The AMHP must also identify the person who is the service user's Nearest Relative (NR) and ensure that they are aware of their rights under the Mental Health Act. The AMHP also has powers of entry and in some circumstances may have to apply for a magistrate's warrant to enter premises to assess a person, who is refusing, or unable to, allow them to gain access. Before making an application for a person to be compulsorily admitted to hospital, it is the AMHP's responsibility to ensure that immediate provision is made to care for any dependent children and/or adults who rely on the person for their care. It is also within the AMHP's role to arrange care for any pets belonging to the person and to ensure that the person's property is left secured (DoH 2007a, DoH 2007b, DoH 2015a).

The process to detain someone under the Mental Health Act and get them into hospital involves an AMHP and two doctors, one of whom should be approved under Section 12 of the Mental Health Act and preferably a doctor who has previous knowledge of the person. If appropriate, after interviewing the person, the doctors provide medical recommendations which means that they are of the opinion that detention in hospital is the most appropriate option to further assess and treat the person's mental disorder. The AMHP also interviews the person and decides independently whether hospital detention is the most appropriate means of providing treatment to address the person's needs. The AMHP must have knowledge of alternative resources and the availability of other appropriate services which could help a person remain in the community and be treated rather than being admitted to hospital. When the AMHP has made the decision to make an application to admit someone to hospital it is the AMHP's responsibility to communicate this information to the person. It is the responsibility of the doctor to organise an appropriate hospital bed, unless other local agreements are in place; and the AMHP's responsibility to organise conveyance to hospital by the most appropriate means. After completing the statutory forms the AMHP is required to accompany the person to hospital wherever possible, and provide an outline report for the hospital upon admission, giving information about the events leading up to the admission and any other relevant information. The AMHP is also required to provide a more extensive report containing details of the assessment and outcome, and give notification to the detained patient, so that the patient can use this information if wishing to make an appeal against detention to a Mental Health Tribunal (DoH 2015a).

## Supervised Community Treatment

Another AMHP function is to consider applications for Supervised Community Treatment (SCT) (see Section 17A – G, Mental Health Act 1983) in respect of discharging patients from detention in hospital onto Community Treatment Orders (CTOs) and agreeing the conditions to be included in the CTO; also approving the extension and revocation of CTOs (DoH 2015a).

Supervised community treatment was introduced through the 2007 amendments to the Mental Health Act 1983 and was one of the most significant changes to mental health law over the last twenty years. Supervised community treatment applies to patients who have been detained on a treatment order of the Mental Health Act 1983 (i.e. Section 3 or unrestricted Part 3 patients). The implications of a patient meeting the relevant criteria are that he or she can be discharged from hospital and treated in the community on what is known as a community treatment order where he/she is subject to mandatory and other conditions to prevent relapse and promote recovery and safe community living. In practice, this means that if his/her mental health deteriorates he/she can be recalled to hospital, treated quickly and when appropriate, discharged back into the community within a short space of time, thus promoting greater freedom and independence and safer community living (Brookes & Brindle 2010, DoH 2015b, Jones 2013). In AMHP practice, when considering least restrictive options, supervised community treatment may be an option which is least disruptive to family life and which may avoid the patient being separated from his/her children, family and carers. Additionally, being on a CTO could mean that a person is able to continue in employment.

The AMHP is also responsible for a number of other statutory functions which include:

● Making applications for Guardianship orders and applications for replacement of unsatisfactory private guardians.

● Preparing and providing social circumstances reports for Mental Health Tribunals.

● Making applications for displacement of Nearest Relative.

● Entering and inspecting premises where someone is believed to be, who is not receiving proper care.

● Applying for a warrant to enter premises to search for and remove a person who is in need of care and living alone.

● Taking into custody a detained patient who has left hospital without leave and returning the patient to hospital (DoH 2015a).

(See Box 19.3 for complete list of functions of AMHPs and refer to *The Reference Guide to the Mental Health Act 1983*, Chapter 30 (DoH 2015b) for further information).

## Box 19.3: The main AMHP functions

● Making applications for admission to hospital for assessment or treatment under part 2.

● The power to convey patients to hospital on the basis of applications for admission.

● Making applications for guardianship under part 2.

● Providing social circumstances reports on patients detained on the basis of an application for admission made by their nearest relative.

● Applying to the county court for the replacement of an unsatisfactory private guardian.

● Confirming that community treatment orders (CTOs) should be made discharging patients from detention in hospital on to CTOs and agreeing the conditions to be included in the CTO.

● Approving the extension of CTOs.

● Approving the revocation of CTOs.

● Being consulted by responsible clinicians before they make reports confirming the detention or CTOs of patients who have been absent without leave for more than 28 days.

● Applying to the county court for the appointment of an acting nearest relative and the displacement of an existing nearest relative.

- Having the right to enter and inspect premises under section 115.

- Applying for warrants to enter premises under section 135.

- The power to take patients into custody and take them to the place they ought to be when they have gone absent without leave (AWOL).

- The power to take and return other patients who have absconded.

(Main AMHP functions, taken from the *Reference Guide to the Mental Health Act 1983*, DoH 2015b.)

# AMHP approval criteria

Local authorities are responsible for the approval of AMHPs and when carrying out statutory duties AMHPs do so on behalf of the local authority, regardless of who they are employed by (Merchant 2007). Although there are local variations, the duration of the AMHP course is approximately six months of full-time study which means that candidates will be expected to be away from their normal workplace during this period. The academic requirements of the course are equivalent to post-graduate level and can count as credits towards a higher degree. In part the course is delivered via university-based sessions which include teaching sessions and facilitated workshops. The primary objective is to enable students to integrate theory and practice and then to consolidate the learning that takes place on the practice placement with that which is gained from the initial university-based teaching sessions. Students are expected to complete a practice placement and will be allocated a practice educator who is a practising AMHP. The AMHP course is assessed by presentation of a synoptic portfolio as required by the Health and Care Professions Council (HCPC 2013) to evidence that the student meets all of the competence requirements based on Schedule 2 to the Mental Health (AMHPs) (Approval) (England) Regulations 2008. The portfolio is made up of a collection of evidence, including written reports providing information of participation in Mental Health Act assessments, case studies and other material to provide evidence about an individual's competence, underpinning knowledge and skills, theoretical perspectives and the consistent application of values.

## Re-approval and AMHP continuing professional development

Local authorities may approve professionals to act as AMHPs for five years at a time, after which they would need to re-submit a portfolio of evidence to gain re-approval to act for a further five years and so on. Approval of AMHPs is conditional on each AMHP completing at least eighteen hours of relevant training per year as agreed with the approving authority (DoH 2015a). When identifying training opportunities the author has found that some training may be relevant to both AMHP and occupational therapy practice. For example, the author recently attended a one-day course on lone working which was relevant not only to AMHP practice but also to working as a community occupational therapist.

The approval criteria for AMHPs can be accessed via: http://www.hcpc-uk.org/assets/docum ents/100414DApprovalcriteriaforapprovedmentalhealthprofessionials(AMHP)programmes.pdf

Box 19.4 summarises the main focus of each of the AMHP competencies and is intended to give occupational therapists a broad overview of what is required in the AMHP competencies.

## Box 19.4: Main focus of the AMHP competencies

### 1. Knowledge

*Legal frameworks*

An AMHP must understand legislation, related codes of practice, national and local policy and guidelines, and be able to apply them in practice. An AMHP must understand the legal position and accountability of AMHPs, employers and the local authority they are acting for in relation to the Mental Health Act 1983/2007. For their role under the Act, AMHPs receive specific training in application of law and are required to pass an examination relating to the law. The AMHP is also required to have a thorough working knowledge of other aspects of the legal framework within which they undertake their duties within health and social care, for example:

● Care Act (2014)

● Children & Families Act (2014)

● Equality Act (2010)

● Mental Capacity Act (2005) and the Deprivation of Liberty Safeguards (DoLS)

● Domestic Violence, Crime & Victims Act (2004)

● Human Rights Act (1998)

● Children Acts (1989 and 2004)

● Police and Criminal Evidence Act (1984).

(DoH 2015b)

The findings of a social work education study (Tew 2002) show that social work education has a much stronger emphasis on knowledge of legislation whereas occupational therapists were perceived to require knowledge of legislation to underpin professional practice. This may indicate that some occupational therapists may find the legal aspects of AMHP training more challenging.

*Mental disorders*

An AMHP needs to have a broad understanding of a range of models of mental disorder and understand the impact of social, physical and developmental factors on mental health and be able to apply this in practice. An AMHP should have an understanding of the implications of mental disorders for service users, their relatives, carers and other professionals and be able to apply this in practice. An AMHP needs to be aware of the

**310**

different types of treatments and interventions available for mental disorders and the impact of these on the service user, their relatives and carers. Understanding of child and adult protection procedures and the needs of children and young people and their families in relation to AMHP practice is also a requirement.

## 2. Autonomous practice

An AMHP should be able to exercise appropriate use of independence, authority and autonomy and recognise, assess and manage effectively the risks related to the role, including risks to the AMHP and other professionals/agencies, the service user, family, friends, carers, neighbours and the general public.

## 3. Informed decision-making

An AMHP should be able to gather, analyse and share information appropriately when making decisions about service users. An AMHP should have the necessary skills to refer to and critically evaluate a range of research which is relevant to evidence-based AMHP practice; and to evaluate critically local and national policy to inform decision-making.

## 4. Equality and diversity

An AMHP should be able to demonstrate sensitivity to factors such as race, gender, age, sexuality, disability, culture, religion and belief and work to identify, challenge and redress discrimination and inequality in AMHP practice. As in most professions, the service users that AMHPs will come into contact with will have a wide range of different qualities, abilities and diverse backgrounds. An AMHP should be able to promote the rights, dignity and self-determination of service users, consistent with the service user's own needs and wishes, and enable them to contribute to the decisions made affecting quality of life and liberty. An AMHP should also be able to demonstrate sensitivity to a service user's needs for personal respect, confidentiality, choice, dignity and privacy.

## 5. Communication

An AMHP should have the ability to communicate advice, instruction, information and professional opinion effectively with people who may be anxious, distressed and volatile; also carers and family members and a wide range of other professionals and colleagues including doctors, nurses, police and ambulance services, advocates and interpreters, both verbally and in the form of written reports, and at legal hearings. The AMHP should also be able to balance and manage the competing requirements of confidentiality and effective information sharing to the benefit of the service user and other persons concerned with the service user's care.

## 6. Collaborative working

An AMHP needs to have a broad knowledge of the roles and responsibilities of other professionals involved in statutory mental health work and also of other mental health services, i.e. community groups, voluntary organisations and advocates. An AMHP should be able to build and sustain effective professional relationships with service users, relatives, carers and other professionals and agencies and work with them to evaluate the outcomes of interventions and identify any unmet needs.

### 7. Assessment and intervention

An AMHP should be able to effectively plan, negotiate and manage all the relevant legal and practical processes to coordinate compulsory admissions to hospital or arrangements for supervised community treatment, and complete all the relevant statutory documentation. Conversely, AMHPs should be able to assess the feasibility of and contribute effectively to the planning of options other than compulsory admission (HCPC 2013).

# Why do we need AMHPs?

## Independent perspective and upholding service user rights

There is evidence to support the theory that some social groups have been disproportionately subject to compulsory powers and that people from these groups have been more likely to be assessed under the Mental Health Act. These include young men, women, people from ethnic minorities, people with schizophrenia or drug addiction. People who are detained also tend to be those who have experienced high levels of social exclusion, poverty, poor housing and unemployment (Hatfield 2008). Additionally, society's sometimes negative and discriminatory attitudes to mental illness, i.e. prejudice, stigma and scapegoating, can marginalise service users so that they are left feeling excluded and powerless (Tew 2002), and more than three-quarters of people with mental health problems have experienced discrimination in some form (Paton 2012). When carrying out statutory duties the AMHP is expected to advocate on behalf of service users, including those who may be victims of social injustices or infringements of their human rights, and ensure their rights are upheld during all stages of statutory procedures (Yianni 2009).

As an autonomous professional an AMHP is responsible for making independent decisions and taking responsibility for their consequences. In practice, this means an AMHP cannot be instructed by a manager, doctor or any other person, to detain someone, and can only be requested to carry out an assessment of someone deemed mentally disordered. The decision regarding whether the person is detained or not is one that is reached by the AMHP using his or her own independent professional judgement after careful consideration of all the available evidence and risk factors and subject to the provision of two medical recommendations as described above. The AMHP, is required to take all the circumstances of a person's situation into account including social context, race, culture, age and gender. For the majority of people, with or without a mental disorder, losing one's liberty must be a frightening thought because it means being separated from family, friends and pets and not being able to continue in caring roles or in employment or education. It is reasonable to believe that the person may feel frightened and disempowered by what is happening to them. It may be the first time they have been admitted to a psychiatric ward, or negative experiences during a past admission may make them feel afraid about going back into hospital. The role of the AMHP is immensely important in ensuring that service users are treated with respect and dignity during all stages of the assessment process and it is reassuring to know that the AMHP's role is to act as independent arbiter on behalf of the service user who is being assessed and provide an independent opinion, which is non-medical and which counterbalances and if necessary challenges the medical model.

In practice, an example of where this may be necessary is when two doctors are recommending a person be compulsorily detained. After considering all aspects of the person's situation, the AMHP may not feel this is the most appropriate and least restrictive method of addressing the person's needs and would be expected to challenge the doctors' recommendations. An AMHP must always consider alternatives to prevent unnecessary hospital admissions and to ensure that the application for detention is appropriate and proportionate. When considering alternatives to hospital detention an AMHP would assess protective factors, e.g. social networks or family relationships which may help to support a mentally unwell person in the community. Alternative treatment options may also include home treatment or other community-based interventions, guardianship, or treatment under the Mental Capacity Act (UK Parliament 2005). The service user may agree to an informal hospital admission which means that he or she is giving his/her consent to go into hospital voluntarily. Discussions with the service user, nearest relative and others involved in his/her care may give an indication of the types of treatment which have worked in the past. An AMHP should have a thorough working knowledge of services in his/her locality, the referral process to these services and their availability, so that he or she is in a strong position to organise these alternatives (Coffey & Hannigan 2013, DoH 2008, DoH 2015b, Rapaport 2006).

Concerns have been widely expressed in social work literature regarding non-social work professionals undertaking the AMHP role and whether they would be able to uphold the independence of the role. As the other non-social work professionals eligible to become AMHPs, i.e. nurses, occupational therapists and psychologists, are in the main from health backgrounds, it has often been assumed that they are in a position of deference to doctors in the medical hierarchy. Hence the worry that they may not be well-equipped to stand up and defend the rights of the service users and challenge doctors' opinions (Barcham 2008, Wellard 2001). The AMHP core competencies identify an ability to articulate and demonstrate in practice the autonomy and authority inherent in the role (HCPC 2013).

From an occupational therapy perspective, occupational therapists are educated to recognise their own prejudices and identify oppression, discrimination, injustice and instances where people are vulnerable. There is awareness in the occupational therapy profession that services might often place undue emphasis on pathology, as opposed to social factors, and of how this can be redressed

(COT 2006). Many occupational therapists often work with service users who are not aware of their rights, or how to secure them and it is part of the occupational therapy role to advocate on their behalf when situations occur where someone is not recognising, or is denying or abusing the rights of others. Occupational therapists work collaboratively with service users and promote their rights by involving them in all decisions about their lives and countering decisions which may discriminate unlawfully against them (Reed & Sanderson 1999). With the above factors in mind, it is apparent that occupational therapists have a number of skills and a wide knowledge base which would be an asset to occupational therapists wishing to train to become AMHPs. On this basis, it is not envisaged that occupational therapists would encounter difficulty meeting the AMHP competencies regarding the independence and autonomy of the role and service user rights.

## Social perspective

One of the key factors about working from a social perspective is the ability to identify social issues that may have contributed to the person becoming mentally unwell, and then to analyse these within a cultural framework of issues such as race, religion, ethnicity and an awareness of how these impact on mental health. By taking into account the social circumstances of the service user, the AMHP may consider less restrictive interventions that provide social support which are underpinned by social approaches, e.g. social inclusion and the Recovery model which recognise the individual within a social context and support the value of social interventions (Hatfield 2008). Tew (2002) describes a social model which locates mental distress in its social context (e.g. unemployment, poor education, unstable family circumstances, substance misuse) and highlights how social roles, for example, work responsibilities or caring roles, may also impact on a person's mental health (as could enforced loss of these roles or being excluded from them). Family dynamics and social identity problems involved in life transitions can also play a role in contributing to social stress, e.g. unrealistic expectations from family members, feeling under-valued, oppression, inequality or abuse.

It has been widely discussed whether non-social work professionals would continue to take a holistic approach and maintain the broad social perspective as social workers do when performing statutory duties and this is regarded as a key concern (Barcham 2008, Revans 2001, Wellard 2001). Hatfield (2008) highlights the importance of preserving the social perspective within the AMHP role. Tew (2002, p. 147) describes holism as a 'process of reclaiming the whole person from the partiality of a purely medical definition', requiring a much deeper level of engagement with service users and their social experience. The AMHP core competencies identify an ability to articulate and demonstrate in practice a critical understanding of the social perspective of mental disorder (HCPC 2013).

Critical analysis of occupational therapy values and working practices establishes that occupational therapists are familiar with the social model of disability and are accustomed to working holistically by taking into account all aspects of a person's situation (Creek 2003, Mayers 1990). The Mayer's Lifestyle Questionnaire (2) (Mayers 2000), Occupational Self Assessment (OSA) (Baron et al. 2006) and the Occupational Circumstances Assessment, Interview and Rating Scale (OCAIRS)

(Forsyth *et al.* 2005) are all examples of standardised assessments used in occupational therapy which reflect the social model of disability. The Lifestyle Performance Model (Velde & Fidler 2002) and the Client-centred Model of Practice (Sumsion 1999) are models of occupational therapy which are underpinned by holism. For occupational therapists, mental health has been defined as 'more than the absence of mental illness; how the individual thinks and feels about her/himself and others; interprets events, communicates and learns; copes with change, stress and conflict; forms and sustains relationships, and participates in her/his social and physical environment' (Creek 2003, p. 55). Occupational therapists are aware of, and able to analyse cultural and lifestyle factors (i.e. age, gender, race, nationality, colour, sexual orientation, level of ability or position in society) and are sensitive to these factors when planning interventions (Creek 2003). Occupational therapists are trained to identify barriers and analyse factors preventing occupational participation, e.g. cultural and lifestyle issues, lack of social networks, environmental factors and the way that some individuals are prevented from participating in activities because they feel excluded, isolated, worthless or lacking in confidence (Finlay 2004, Kielhofner 2002). An analysis carried out by Alsop and Vigars (1998) in relation to social work and occupational therapy practice identified that knowledge, skills and values were very similar for both professions and were found to be carried out from a similar philosophical perspective. Empowerment was identified as a strong guiding principle for both professions, as well as autonomy, working in collaboration with service users and working holistically. Many shared and overlapping values were identified between social work and occupational therapy and shared ways of working, e.g. use of social model of disability, holism. This gives a good indication that occupational therapists should not encounter any difficulty meeting the AMHP competencies which relate to the social perspective nor applying these in practice.

## Ethical dilemmas

Ethical dilemmas faced by AMHPs when performing statutory duties have been widely discussed (Hatfield 2008, Wellard 2001, Yianni 2009). Shortage of beds within mental health services is a contentious and ongoing issue. The availability of inpatient psychiatric beds was highlighted in a practice survey of AMHP leads over 152 local social services authorities undertaken by the College of Social Work in 2013 (CSW 2013). Concerns were reported both at assessment and admission stages with admissions being delayed due to difficulties finding an appropriate bed resulting in increased risk to the patient, family/carers, members of the public and professionals involved. What is most concerning is that 16.5 per cent of respondents stated that in one or more cases an individual had been detained because an informal admission to psychiatric inpatient care was unavailable. This means that a person has been detained for reasons other than for their health, safety or protection of others which are the criteria for formal detention under the Mental Health Act. In my own practice as an AMHP I have encountered situations where an out-of-area bed has had to be sought because of bed shortages locally. This has resulted in mentally distressed patients being conveyed and admitted to hospitals which are often over 100 miles away. I believe that the furthest distance a patient has had to travel to an out-of-area bed is 370 miles, a journey which took six hours (McNicoll 2015). Occupational therapists contemplating becoming AMHPs should have an awareness of ethical issues and consider how they might feel if they had to make decisions which they felt were in conflict with their professional values or where there are situations of competing interests.

Balancing the needs of the service user alongside those of the wider public is a recurrent theme (Campbell 2010), and AMHPs often have to make highly complex decisions which involve competing needs. On many occasions situations arise where the value of a person's right to freedom is overridden by the competing value of his/her need for protection and treatment; or the need for public safety, and skill is required to uphold service user rights while protecting others from the danger their mental illness may cause (Lepping 2007, Yianni 2009). The power imbalance between the AMHP and the service user is also a widely discussed theme as it is inevitable that there is considerable imbalance of power when one individual has the power to enforce a decision on behalf of another (Chan 2002). Occupational therapists considering becoming AMHPs would be wise to consider whether they would be comfortable exerting some of the powers associated with the role and the level of complexity of judgement associated with some of the decisions AMHPs are required to make.

For occupational therapists contemplating becoming an AMHP to gain a more in-depth understanding of the difficulties, ethical considerations and dilemmas faced by AMHPs and a clearer picture of what the daily life of an AMHP is like, I would recommend reading Sandra Dwyer's paper 'Walking the tightrope of a Mental Health Act assessment' (Dwyer 2012). Although the paper is written from a social work perspective, as a practising AMHP and occupational therapist, I have experienced situations similar to most of those that are discussed. One example is the inaccuracy or dearth of information often provided on Mental Health Act assessment referrals which makes the information gathering process even more difficult, when there are often time limitations as this is a crisis situation and action is required. Managing the emotions of others, including relatives and friends of the service user who may be crying and distressed, or angry and resentful that their loved one has been sectioned, alongside managing the emotions of the mentally ill person who may be becoming increasingly distressed can be challenging.

I have experienced a situation where the service user blamed her son for the fact that she had been sectioned and proceeded to throw all her son's belongings out into the street. In these types of circumstances the AMHP's focus will be on trying to maintain the service user's privacy and dignity from the neighbours, who may be looking out of their windows or who may have even approached the AMHP to ask what is happening. Long waiting times for ambulances is an issue and though this is not always the case, most AMHPs will have experienced this. I have often had to wait in the service user's home for four hours or more for an ambulance to arrive. These situations are difficult because the service user and family may not want the AMHP to be there. It is true that the AMHP's car may sometimes be the only safe place in tense situations and I have spent a large amount of time in my car, cold, tired and hungry, waiting for an ambulance to arrive to convey someone to hospital. On many occasions I have not arrived home until after midnight, having been on AMHP duty since nine that morning, and have then had to get up for work the next morning as usual. Although police involvement in conveying someone to hospital is a last resort it is often necessary due to levels of risk; Dwyer (2012) describes the barbarity of forcing someone to leave their home. I have experienced situations where service users have had to be physically restrained by the police and one occasion when the use of handcuffs was required because the person was refusing to go into hospital after being sectioned and was being physically aggressive. When inside the police van the person harmed himself by hitting his head repeatedly against the side of the vehicle, his mental distress and frustration at the situation he found himself in was so great. Some service users regard being sectioned as evidence that they have done something wrong and are being punished by being taken to hospital against their will. I have been involved in assessments where the service user has actually said words to this effect and these situations can be very difficult to deal with because they emphasise the power imbalance between the AMHP and the person they have sectioned. When assessing older people, with dementia for example, it should be borne in mind that the person may be leaving their home for the last time, as long-term care may be the most appropriate option after being discharged from hospital. Occupational therapists thinking about becoming AMHPs should consider how these types of situations might affect them and what skills they would use to manage them effectively.

## Conclusion

The AMHP role is complex, and without doubt the most demanding and challenging role in community mental health. As such, it is recognised and acknowledged within health and social care services as a senior and exacting role. Uptake of the role by occupational therapists has been low (Smyth 2013, Knott & Bannigan 2013). The College of Occupational Therapists cites the reasons for this as being due to education providers making entry to AMHP courses difficult for occupational therapists, work agencies refusing to accept AMHP trained occupational therapists and social work colleagues expressing doubt and disbelief that an occupational therapist could undertake the AMHP role; and the College of Occupational Therapists regards these reasons as unfair. As an occupational therapist-AMHP I have experienced negative attitudes from social work colleagues but none of the other difficulties described above. A positive view of an occupational therapist undertaking AMHP training can be found in De-Feu's 2012 paper. From a knowledge and skills perspective, most occupational therapists should not encounter any difficulty during AMHP training. The course is challenging, as academic standards are high and academic abilities will vary, as with professionals from all disciplines. From a values perspective, there is coherence between social work and occupational therapy values (Knott & Bannigan 2013) so it is not envisaged that this will cause any more difficulty to occupational therapists than it would do to social workers. Practice as an AMHP offers the opportunity to work autonomously and take responsibility for making independent decisions based on professional judgement which some occupational therapists may regard as an incentive. The AMHP is rewarded in monetary terms, either by increments to their basic pay or via a separate monthly payment; however, the financial incentive for becoming an AMHP is relatively small. From a job satisfaction point of view, it is rewarding to know that by sectioning someone you may have saved their life, and although most service users don't think so at the time they are being detained, some may even thank you afterwards for intervening and removing them from situations in which they were at risk themselves and may have been causing risks to others.

## Deciding whether to train to become an AMHP

If after reading this chapter, you are still considering whether to become an AMHP, undertaking any of the following activities may help to provide a broader perspective and deeper insight into the role for occupational therapists who are unsure whether this is the right career choice for them. Alternatively, if as an occupational therapist you have already made the decision to apply for AMHP training, some of the ideas in Box 19.5 may prove useful in preparing for the course.

**Box 19.5: Ideas for preparation for/deciding whether to undertake the AMHP course**

- Shadow AMHPs who are carrying out Mental Health Act assessments. Aim to shadow assessments in a variety of settings, e.g. service users' homes, hospitals, police stations, care homes, and with different client groups, e.g. older people, adults, children and adolescents.

- Learn more about Community Treatment Orders and how these are put in place by shadowing an AMHP and discussing the process.

- Attend a Mental Health Tribunal or Hospital Managers' hearing.

- Find out if your local university offers a pre-AMHP foundation course to assist potential candidates in familiarising themselves with the current academic requirements and other aspects of the course, e.g. building knowledge of social perspectives on mental health.

- Discuss the course requirements with your local AMHP lead or with AMHPs who have recently completed the course, particularly occupational therapist AMHPs (if you can find one!).

- Discuss your thoughts about training to become an AMHP with other AMHPs to get an idea of how the role impacts on them carrying out their normal duties, for example – how many times are they expected to act as AMHP per week on the duty rota, do they carry a reduced caseload and how does this impact on the rest of the team?

- Arrange to spend some time in different mental health settings, e.g. forensic, eating disorders, acute wards, autism services, assertive outreach (wherever you feel you are lacking knowledge and experience) to gain an understanding of the needs of different groups of mental health service users and how these are managed.

- Develop your knowledge of child and adult protection procedures and the needs of children and young people with mental health issues. Find out more about the services for children and young people in your local area.

- Raise your awareness of the services in your area which may help to keep a person out of hospital, e.g. Intensive Community Treatment teams and other community services.

- Develop your knowledge of other relevant legislation, e.g. the Mental Capacity Act 2005 and Deprivation of Liberty Safeguards (DoLS).

- Become involved with voluntary sector groups, e.g. Mind, to learn more about their work and service user perspectives on mental health issues.

- Spend some time with an Independent Mental Health Advocate (IMHA) to learn more about their role in relation to the Mental Health Act. (Note: the IMHA role is another role related to the Mental Health Act which is open to occupational therapists and which utilises their advocacy strength.)

- Find out more about issues related to drugs and alcohol and their impact on mental health. Spend some time with your local drug and alcohol service to find out more about their work.

- Think about your own work–life balance and your roles and responsibilities outside work and how being an AMHP might impact on them.

# Useful resources

- Department of Health (2013) *Code of Practice: Mental Health Act 1983*. London: TSO.
- Suggested further reading to gain a picture of what life is like from a mental health service user's perspective:
  - Filer, N. (2014). *The Shock of the Fall*. London: The Borough Press.
  - O'Donoghue, J. (2009). *Sectioned – A Life Interrupted*. London: John Murray.
  - Sanghera, S. (2009). *The Boy with the Top Knot*. London: Penguin.

# References

Alsop, A. & Vigars C. (1998). Shared learning: joint training or dual qualification in occupational therapy and social work: a feasibility study. *British Journal of Occupational Therapy* **61** (4), 146–152.

Barcham, C. (2008). From ASW to AMHP. *Community Care.* http://www.communitycare.co.uk/2008/10/28/from-asw-to-amhp/ (last accessed: 30.11.2015).

Baron, K., Kielhofner, G., Lyenger, A., Goldammer, V. & Wolenski, J. (2006). *The Occupational Self Assessment (OSA). Version 2.2.* Chicago: Model of Human Occupation Clearinghouse, Department of Occupational Therapy, College of Applied Health Sciences, University of Illinois.

Brookes, G. & Brindle, N. (2010). Compulsion in the community? The introduction of supervised community treatment. *Advances in Psychiatric Treatment* **16** (4), 245–252.

Campbell, J. (2010). Deciding to detain: the use of compulsory mental health law by UK social workers. *British Journal of Social Work* **40** (1), 328–334.

Chan, P. (2002). In whose best interests? An examination of ethics of the UK government's white paper 'Reforming the Mental Health Act'. *Journal of Psychiatric and Mental Health Nursing* **9** (4), 399–404.

Coffey, M. & Hannigan, B. (2013). New roles for nurses as AMHPs. *International Journal of Nursing Studies* **50** (10), 1423–1430.

College of Occupational Therapists (2006). *Recovering Ordinary Lives: the Strategy for Occupational Therapy in Mental Health Services 2007–2017 – a vision for the next ten years*. London: COT.

College of Social Work (2013). *AMHP Survey 2013*. London: CSW.

Creek, J. (2003). *Occupational Therapy Defined as a Complex Intervention*. London: COT.

De-Feu, M. (2012). What did the OT say to the AMHP … *Professional Social Work* (June), 14–15.

Department of Health (2007a). *New Ways of Working for Everyone – a Best Practice Implementation Guide*. London: TSO.

Department of Health (2007b). *National Institute for Mental Health in England/Care Services Improvement Partnership: Preparing for Change: understanding how the amendments to the Mental Health Act 1983 will affect the practice of ASWs and RMOs.* London: TSO.

Department of Health (2008). *National Institute for Mental Health in England/Care Services Improvement Partnership: Workbook to support implementation of the Mental Health Act 1983 as amended by the Mental Health Act 2007.* London: TSO.

Department of Health (2015a). *Mental Health Act 1983: Code of Practice*. London: TSO.

Department of Health (2015b). *Reference Guide to the Mental Health Act*. London: TSO.

Dwyer, S. (2012). Walking the tightrope of a mental health act assessment. *Journal of Social Work Practice* **26** (3), 341–353.

Finlay, L. (2004). *The Practice of Psychosocial Occupational Therapy,* 3rd edn. Cheltenham: Nelson Thornes.

Forsyth, K., Deshpande, S., Kielhofner, G., Henriksson, C., Haglund, L., Olson, L., Skinner, S. & Kulkarni S. (2005). *The Occupational Circumstances Assessment, Interview and Rating Scale (OCAIRS).* Chicago: Model of Human Occupation Clearing House, Department of Occupational Therapy, College of Applied Health Sciences, University of Illinois.

Hall, I. & Ali, A. (2009). Changes to the Mental Health and Mental Capacity Acts: implications for patients and professionals. *Psychiatric Bulletin* **33** (6), 226–230.

Hatfield, B. (2008). Powers to detain under mental health legislation in England and the role of the approved social worker: an analysis of patterns and trends under the 1983 Mental Health Act in six local authorities. *British Journal of Social Work* **38** (8), 1553–1571.

Health and Care Professions Council (2013). *Approval Criteria for Approved Mental Health Professional (AMHP) Programmes.* London: Health and Care Professions Council. http://www/hcpc-uk.org (last accessed: 22.2.2016).

Jones, R. (2013). *Mental Health Act Manual,* 16th edn. London: Sweet & Maxwell.

Kielhofner, G. (2002c). *Dimensions of doing in Model of Human Occupation, theory and application,* 3rd edn. Baltimore, MD: Lippincott, Williams and Wilkins.

Knott, G. & Bannigan, K. (2013). A critical review of the approved mental health professional role and occupational therapy. *British Journal of Occupational Therapy* **76** (3), 118–126.

Lepping, P. (2007). Ethical analysis of the new proposed mental health legislation in England and Wales. *Philosophy, Ethics and Humanities in Medicine* **2** (5), 5–9.

McKay, E., Craik, C., Lim, K.H. & Richards, G. (2008). *Advancing Occupational Therapy in Mental Health Practice.* New Jersey: Wiley-Blackwell.

McNicoll, A. (2015). *Mental health patients sent hundreds of miles for beds as out of area placements rise 23 percent. Community Care.* http://www.communitycare.co.uk (last accessed: 22.2.2016).

Mayers, C.A. (1990). A philosophy unique to occupational therapy. *British Journal of Occupational Therapy* **53** (9), 379–380.

Mayers, C.A. (2000). The Lifestyle Questionnaire (2). School of Professional Health Studies: York St. John College.

Merchant, C. (2007). Matching skills to needs. *Mental Health Today* (April) 23–25.

Mind (The National Association for Mental Health) (2011). *Mind Rights Guide 1: Civil Admission to Hospital.* http://www.mind.org.uk (last accessed: 1.2.2016).

Ministry of Justice (2007). *Mental Capacity Act 2005: Code of Practice.* London: TSO.

Paton, N. (2012). Miliband unveils labour plans to address mental health problems. *Occupational Health* **64** (12), 7.

Rapaport, J. (2006). New roles in mental health: the creation of the approved mental health practitioner. *Journal of Integrated Care* **14** (5), 37–46.

Rapaport, J. & Manthorpe, J. (2008). Putting it into practice: will the new mental health act slow down or accelerate integrated working? *Journal of Integrated Care* **16** (4), 22–29.

Reed, K.L. & Sanderson, S.N. (1999). *Concepts of Occupational Therapy*, 4th edn. Philadelphia: Lippincott, Williams and Wilkins.

Revans, L. (2001). Social workers fight to retain role in mental health assessments. *Community Care* http://www.communitycare.co.uk (last accessed: 30.11.2015).

Smyth, G. (2013) *OT AMHPs face 'catalogue of prejudice and misunderstanding'.* London: College of Occupational Therapists. https://www.cot.co.uk/ (last accessed: 22.2.2016).

Sumsion, T. (1999). *Client-centred Practice in Occupational Therapy: a Guide to Implementation.* Edinburgh: Churchill Livingstone.

Tew, J. (2002). Going social: championing a holistic model of mental distress within professional education. *Social Work Education* **21** (2), 143–155.

United Kingdom Parliament (1983/2007). *Mental Health Act.* London: TSO.

United Kingdom Parliament (2005). *Mental Capacity Act.* London: TSO.

Velde, B.P. & Fidler, G.S. (2002). *Lifestyle Performance: A model for Engaging the Power of Occupation.* Thorofare NJ: Slack.

Wellard, S. (2001). Reform of role leads to independence worries. *Community Care* http://www.communitycare.co.uk (last accessed: 30.11.2015).

Yianni, C. (2009). Aces high: my control trumps your care. *Ethics and Social Welfare* **3** (3), 337–343.

# Chapter 20

# Roles associated with mental capacity and the Deprivation of Liberty Safeguards

Julie Carr and Jane Clewes

## Introduction

This chapter outlines the extended role of Best Interests Assessor (BIA) which occupational therapists can undertake following specific training for the role. Other associated roles are included, and a general overview of the role of mental capacity and the Deprivation of Liberty Safeguards (DoLS) is given.

## Key points

- Mental capacity should be considered in all areas of clinical practice, and all healthcare professionals should be able to undertake decision-specific assessments of mental capacity.

- Occupational therapists make good BIAs as they are inherently client-centred, creative problem-solvers and pragmatic, as well as holding beliefs and philosophies which are compatible with/similar to the principles of the Mental Capacity Act.

- The core and unique knowledge of the occupational therapist regarding activity analysis offers very valuable insights into the formulation which takes place when choosing between care and accommodation options for a person: they can predict and transfer information about the person to understand the subtleties between one environment and another impacting on the complexity of the way a person functions.

## Occupational therapists and the Mental Capacity Act (2005)

All occupational therapists need to develop a working knowledge of the Mental Capacity Act (UK Parliament 2005), including its five principles (which coincide well with the philosophy and priorities

**323**

of occupational therapy). Occupational therapists make skilled and natural advocates, and it is within living memory that occupational therapy was the discipline that was tasked with undertaking an advocacy role for patients/clients. Occupational therapists think independently and are client-centric and are familiar with negotiating the space between the forces of the rest of the MDT (multi-disciplinary team)/organisation and the preferences of the person in order to do this. Occupational therapists are ideally suited to roles such as discharge facilitator/coordinator with inpatient elderly (COT 2016) where the guidelines of the National Institute for Health and Care Excellence (NICE 2015) recommend increased person-centred care, communication and information sharing, and coordination and planning of the discharge process. In today's world of pressures on beds, occupational therapists are, perhaps, the discipline most likely to retain some semblance of common sense and ability to work with a humanistic approach (thus achieving the outputs which are within the principles of the Mental Capacity Act 2005).

The role of BIA is relatively new. It is open to social workers, nurses, occupational therapists, psychologists and medics. The role was introduced with the DoLS amendments in 2007 to the Mental Capacity Act 2005, being found at SI 2008/1858, regulation 5 legislation. To be a BIA requires two years of post-registration experience in one of the identified professions (social work, nursing, medic, occupational therapist and psychologist); to be registered with the appropriate professional body and not suspended from the register; to obtain an accredited qualification; to become recognised (endorsed) by the Supervisory Body (SB) who instruct the BIA to undertake the identified DoLS assessments; and to complete annual update training as evidence of ongoing knowledge and competency. At the time of writing, the Law Commission has submitted in their consultation report a recommendation for the renaming of the role from 'BIA' to 'Approved Mental Capacity Professional' (AMCP or AMCaP) (Law Commission 2015).

A BIA is an independent assessor who brackets off any bias from political pressures of their employer or commissioner when they undertake the DoLS assessment. They take an objective stance in their examination of the case. The role draws heavily on clinical experience and knowledge. Occupational therapists are ideally suited to the role due to their client-centred, empowering, empathetic stance. If the reader is:

● an occupational therapist from any field who is looking around for a new challenge/direction

● an occupational therapist who is thinking of embarking on a BIA course

● just starting to study on a BIA course

or

● working with a population where they need to understand what a DoLS involves,

then this chapter will be of interest.

The authors have both practised as BIAs for some years now. They enjoy this work and would strongly recommend it to occupational therapists as something that fits well with the occupational therapy philosophy and skill set. They would urge occupational therapists to take up the opportunity of training to become a BIA for reasons of job satisfaction, service user empowerment, and to positively promote the profession of occupational therapists. It could be said that an occupational therapist already has most of the skills to undertake the work of a BIA but would need to be trained in order to gain knowledge of the processes and legislation involved in the role.

# Brief summary of the evolution of Deprivation of Liberty Safeguards

## The legislation

Over the years there is a wide background of legislation which addresses the autonomy and rights of the person. Most societies worldwide are developing a shared understanding and increased recognition of equality which includes within it an emphasis upon respecting others. In comparatively modern times within the UK, mainstream slavery has been abolished, women secured the vote and equal opportunities have become a legal framework for employers to adhere to. During the Second World War there were atrocities carried out whereby humans were forced to submit without voluntary consent to having their body/person experimented on. This gave rise to the Nuremberg Code (National Institute of Health 1949) which was superseded later by the World Medical Association Declaration of Helsinki (DoH 2008). United Kingdom law has grown in recent decades considerably, and we now have the Human Rights Act (1998), the Mental Capacity Act (2005), a revised Mental Health Act (2007), and updated social care legislation (the Care Act 2014). In future years, who knows what may develop? The United Nations Convention on the Rights of Persons with Disabilities (UNCRPD) (Geneva) are currently reviewing practices such as the UK's Mental Health Act (1983/2007) and DoLS, and may deem them to be too patriarchal, suggesting they be revised to reflect a move from substitute decision making to supported decision making.

The right to liberty is enshrined in English Law, with the earliest record of this being found in Magna Carta and quoted in a speech by the Right Honourable the Lord Chief Justice in a speech he delivered in 2012:

> No free man shall be seized or imprisoned, or stripped of his rights or possessions, or outlawed or exiled, or deprived of his standing in any other way, nor will we proceed with force against him, or send others to do so, except by the lawful judgement of his equals or by the law of the land.
>
> (Lord Chief Justice 2012)

More recently, following the atrocities committed during the Second World War, a treaty known formally as the Convention for the Protection of Human Rights and Fundamental Freedoms was drafted by the newly formed Council of Europe. It was signed by all member states of which Britain was one and the convention entered into force on 03 September 1953. This Treaty is now known as the European Convention for Human Rights (ECHR). The Human Rights Act 1998 (c42) received Royal Assent on 9 November 1998, and mostly came into force on 2 October 2000. The aim of this Act was to incorporate the ECHR into domestic law. All new Acts of Parliament must be compliant with the requirements of the Human Rights Act 1998.

In 2004 a long running case (HL v UK (ECtHR; 2004) 40 EHHR 761) was brought before the European Court in Strasburg, contending that the applicant had been deprived of his liberty. The court found that HL had indeed been deprived of his liberty and that English Law was not compatible with the ECHR in that there was no legal provision to detain a person who lacked capacity to consent to the circumstances of his care and treatment and was essentially compliant. The conclusion was that a legal remedy was required.

Article 5 Human Rights Act 1998 shows its relationship to Magna Carta, stating that:

> **Art.5 (1) Everyone has the right to liberty and security of person. No one shall be deprived of his liberty save in the following cases and in accordance with a procedure prescribed by law.**
>
> (UK Parliament 1998)

At this time the Mental Capacity Bill (c9) was too far progressed to incorporate a provision for the incapacitated compliant patient and therefore it proceeded, receiving Royal Assent in 2005 and was enacted in 2007. The remedy to the gap in law which became known as 'The Bournewood Gap' was found through the vehicle of the amendments to the Mental Health Act 1983 (c20) which created the Deprivation of Liberty Safeguard as an amendment to the Mental Capacity Act 2005.

## Neary and the Bournewood Gap

Steven Neary is a young man with a learning disability who was cared for at home primarily by his father. When Mr Neary became unwell with flu, Steven was admitted to a known unit for a period of respite to allow his father to recover. From this unit Steven was moved to long-term placement in 24-hour care and Mr Neary's contact was limited. Steven was made subject to a DoLS authorisation. Following 18 months of contesting the authorisation, the case was heard in June 2011 by Jackson J. at the Royal Courts of Justice. Jackson J. found that Hillingdon Borough had:

- unlawfully breached Steven's Art. 8 rights
- unlawfully breached Steven's Art. 5 (1) rights
- unlawfully breached Steven's Art. 5 (4) rights
- deprived Steven of his liberty without lawful authority under Schedule A1 Mental Capacity Act 2005.

Steven Neary reacted with distress when there was a different driver than usual when he boarded the dedicated bus to travel to his day care. When he arrived at the day centre, the care staff initiated arrangements for him to be admitted to the psychiatric hospital. Steven remained in the hospital for a long time, and when his family asked why he was not returning home the hospital team said that he needed to remain there still. Steven was not on a Mental Health Act (1983/2007) Section. Steven's father took this to the Court of Protection where it was found that Steven was unlawfully deprived of his liberty.

Chapter 2 of the DoLS Code of Practice (Ministry of Justice 2008) provides a concise synopsis of the case of HL, who it was determined had been unlawfully deprived of his liberty at Bournewood Hospital. Essentially the ECtHR considered the impact of HL's admission on his Art. 5 rights. In this case they determined that by exercising 'complete and effective control over his care and movements' (2.22 Code of Practice) and that the evidence of consultant psychiatrist was that had HL 'resisted admission or tried to leave thereafter, she would have prevented him from doing so and would have considered his involuntary committal under S.3 of the 1983 Act'.

The Court concluded that '[a]ccordingly, the concrete situation was that the applicant was under continuous supervision and control and was not free to leave'. As such the court found that HL's Art.5 rights had been breached. The DoLS were developed in response to this matter and focused initially on addressing the Art. 5(1) issues of his right to liberty, and Art. 5(4) rights to a speedy review of detention by a court.

The key practice change from this landmark case was the raised profile of the role and importance of a person's Art. 8 rights to a private and family life within the considerations for a DoLS authorisation. A much greater emphasis was placed on the views of those consulted and DoLS became a balancing act between Art. 5 and Art. 8 Human Rights Act 1998.

More recently, a change through case law has created an emphasis which is now required to be based upon the person's own wishes: Re Wye Valley NHS Trust v Mr B [2015] EWCOP 60 (Peter Jackson J). When weighing up what is in the person's best interests, a heavier weighting than before this case should be placed on the person's own wishes (especially when longstanding). This may lead to an increase in cases being taken to the Court of Protection.

## The Supreme Court Judgement: Lady Hale and 'the acid test'

In March 2014 the cases of P v Cheshire West and Chester Council and P&Q v Surrey County Council resulted in a significant piece of case law which increased the volume of DoLS cases wholesale. The judge, Lady Hale, defined a deprivation of liberty (DoL) as applying to *everyone* who lacks capacity to decide on their own care and accommodation in a care/nursing home or hospital whether they are stating objections to their deprivation or not. She ruled that whether it was the norm for someone with the person's disability or condition to be subjected to a level of control, supervision and restriction or not, they were still being deprived of their liberty. The 'acid test' included that if the person was to walk out of the door they would, for reasons of their safety, be stopped from doing so. Until this point, DoLS authorisations were generally limited to being sought for those people who lacked capacity to consent to being resident at a care/nursing home or hospital and were also objecting to this by saying that they wished to leave or through their behaviour such as trying to get out of the door or abscond. It had not accounted for those people who are often referred to as 'the pleasantly demented', i.e. people who state or demonstrate no objection to their residency at a care/nursing home or hospital. This in many ways made sense as, just because someone is not objecting to their residency, it does not mean that if they were aware/able to they wouldn't object.

> Was he free? Was he happy? The question is absurd:
> Had anything been wrong, we should certainly have heard.
>
> (W.H. Auden, *The Unknown Citizen* 1942)

If taken in the context of DoLS, this could be interpreted to mean that people can be compliant, coerced and/or unaware of their lack of freedom and agency, or all three. The poem draws on the idea of a standardising bureaucratic organisation viewing the person as average, non-individual and arbitrary (Haffenden 1983).

# The training to become a Best Interests Assessor

Each locality will have its own arrangements for recruiting and training BIAs. Since the Local Authority (LA) has an obligation to undertake DoLS assessments and authorisations, they will often provide the funding for people to train. The selection process for acceptance for sponsorship to attend the training for each LA will vary, but it might include an interview process, and even a written piece as part of the application (such as a statement of why the candidate wants to undertake the role and training, or even an actual marked assignment to test whether the applicant can work and clinically reason to Masters level (M-level)). The local policy might include the need for the trainee's current manager to agree to them doing the training, and for them to be released on the days when the training and shadowing experience takes place. It would also be at the discretion of each manager whether any additional study time is approved. Part of a manager's consideration regarding whether to authorise the release of their staff member might be whether they will be able to release them to go to work on a rota once they are trained and endorsed. This would depend on how funding takes place at the locality.

The training course is usually an M-level module; some courses are run at H-level. Entry requirements may be different – some universities demand evidence of recent study, others may require a written assignment to a set question/essay title. It might be offered as a stand-alone module or as part of a full Masters degree course such as Adult Safeguarding. Typically, the student attends six to ten full days of training at the university, and has days where they are 'on fieldwork placement' when they shadow a practising BIA. There will be a number of assessed assignments to pass, which are often applied in nature such as focusing on a case study; they may also include the submission of a reflective portfolio or a presentation of a case to a panel who then ask questions.

The training covers the Mental Capacity Act (2005), the related legislation, and how to undertake a DoLS in practice.

Once qualified, the BIA is usually put through a process of endorsement for the LA they are to practise for. This could take the form of carrying out a couple of DoLS assessments under the supervision of an endorsed BIA; their reports are then submitted for review and an endorsement letter is supplied. The BIA has to undertake a specified minimum of practice per year as well as a minimum number of hours in update training per year in order to continue to practise; every five years they submit a portfolio of experience, feedback, training log and reflective written assignments (not dissimilar to those for occupational therapists with the HCPC) in order to be reaccredited.

# Working as a Best Interests Assessor

Again, each locality makes its own arrangements for securing sufficient DoLS assessors for its population. There could be one or a range of strategies, such as: (a) having a number of trained BIAs within the organisation who operate on a rota basis where they undertake a day or two each month out from their main role in order to carry out DoLS assessments; (b) set posts with part-time or full-time BIAs employed. Other localities might utilise bank or agency staff, or BIAs who are self-employed – in these cases there may be a cost-per-case payment instead of a payment by the number of hours.

## What does a DoLS assessment comprise?

Every Managing Authority (MA) (residential care or nursing home licensee, the manager of a hospital and, more recently (DoH 2014), the licensees of community supported living placements) has a responsibility to undertake regular mental capacity assessments with each of their residents around the decision of whether to remain at that residence and receive the care therein (as per care plans). On an occasion that they deem a resident to have lost the capacity (or, on admission to the unit when the assessment is done the person is deemed not to hold the capacity) regarding this decision, they must place an urgent (seven days) DoLS authorisation on the person. The person is known as the 'Relevant Person' or 'RP'. At the same time, they apply to the LA (the local DoLS team) for a DoLS assessment to take place with a view to placing a 'standard authorisation' on the RP. The LA can extend the duration of the urgent DoLS authorisation a further seven days if there is good reason to do so. The MA must also ensure that they make a written request for a further standard authorisation for each of their residents who are already subject to a DoLS authorisation in good time (three weeks ahead) before the current authorisation expires.

There are six assessments within the process of the DoLS' 'Best Interests Assessment':

- Age
- No refusals

- Mental capacity
- Mental health
- Eligibility
- Deprivation.

Each DoLS assessment must be undertaken by at least two clinicians who have been accredited to do so.

A BIA is allocated to lead the DoLS assessment. They are responsible for arranging that a Section 12 approved doctor is asked to undertake (a) a mental health assessment; and (b) an eligibility assessment. The Section 12 approved doctor in some localities is the person who carries out the capacity assessment, but in other localities it is the BIA who does the capacity assessment.

The mental health assessment seeks to determine whether the RP has an impairment of, or disturbance in, the functioning of the mind or brain. This can be of a temporary or permanent nature. There does not need to be a formal diagnosis in place, the doctor can assess for e.g. 'cognitive impairment' for people who may have declined a memory clinic assessment. The mental health assessor also assesses and reports on the ways in which being deprived of liberty is likely to affect their mental health. The Section 12 approved doctor usually undertakes the eligibility assessment too: this is to make sure that the RP is not currently subject to any conflicting conditions under the Mental Health Act (1983/2007) or whether the issue in hand should be something more appropriately dealt with through assessment and treatment under the Mental Health Act (1983/2007). Either the Section 12 approved doctor or the BIA undertake the capacity assessment (depending on local arrangements).

The BIA makes sure that the person is aged 18 or over (age assessment). They check whether there are any conflicting authorities in place, such as whether the RP has an Advance Decision, Power of Attorney for health and welfare, or deputee (no refusals assessment).

The BIA gathers supporting information for their best interests assessment. They examine written records (care plans, risk assessments, reports etc.), interview staff who are involved in the RP's care (carer staff, nursing, social work, therapists, etc.). They speak to friends and family members. They interview the RP themselves, taking care to ensure full opportunity for their participation in the process; and if there is the need, the BIA requests an independent advocate (a paid representative or Independent Mental Capacity Advocate (IMCA)) is appointed to support the RP and speak on their behalf. The BIA needs to gather information on risks (likelihood, severity, consequences etc.), what the care needs are, whether the RP is objecting to being there or to any part of their residence or care.

The BIA establishes what the controls and levels of supervision are (locked door, telecare, one-to-one, cot sides, sedative medicines, etc.). They determine whether a deprivation is taking place, as defined in the legislation. They produce a detailed report giving their reasons for their conclusions and taking into account everyone's views (including the advocate/IMCA's).

The six parts to the DoLS assessment along with the MA's request are submitted to the LA who review them and give authorisation to the DoLS. The LA then issue a summary report to the MA, the RP and the people involved.

## Assessing capacity

All health professionals should be able to assess a person's capacity. The Mental Capacity Act (2005) gives three principles to apply:

- A person must be assumed to have capacity unless shown otherwise;
- All practicable steps should have been taken to help the person make the decision (demonstrate capacity);
- A person with capacity can make an unwise decision if they so wish (Mughal & Richards 2015, p. 8).

Remember, assessing capacity is *decision specific*, so the first thing to do is to specify the decision to be made. If you see a comment in a set of case notes with a vague 'does not have capacity' which is not accompanied by a statement of what it is that the person does not have capacity to decide, then you don't know whether this is referring to the person not having capacity to choose between a cheese or ham sandwich or whether to declare war on penguins! The second thing to do is to *tell the person* what the decision being made is, and what the *salient points* of that decision are (e.g. whether to move into a care home or return home with a social care package, and the potential harm is that a further fall risking severe injury is very likely). Capacity assessments are also *time specific*.

The DoLS capacity assessment uses a 'two-stage' process. First, they should have an impairment or disturbance of the mind or brain, which can be temporary or permanent (e.g. acute confusional state such as UTI; dementia; personality disorder; eating disorder; psychosis; brain injury; learning disability; hyponatremia; kidney failure), and does not necessarily have to be a formally diagnosed condition – it may be that the person has clearly observable signs of cognitive impairment. Secondly, the functional assessment: this is where the assessor finds out whether the mind/brain impairment/disturbance is to the degree that it is preventing the person undertaking the decision at hand. Does the person *understand* the salient points? Do they *retain* the information (for long enough to undertake the decision)? And, do they *use* the information when processing their decision? Then, a 'causative nexus' should be stated to link a lack of capacity to the mind/brain impairment/disturbance.

## Going to court

Just as people detained in prison have the right to appeal, and people detained under the MHA have the right to a tribunal, people subject to a DoLS have the right to representation to the Court of Protection. There are occasions when the BIA will have to attend court. This is the Court of Protection, and it is here that issues of disagreement (appeal) are scrutinised, and instances when a court decision over and above a DoLS authorisation is required (e.g. a 2IA application, UK Government 2014). The RP has the right to challenge the DoLS, and the RPR or IMCA can support them to take it to court, or can do so on their behalf if they are not able to engage in the process. The BIA might themselves decide that the issue requires a court ruling.

## Box 20.1: Case study – contact with family members

An RP with a mild learning disability has a childhood history of abuse. He was removed as a child from the family home where he had been neglected, physically abused and subjected to witnessing constant discord within the home which often turned to violence. He currently resides in a residential group home where he is gaining in confidence and having positive experiences. His father has found out where he lives and approached the home, asking to see the RP. The staff at the home are reluctant to allow this. They submit a DoLS request.

The BIA gives guidance on the process. The BIA undertook a capacity assessment where they deemed the RP not to have capacity specifically regarding the decision about whether to have contact with their father. The BIA then requests that a best interests meeting is set up, with representatives there including the RP, the RP's key worker and care home manager, a paid independent representative (advocate, who should meet the RP prior to the meeting), and the RP's social worker (or, if there is no current social worker, they request that one is allocated). The best interests meeting takes place and everyone except the RP agrees that there should be no contact between the RP and their father. The BIA completes the DoLS authorisation report placing the condition that there should be no contact between RP and father. This is a restriction – without the DoLS authorisation, the RP would have the right to family life and the freedom to be in contact with people of their choosing (HRA Article 8).

# Occupational therapists as DoLS assessors

Occupational therapists are essentially trained to 'do with' rather than 'do to', so that the therapeutic intervention becomes an opportunity to 'partner' the person (Townsend et al. 2002). Through partnership they facilitate the person towards personal growth and furthering their 'life-career rainbow' (Wright & Sugarman 2009, p. 16). The occupational therapist uses empathy, placing themselves in the shoes of the person and understanding the dynamics of culture, society, family, institutions, biology, temporal stage, developmental stage, etc. Sumsion (1999) describes how occupational therapists consider the interplay between the person and the 'cultural, economic, legal, physical, political and social environments' (p. 21). This empathy gives the occupational therapist a ready appreciation of the spiritual centre of the person, which is emphasised as an important attribute for the BIA; for example, McColl (2003) found in her research that:

**occupational therapists use four themes to define spirituality and to recognise the spiritual component in their clients. These four characteristics were positive energy, connections to the self and others, awareness of a higher power, and subscription to a particular belief system.** (p. 51)

Core to being an occupational therapist is the use of client-centred practice (Townsend *et al.* 2002) and enablement (Christiansen & Townsend 2004). Chapter 2 of the Mental Capacity Act (2005) Code of Practice (Ministry of Justice 2007) sets out the statutory principles of the Act. Principle 4 states '[a]n act done, or decision made, under this Act for or on behalf of a person who lacks capacity must be done, or made, in his best interests' (Ministry of Justice 2007, p. 19). But how can anybody be sure of knowing what is in someone's best interests? This powerful role – to decide something which is going to have a significant impact on someone else's life – might at first feel like 'playing at being God'. Such an authority over others does not sit easily with the occupational therapist – the occupational therapist wishes to empower and enable the person themselves to make decisions (COT 2015, Serrett 1985). This is generally held to be useful and 'right' in so many ways: (a) when the person themselves makes a decision, they are much more likely to feel comfortable with it and stick to it than if it were made for them (Coulter 2003); (b) a decision facilitated by a guide who provides clarity and depth as well as negating any coercion is more 'true' (Career Cornerstone Center 2016). The occupational therapist, as an Approved Mental Health Professional (AMHP) (see Chapter 19), might in some situations find compromises in the AMHP role and conflicts between their AMHP and occupational therapist roles. However, all that said, it is the authors' assertion that it is *because* occupational therapists are so client-centred and empathetic that they are so ideal for the role of BIA: they embody the 'being a deputy' for the RP in making those decisions which the RP cannot themselves take.

Notwithstanding the qualities of client-centredness and empathy, the occupational therapist is also very used to dealing with taking risks; they handle therapeutic risk taking on a daily basis. The statutory organisations such as the NHS and LA are increasingly risk averse in the current climate of governance, and yet occupational therapists continue to challenge these values by presenting the whole picture of the service user where they recognise the longer-term benefits of living with risks (e.g. Reich *et al.* 1998).

Activity analysis (also known as 'task analysis') is fundamental to how occupational therapists' clinical reasoning is informed. It can be defined as:

**Breaking up an activity into the components that influence how it is chosen, organised and carried out in interaction with the environment.**

(Consensus definition from a European Network of Occupational Therapy in Higher Education (ENOTHE) working group as detailed in Creek 2010, p. 25)

The occupational therapist is skilled in breaking a task into its sequence of steps, breaking it down into sub-tasks and understanding how motor, cognitive, process, interactive skills are all used at each stage (Creek 2010). It is reductive and atomistic (Hagedorn 2001), and this is the way in which occupational therapists assess and measure performance. The occupational therapist understands how deficits in one skill domain might be compensated for by using strengths in another skill domain such as is described by the Assessment of Motor and Process Skills (AMPS), a standardised measurement tool (Robinson & Lumb 1997). The occupational therapist then uses clinical reasoning skills to contextualise the individual, the task, the occupation within their environment: they undertake a process of consideration of the whole; this is a complex intervention (Creek 2003).

The occupational therapist who is a BIA is able to use this skill of activity analysis in their assessment of the RP's mental capacity. They are able to break down the components of rehearsal memory (Jarrold & Hall 2013) and notice how the elements of a conversation utilise this facility. They can compensate for a poor short-term memory through the creative use of aids (e.g. AOTA 2012).

The occupational therapist will appreciate that risks to the body (such as are typically reasons given for authorisation of a DoLS – risks such as malnutrition, falls, self-neglect) are not necessarily more important than some other risks. A life which is safe but without purpose or occupational balance (Reed & Sanderson 1999) could be to many a life not worth living (Parker 1986). Creek (2010) emphasises the primary need of a person to engage in occupation, giving the definition of occupational deprivation from Christiansen and Townsend (2004):

> **Occupational deprivation: A state of prolonged preclusion from engagement in occupations of necessity or meaning due to factors outside the control of an individual, such as through geographic isolation, incarceration or disability.** (p. 278, our italics)

The DoLS can, in fact, empower the RP through routes such as use of the IMCA, and through the setting of conditions onto the DoLS authorisation, where quality of life issues are addressed. In the experience of the authors, there have been occasions where RPs in nursing homes have benefited from conditions being placed on their DoLS which support the securing of resources and supplying of activities for mental stimulation and engagement in purposeful relationships. Kronenberg and Pollard (2005) might go as far as to describe a person with poor cognitive function residing in an EMI nursing home as being at risk of occupational apartheid, where:

> **people experiencing disabling conditions find themselves in a situation where their personal participation in daily life is limited or denied through broader factors than physical or cognitive disability [which suggests that] socio-political conditions themselves can be the principal barrier to access. [They note that o]ccupational apartheid therefore describes circumstances which go beyond the description of occupational deprivation: 'a state of preclusion from engagement in occupations of necessity and/or meaning due to factors that stand outside the immediate control of the individual', ... although occupational deprivation may be a contributing factor to or a product of occupational apartheid.** (p. 59)

Thus a further 'layer' of complexity around the RP's situation is considered by the BIA who is an occupational therapist.

# Mental health professional working in elderly services at a DGH (e.g. liaison psychiatry)

Working as an occupational therapist, or perhaps with a generic title such as mental health professional or discharge coordinator, in a district general hospital on elderly wards would currently offer a ripe opportunity for role/job development in the area of DoLS. By taking on a lead role around those patients who are presenting with a lack of mental capacity to undertake decisions around their own care and accommodation, the occupational therapist is well equipped already (without necessarily training to become a BIA as such) in coordinating their discharge plans and arrangements. There are roles around (a) staff training about DoLS; (b) coordination of best interests decision meetings; (c) initiating referrals for advocates/IMCAs; (d) advising family about the role of DoLS and associated legislation (e.g. Power of Attorney).

Hospital staff are very busy with multiple roles already, and with the ever evolving landscape of the Mental Capacity Act (2005), it could prove an efficient use of resources if there was someone such as an occupational therapist dedicated to overseeing and facilitating DoLS. It is considered best practice that the BIA is involved at an early stage of decision making in a person's care planning so that the RP can be sure (a) to have had good representation during the planning; (b) family members/ friends involved can have access to support (e.g. paid advocates to assist the RPR; e.g. for family/ friends to have been fully informed regarding the role of the Mental Capacity Act 2005/DoLS); and (c) that the RP is not placed somewhere without full consideration of alternatives and possible lesser restrictive options having taken place.

To illustrate how this role might impact on practice, consider the following case study (Box 20.2).

## Box 20.2: Case study – 'duty of care'

Mr and Mrs A are an elderly couple. Mr A's memory has been deteriorating and Mrs A has been caring for him at home and ensuring his safety there, despite her own recent news that she has a progressive cancer and her life expectancy is about 12 to 18 months. Mr A is admitted with a severe chest infection to the local DGH. During his admission, his cognitive function deteriorates to the point where the ward staff deem it too risky to send him home. There is a meeting called – Mrs A attends and is met with a room full of professionals (sister, key nurse, physiotherapist, occupational therapist, mental health professional, and discharge coordinator). Mrs A wants her husband to return home with her so that they can both enjoy the few months of reasonable quality life they have left. The meeting upsets

Mrs A; she finds that she is unheard, that the staff repeat the fact that they have a duty of care so can't let Mr A go home, and nothing is progressed.

This meeting would have benefited enormously from a coordinator who could have briefed the individuals attending beforehand, asked each person to prepare a report and specifying what to include (evidence of risks, likelihood of risks, severity of the consequences of risks), asked some of the staff to undertake additional work (e.g. asked for a report on the possibilities for telecare, respite care, a 'double placement' where both Mr and Mrs A could go into residential care together), chaired the meeting so that everyone had their say, appointed an advocate for Mr A, appointed a paid representative to support Mrs A through the process, specified what the decision was, etc.

# Training roles

There is significant potential for both formal and informal teaching roles associated with the Mental Capacity Act (2005) and DoLS to be developed. The practising clinical occupational therapist, taking a holistic stance and being trained in assessment of mental processing skills, is ideally placed to develop an expertise and role around this subject. Opportunities can be sought to develop a special interest in the DoLS and to be the 'expert' within the team where a clinical occupational therapist is working. There are also more formal teaching roles increasingly required around the subject of DoLS, with the increase in number of DoLS and the increasing range/quantity of Managing Authorities (MAs) (an MA is the organisation licensed to provide care and residency, such as a care/nursing home or hospital) where staff are required to complete DoLS training as mandatory (e.g. the addition of the community supported living placements as now requiring DoLS).

# The Independent Mental Capacity Advocate (IMCA)

Any role in advocacy, whether it is for a specific concern (e.g. housing needs), as a support to getting a person's own voice heard, on behalf of a group (e.g. the Lesbian, Gay, Bisexual and Transgender (LGBT) community), or associated with the Mental Capacity Act (2005) or Mental Health Act (1983/2007), is something which an occupational therapist will be well suited to undertake. The role of the occupational therapist clinician has always included an element of advocacy (Dhillon et al. 2010), more so in some eras, and perhaps with the current access to specific and independent advocates less so currently.

The Mental Capacity Act (2005) specifies that advocates should be available to people who are subject to a DoLS, it being their right to 'a voice' and an appeal. Most RPs who are under a DoLS have a relative or friend who is suitable for and willing to undertake the role of RPR. However, some RPs do not have living relatives or friends, or if someone has been identified, there might be a clash of interests, thus rendering the potential RPR unsuitable. In cases where there is no one suitable to become the RPR, or for specific decisions that need to be made, a request is made for an IMCA or a paid representative. These advocates are usually provided by organisations within the third sector, recognising the need to maintain the advocate's loyalties as independent from an organisation such as the NHS or LA so that conflicts of interest can be avoided. It is the responsibility of the LA to ensure provision of such advocacy, and the LA will usually have contracts with these organisations.

The role of the IMCA involves getting to know the RP, their history, their own views and values. The IMCA visits the RP and raises concerns with relevant staff members. They glean information about their progress from speaking to others such as care staff. The IMCA can make a request for a DoLS to be reviewed if an issue requiring this is raised. The IMCA will at times have to initiate appeals at the Court of Protection on behalf of the RP. When a BIA undertakes a DoLS assessment and the RP has an IMCA, the BIA will address all the points made by the IMCA in their report.

## Thoughts for the future

The roles for occupational therapists around the Mental Capacity Act (2005) are currently being devised and present as exciting opportunities. The occupational therapist should give serious consideration to taking up a role within this field if they are interested in contributing to society through operating and influencing this part of the law. For those who take up posts which are designated specific BIA work, there could be opportunities to become involved in research, development, and play a part in influencing the next stages of how practice evolves around the DoLS. The reader is urged to at least seek to shadow a DoLS assessment taking place as a part of their own Continuing Professional Development (CPD).

In a society currently facing increasingly limited state funding of welfare there is a possibility that DoLS may be implemented in the community in people's own homes. Unless research produces the well anticipated strides in the prevention of dementias soon, the use of assistive technology and telecare to maintain the growing population of elderly people with cognitive impairment in their own homes for longer periods is likely. This poses an important issue for occupational therapists' consideration: after a point, does the use of assistive technology and telecare provide people with a false sense of security about a person being maintained in their own home? Whilst these are fabulous tools for use when the situation is suitable, without the expert understanding of the complexity of risk and function, significant dangers might be overlooked, or people might be placed in 24-hour care when not necessary were assistive technology to be used. Occupational therapists are particularly well placed to carry out assessments of risk for individuals; they understand function and the complexity of how different skill areas interplay within the person and environment. Risk in such circumstances is non-linear in its prediction; it is not a straightforward assessment. There is a danger that services other than occupational therapists will utilise assistive technology tools too simplistically so that risk is actually increased if there is not a full appreciation of people's functional processes.

# Useful resources

- 39 Essex Chambers: http://www.39essex.com
- College of Occupational Therapists (2016) *Care Act 2014: Guidance for Occupational Therapists: Wellbeing.* London: COT.
- http://daisyboggconsultancy.co.uk
- E-network of people interested in occupational therapists being AMHPs and BIAs: email cleweshj@gmail.com
- The Law Commission: http://www.lawcom.gov.uk/
- The Law Society: http://www.lawsociety.org.uk
- http://www.mentalcapacitylawandpolicy.org.uk/
- Mughal, A.F. & Richards, S. (2015) *The Deprivation of Liberty Safeguards (DoLS) Handbook.* Camden, London: BooksWise.
- Office of the public guardian: https://www.gov.uk/government/organisations/office-of-the-public-guardian

# References

American Occupational Therapy Association (2012). *Dementia and the Role of Occupational Therapy.* Bethesda, Maryland: AOTA.

Auden, W.H. (1942). *Another Time.* London: Random House.

Career Cornerstone Center (2016). *Occupational Therapist.* http://www.careercornerstone.org (last accessed: 19.2.2016).

Christiansen, C.H. & Townsend, E.A. (2004). *Introduction to Occupation: the Art and Science of Living.* Upper Saddle River, NH: Prentice Hall.

College of Occupational Therapists (2015). *Code of Ethics and Professional Conduct: College of Occupational Therapists.* London: COT.

College of Occupational Therapists (2016) News: Nice recommends creation of discharge coordinator position. *OT News* **24** (1), 10.

Coulter, A. (2003). *The Autonomous Patient: Ending Paternalism in Medical Care.* London: TSO.

Creek, J. (2003). *Occupational Therapy Defined as a Complex Intervention.* London: COT.

Creek, J. (2010). *The Core Concepts of Occupational Therapy: a Dynamic Framework for Practice.* London: Jessica Kingsley Publishers.

Department of Health (2008). *World Medical Association Declaration of Helsinki: Ethical Principles for Medical Research Involving Human Subjects.* London: TSO.

Department of Health (2014). *Letter: Deprivation of Liberty Safeguards (DoLS) 28th March 2014.* http://www.cqc.org.uk (last accessed 19.2.2016).

Dhillon, S.K., Wilkins, S., Law, M.C., Steward, D.A. & Tremblay, M. (2010). Advocacy in occupational therapy: exploring clinicians' reasons and experiences of advocacy. *Canadian Journal of Occupational Therapy* **77** (4), 241–248.

Haffenden, J. (1983). *W.H. Auden.* London: Routledge.

Hagedorn, R. (2001). *Foundations for Practice in Occupational Therapy,* 3rd edn. Edinburgh: Churchill Livingstone.

Jarrold, C. & Hall, D. (2013). The development of rehearsal in verbal short-term memory. *Child Development Perspectives* **7** (3), 182–186.

Kronenberg, F. & Pollard, N. (eds) (2005). 'Overcoming Occupational Apartheid: a Preliminary Exploration of the Political Nature of Occupational Therapy' in *Occupational Therapy Without Borders: Learning from the Spirit of Survivors,* eds. F. Kronenberg, S.S. Algado & N. Pollard. London: Elsevier, Churchill Livingstone.

Law Commission (2015). *Mental Capacity and Deprivation of Liberty Consultation Paper.* http://lawcom.gov.uk (last accessed: 19.2.2016).

Lord Chief Justice (2012). *Magna Carta.* http://templechurch.com (last accessed: 25.1.2016).

McColl, M.A. (2003). *Spirituality and Occupational Therapy.* Ottawa, Ontario: Canadian Association of Occupational Therapists.

Ministry of Justice (2007). *Mental Capacity Act 2005: Code of Practice.* London: TSO.

Ministry of Justice (2008). *Mental Capacity Act 2005: Deprivation of Liberty Safeguards: Code of Practice to supplement the main Mental Capacity Act 2005 Code of Practice.* London: TSO.

Mughal, A.F. & Richards, S. (2015). *Deprivation of Liberty Safeguards (DoLS) Handbook.* Croydon, London: BooksWise.

National Institute for Health and Care Excellence (2015) *Transition Between Inpatient Hospital Settings and Community or Care Home Settings for Adults with Social Care Needs.* http://www.nice.org.uk/guidance/NG27 (last accessed: 24.1.2016).

National Institute of Health (1949) *Trials of War Criminals before the Nuremberg Military Tribunals under Control Council Law No. 10.* Washington, D.C.: U.S. Government Printing Office. htttp://www.nih.gov/guidelines/nuremberg.pdf (last accessed: 9.12.2010).

Parker, J. (1986). A life worth living. *British Journal of Occupational Therapy* **49** (11), 362–364.

Reed, K.L. & Sanderson, S.N. (1999). *Concepts of Occupational Therapy,* 3rd edn. Philadelphia, PA: Lippincott Williams & Wilkins.

Reich, S., Eastwood, C., Tilling, K. & Hopper, A. (1998). Clinical decision making, risk and occupational therapy. *Health & Social Care in the Community* **6** (1), 47–54.

Robinson, S. & Lumb, A. (1997). Use of the AMPS to evaluate older adults with mental health problems. *British Journal of Therapy and Rehabilitation* **4** (10), 541–545.

Serrett, K.D. (1985). *Philosophical and Historical Roots of Occupational Therapy.* London: Haworth Press.

Sumsion, T. (1999). 'Environmental Considerations' in Client-centred Practice in *Occupational Therapy: a Guide to Implementation*, ed. T. Sumsion. London: Churchill Livingstone.

Townsend, E., Stanton, S., Law, M., Polatajkon, H., & Baptiste, S. (2002). *Enabling Occupation: an Occupational Therapy Perspective*, Revised edition. Ottawa: Canadian Association of Occupational Therapists.

United Kingdom Government (2014). *Practice Direction – Deprivation of Liberty. Practice Direction A – Deprivation of Liberty Applications.* http://www.judiciary.gov.uk (last accessed: 19.2.2016).

United Kingdom Parliament (1998). *Human Rights Act.* London: TSO.

United Kingdom Parliament (2005). *Mental Capacity Act.* London: TSO.

Wright, R. & Sugarman, L. (2009). *Occupational Therapy and Life Course Development: a Workbook for Professional Practice.* Chichester: Wiley-Blackwell.

# Chapter 21

# The occupational therapist as an advanced practitioner

## Kim Atkinson

## Introduction

This chapter will explore the factors which have shaped the development of advanced practice and how these inform the current situation. It will outline the current definition of this level of practice and look at the underpinning principles of advanced practice and the common features of these roles. The final part of the chapter will offer a review of some of the issues for organisations and occupational therapy for the ongoing development and success of advanced practitioner posts.

## Key points

- Advanced practice is a level of practice, not a specific role.

- Advanced practice roles could be in research, education, management and leadership or clinical practice. Only those in clinical practice need to use the title 'advanced practitioner'.

- Advanced practice is not just about extending professional boundaries; it provides an opportunity for new and innovative approaches to practice and service delivery, increasing the efficiency and effectiveness of services.

- Advanced practitioner roles contain the four pillars of practice: clinical, leadership, facilitation of learning and research and development but they will be present in varying degrees depending on the role.

- Advanced practitioners are autonomous practitioners with a high level of skill in critical thinking, decision making and problem solving supported by a strong value base. Improving practice and demonstrable impact is inherent in their role.

# Advanced practice and occupational therapy

Advanced practice is a highly skilled, rich and multi-faceted level of practice. Hearing people at this level talk about their work, or indeed having the opportunity to observe them in practice, is quite humbling. It is akin to listening to or observing someone who is a true master of their trade; the ease with which they approach practice looks effortless, yet the skill, knowledge and mastery involved is very evident. Advanced practice is a feature of remodelling the traditional models of healthcare delivery. The drivers of this remodelling have been a need for efficiency with increasing demand outstripping supply, shortage of some professional groups, increased prevalence of complex and chronic health conditions and a cultural shift towards patient-centred care. The role of the advanced practitioner is not a new concept but within occupational therapy the meaning of this level of practice, where it sits within the professional structures and what these roles contribute to healthcare, is still being developed. Within all health professions, there is ambiguity around advanced practice; this arises from historical notions of what it is, as well as the modern context for this level of practice. Some professions, notably nursing, and in the allied health professions physiotherapy and radiography, have a longer history with advanced practice. The advantage of this for occupational therapy is that their experience can be drawn upon. Occupational therapy is a profession which is at last being recognised as having a great deal to contribute to meeting the demands of modern health and social care. The opportunities that advanced practice provides will support the ongoing development of high impact practice and professional strengthening.

# Context of development

The past 20 years in healthcare have seen an emergence of additions to the professional title, for example, 'specialist' or 'highly specialist occupational therapist', 'clinical nurse specialist' and 'extended scope physiotherapist' as well as 'advanced practitioner', the subject of this chapter. These titles are unhelpful because they tell the public, and other health professionals, very little about the knowledge and skill set of the individual and how that differs from a practitioner without such additions to their title. This is important to employers and those concerned with the standard of professional practice, including our service users. Clarity of expectation around the knowledge and skill set of someone in clinical practice is essential in understanding the scope of practice, the level of autonomy and, in essence, every aspect of the governance of a role.

Advanced practice is an evolving concept first developed in nursing in rural parts of the USA in response to need. Efforts were made on an international basis through the World Health Organisation (WHO), who recognised the untapped potential of nursing, to demonstrate how nursing, through working beyond traditional professional boundaries, could provide solutions to specific local health needs (McGee 2009). Advanced practice roles are not simply about extending professional boundaries into the remit that has traditionally sat within another professional group such as medicine, although they may incorporate some aspects of this. These roles provide an opportunity for new directions, new approaches to delivering healthcare and unique skill sets that enable professional roles to meet modern healthcare needs (McGee 2009). Advanced practice has inevitably challenged professional boundaries, the pre-eminence of doctors is no longer viable and care pathways no longer hold doctors at the centre of all clinical decisions. It is recognised that a range of professionals have expertise which can streamline the patient experience. In addition, patient-centred care has driven a need to find new ways of working. Advanced practitioners, with their skill set, are well placed to support this process. They have clinical expertise from a diverse range of areas, they can lead, shape development and manage change and they are able to work beyond the usual professional boundaries to support the patient experience (McGee 2009, Saxon *et al.* 2014).

Inevitably, much of the developmental context for advanced practice must be drawn from the experience of the nursing profession because they have the longest history with this. In the late 1990s the United Kingdom Central Council for Nursing, Midwifery and Health Visiting (UKCC) recognised lack of clarity about practice beyond that of initial registration on the part of both the profession and among employers. There was no consensus on terms used in reference to higher level practice such as 'advanced', 'specialist', 'expert' and no consensus on what preparation in terms of education and skill attainment a practitioner needed for these different types of higher level practice. At this time the UKCC did a piece of work involving a wide ranging consultation and development exercise across the UK where they achieved a standard for higher level practice which was later adopted by employers to facilitate the development of nurse consultant posts (McGee 2009).

Changes in the focus of healthcare delivery also played a part in opening the way for forms of advanced practice. The health reforms of the late 1990s and early 2000 set a foundation for patient-centred care which was more inclusive of community-based practice, health promotion, working with communities to support healthy lifestyles, and a more fluid and responsive approach to meeting the healthcare needs of populations. These reforms facilitated changes to traditional patterns of working, providing opportunities for the professions to be creative about how services could be provided including more services led by non-medical practitioners. Such healthcare reforms required a workforce that was fit to meet the challenges and opportunities of the brave new world. These changes were further supported by Agenda for Change (DoH 2007) which provided a career structure with appropriate pay which supported experienced practitioners staying in clinical roles. In addition, developments at this time also led to the introduction of the consultant therapist, although time has shown this role to be rather underutilised. Pre-registration courses were linked to academic institutions to raise their academic standing, and courses were developed which had both academic and professional credibility. Moving professional education for the allied health professions into universities provided a basis to develop coherent post-registration education, thus supporting higher level practice roles such as those of non-medical consultant and advanced practitioner (DoH 2000, McGee 2009).

Such a review of the development of advanced practice can tell us something about how we have arrived at where we are today. The current landscape of advanced practice could be seen in one of two ways. The first view could be as an attempt to pull together and place some order around a series of developments and expansions of job roles and as a response to anxieties in the modern context about how we govern these roles. The second view of the existing landscape could be perceived as a very positive attempt by professions to creatively evaluate what they may be able to offer in the modern healthcare context, building on the increased professional maturity of all health professions. The reality is that the current position of advanced practice, and the shape that it will take from this point in its development, will actually be determined by a combination of both of these views; they both apply and are relevant to the agendas we face in modern healthcare.

# Defining advanced practice

In 2002 the International Council for Nurses recommended that each country should produce specific legal and regulatory mechanisms to ensure that the title 'advanced practitioner' was protected and to allow nurses to perform activities outside the scope of current regulations governing their practice (McGee 2009). Fifteen years on we are beginning to make some headway with this in the UK. We have seen that advanced practice has not had a linear development, it has been shaped by many factors and its emergence has been rather piecemeal; hence the matter of definition is quite difficult as true consensus does not exist in either the literature or in practice. In Wales I was involved in a piece of work establishing a framework for advanced practice to contribute to the process of consensus (National Leadership and Innovation Agency for Healthcare (NLIAH) 2010). This was a piece of work specifically for Wales, and it succeeded in achieving a position where a benchmark for advanced practice exists. This benchmark offered definition to these roles, identified the common components and qualities which would need to be present in all advanced practice roles and provided guidance for organisations on their development and governance. The framework also directs that unless the components of the framework are demonstrated within a role, the title of 'advanced practitioner' cannot be used. Similar work to that completed in Wales had already been implemented in Scotland (Scottish Government 2008) and the Welsh initiative drew heavily upon this. England has followed through its authorities and again the documents they have produced to support this draw heavily upon, rather than build upon, the work already completed in Scotland and Wales. All the frameworks for advanced practice are consistent in clearly indicating that advanced practice is a level of practice and not a specific role (Health Education East Midlands 2014, NLIAH 2010, Scottish Government 2008).

Practitioners functioning at an advanced level may be in research, education or management and leadership roles as well as clinical roles but the title 'advanced practitioner' need only be applied to those roles with a predominantly clinical focus (NLIAH 2010). It should also be noted that advanced practice refers to the job role and not the person occupying the role; a role needs to be defined as at advanced level and then the post holder is required to demonstrate the skills and knowledge for appointment into the role and then go on to deliver the remit required of the role. It is also worth noting that what constitutes advanced practice needs to be understood in the context of the time. What is advanced practice now may be considered rather mainstream in ten years; advanced practice is dynamic (CHRE 2009).

The term 'advanced practice' could be used to refer to all practice roles above the level of initial practice. It could include specialists working in a defined area of clinical practice as well as expert practitioners demonstrating a higher level of knowledge and skill including those occupying non-medical consultant roles. In obtaining a good understanding of what advanced practice is, it is useful to unravel two terms: 'advanced' and 'specialist'. If we consider Benner's stages of clinical competence (Benner 1984) from novice practitioner to expert practitioner, 'advanced practice' sits on that continuum reflecting a benchmark on the career development ladder. This is outlined in the *Career Framework for Health* (Skills for Health 2010) which was developed as a way of expressing workforce roles recognising skills and competence. There are nine levels on the framework. These start at level one where the employee would demonstrate basic general knowledge and be expected to perform a limited number of straightforward tasks under direct supervision. The highest level is nine where the employee will have responsibility for the development and delivery of services to whole populations, requiring extensive knowledge at the forefront of their field. In contrast, advanced practice sits at level seven on the career framework and people at this level are expected to engage critically with knowledge related to their field and its boundaries with other fields; they are also expected to be innovative and have responsibility for developing and changing practice and/or services in complex settings (Skills for Health 2010).

A specialist role refers to a skill set or a specific context. So, we could have a novice practitioner working in a specialist area or an advanced practitioner working in a specialist area. These two practitioners would be bringing a very different skill set and fulfilling very different roles. This view is reflected in a position statement issued by the Department of Health (2010) as well as the frameworks developed within the three countries referred to above. These all describe advanced practice as a '*level of practice*', not a speciality or role, and they state that there are common features of this level of practice regardless of professional group, clinical setting or client group (Cox *et al.* 2012, DoH 2010).

To summarise, advanced practice is a level of practice characterised by high levels of skill and competence; specialist skills do not, in themselves, characterise an advanced level of practice. Only those occupying predominantly clinical roles need to use the title advanced practitioner and this title refers to the job role and not the person occupying that role (NLIAH 2010).

# Underpinning principles of advanced practice

Advanced practice does not relate to a specific role or clinical area; it is more a concept around a defined level of practice. For a concept to be useful operationally it needs further definition, and this is offered within the literature as a description of the underpinning principles of advanced practice. These are the principles which would be present in every advanced practitioner role and it is the description of these principles which support understanding advanced practice as a level of practice.

The underpinning principles of advanced practice are:

- Autonomous practice
- Critical thinking
- High level decision making and problem solving
- Values-based care
- Improving practice.

(McGee 2009, p. 40)

Having been party to many discussions about advanced practice posts I would suggest a sixth principle:

- Impact.

These six principles are very inter-related but it is useful to attempt to separate them in order to drill down to what is the essence of advanced practice.

# Autonomous practice

Advanced practitioners are autonomous practitioners. In occupational therapy we are very familiar with this as a concept. Generally it is not a quality which vexes us because we are autonomous practitioners from the moment we become state registered. This means we are responsible and accountable for the work that we do. We are able to accept or decline referrals, assess, plan and deliver interventions, and review and discharge a patient without reference to a medical practitioner. Of course what each therapist brings to their practice will vary according to their level of experience and expertise. In addition to this, organisations place mechanisms around an individual practitioner to support autonomy; these mechanisms include supervision, placing appropriately experienced staff in certain job roles and providing training opportunities.

For an advanced practitioner in occupational therapy, autonomous practice takes a higher level. As well as the likelihood of being the only occupational therapist within the team, the advanced practitioner is likely to require a unique skill set to meet the demands of the role. Advanced practice also requires the ability to introduce and take the lead on innovating new practices and working methods (McGee 2009). The advanced practitioner will need to use and develop skills beyond their core skill set. To achieve this they will need to be autonomous in defining what their learning needs are and how best to meet those needs, often utilising non-traditional resources and uniquely synthesising learning to apply it to the advanced role requiring highly developed skills in critical appraisal. The advanced practice role is also likely to involve developing pathways across the usual boundaries; this will require the development of protocols to support practice. High levels of competence in interpersonal relationships and leadership skills will be required in order to drive through and sustain such change in traditional working practices.

The advanced practitioner will need to be fully conscious of the implications of their role; they will need to be explicit about these and able to work autonomously with their organisation to ensure the governance of the role. Because of the uniqueness of the role the employing organisation will be able to offer the practitioner less support through the usual mechanisms of supervision and training for example. Practising beyond the core skill base may also mean that the professional body does not indemnify the practice of the advanced practitioner (McGee 2009); the employing organisation needs to be clear about its liabilities and governance at this level of practice.

By their nature, practitioners in advanced practice roles will bring with them extensive knowledge and experience gathered over a number of years of practice in a range of settings. They will have held senior positions en route to their advanced practice role and they will have studied at a higher level, gaining academic qualifications to support their advanced role. All of these factors develop the professional maturity of the individual and significantly contribute to their ability to function at an advanced level.

# Critical thinking

Critical thinking is the ability to 'think, question and reason' (McGee 2009, p. 194). The advanced practitioner will inevitably come to the role with a high level of clinical skill gained from many years of experience in professional practice across a range of settings. Critical thinking is the process of taking existing and new knowledge and experience and actively engaging with it to analyse and synthesise its relevance to the current situation to support decision making. The advanced practitioner will need the skills to interrogate such knowledge and experience to identify if it is accurate and unbiased, the most up-to-date and whether it is genuinely applicable to the current situation. If it is knowledge gained from research or evidence the advanced practitioner needs to use critical thinking skills to form an opinion on its credibility, its methods and findings, and needs to analyse how it supports their own context of practice. Without critical thinking the advanced practitioner cannot be an autonomous practitioner nor monitor the quality of their own practice or engage in a cycle of continuous improvement (Cox et al. 2012). Critical thinking is a very significant underpinning principle in advanced practice because it is so important in supporting these roles in terms of their effectiveness and their governance. It is because of the centrality of critical thinking to advanced practice that this level of practice needs to be supported by Masters level education as it is within this level of education that critical thinking skills are really honed.

# High level decision making and problem solving

High level decision making and problem solving are supported by high level critical thinking. In high level clinical decision making, the advanced practitioner is synthesising knowledge, drawing upon their clinical expertise, weighing this in light of the individual set of circumstances and the resources available. They analyse these factors and use this thinking to make decisions which are reasoned and therefore ones for which they can be accountable. Reflection is an important strategy within this. Reflection in action (Schon 1991) supports the advanced practitioner both in their decision making and problem solving, and in the process of monitoring the quality of practice and continuously improving. Within occupational therapy we tend to view the two principles of critical thinking and decision making as one concept: that of clinical reasoning. Pre-registration education within the profession has been shaped through methods such as problem-based learning to enhance the ability of new practitioners in clinical reasoning as it is vital for autonomous practice at the registration level. Again for advanced practitioners this will be taken to a higher level through Masters level education where the emphasis on evidence and the critical examination of evidence, from all sources (literature, experience, what we are being told), is taken to a higher level and used.

# Values-based care

Values-based care has always existed but it is receiving increased attention in modern healthcare where values as well as evidence are seen as important in underpinning effective decision making. This work has been led by Oxford University and has been used to underpin many policy frameworks especially in the field of mental health practice (Collaborating Centre for Values-Based Practice in Health and Social Care 2016). Values-based care requires the practitioner to be highly aware of their own values and also to give weight to the values of the patient in supporting clinical decision making. Values-based practice supports balanced decision making on the premise of mutual respect for differences of values (Collaborating Centre for Values-based Practice in Health and Social Care 2016). Within occupational therapy this sits very comfortably with us as it is heavily reflected in the core values and beliefs of our profession; for example, the Canadian Association of Occupational Therapists (CAOT) (2016) states that occupational therapists believe that: 'every person has the right to make choices about life; every person has the right to self-determination, and every person is unique'. Values-based practice also supports the work of the advanced practitioner within the multi-disciplinary team. An advanced practice occupational therapist may well be the only occupational therapist within the team. He or she in an advanced practice role will also be 'pushing the boundaries' of their practice and their contribution to pathways of care beyond traditional routes and this requires effective communication and interpersonal skills. Practitioners are socialised into the values of their own profession, each bringing something different to the table which is often a huge advantage but can also, on occasions, provide barriers to new ways of working. An in-depth awareness of one's own values, as well as an ability to recognise and use the values of the team members, will support this process of embedding new ways of working.

# Improving practice

Having considered the development of advanced practice, it is evident that practice at this level is inherently about improving practice and thus improving the experience of the people who use our services. In addition to this, if we see advanced practitioner roles as a new direction and as a positive opportunity to creatively evaluate what professional groups could offer in the modern healthcare context, it is evident that advanced practice has much to offer. Advanced practice roles have the potential to deliver innovative models of service delivery, streamline pathways for service users, and meet the current agenda around prudence in healthcare (Welsh Government 2016). We have already discussed how the advanced practitioner is a critical consumer of evidence and research to develop and shape their own practice. They will also be a researcher and will actively contribute to the evidence base of their field of practice. As a good communicator they will be effective in disseminating their work, thus enhancing its impact. Advanced practitioners are the senior practitioners within their organisations; they will be in positions of influence and will have an opportunity to mentor and lead, thus having a wide influence on shaping practice.

# Impact

I took the liberty of adding a sixth principle of advanced practice to those widely provided within the literature. I added the principle of 'impact'. In my work with advanced practice at various levels, as a member of the working party developing the framework for Wales, as a lead on implementing advanced practice within my own organisation, and as a professional leader for an occupational therapy service, it has been very evident to me that impact is a key principle of this level of practice. Before an advanced practice role is established, organisations should identify how the impact of the role will be measured and this should focus on factors such as safety, efficiency, organisational impact, acceptance, satisfaction, costs and role transfer (NLIAH, 2010). It is essential that the impact of any advanced practice role is measurable, made evident and is communicated. Measures of impact should be chosen which evaluate the service from the perspective of all the stakeholders including service users, clinicians and that of the healthcare organisation (Comans *et al.* 2011). It is on the issue of impact that the other five principles (of autonomy, critical thinking, high level decision making and problem solving, values-based care and improving practice) come together. Impact is evident in the successful performance of all these roles. Advanced practitioner posts are expensive and while they provide solutions for organisations they also provide challenges. These challenges may come in many forms: governance, professional values and workforce issues. The motivation to sustain and nourish these roles, despite these challenges, will depend upon their demonstrable impact.

# The pillars of advanced practice

We have already stated that advanced practice relates to a level of practice, not a specific job, and practitioners could be working at an advanced level in many fields of practice. It is only those working in a predominantly clinical role who need to call themselves 'Advanced Practitioner' (NLIAH 2010). The four pillars of practice can be used to help further our understanding of advanced practice. They are outlined in the *Post Registration Career Development Framework for Nurses, Midwives and Allied Health Professionals* (NHS Education for Scotland 2016).

The pillars are:

- Clinical practice
- Leadership
- Facilitation of learning
- Evidence, research and development.

Each of the four pillars needs to be present within the practice of someone working at advanced level. So every role at this level of practice will have a clinical element, some leadership, an educational element and a research/development element. All people in advanced level roles will have the same level of skill and knowledge and be able to make high level decisions of similar complexity and responsibility. This is often referred to as 'Masters level thinking'. Advanced practice is underpinned by knowledge and thinking at this level and people in advanced practitioner posts need to demonstrate Masters level education to support their role. Advanced level practice can apply to people working in clinical, research, education or managerial/leadership roles. Depending on what their role is, the height of the four pillars of practice will vary. For example, someone at level seven of the post-registration career framework may occupy a largely managerial/leadership role in which case this pillar of practice would dominate in their role profile, but they may hold a tiny clinical caseload so the clinical pillar may be their smallest with the educational and research pillars sitting somewhere between. For those calling themselves an advanced practitioner, the clinical pillar will always be the most dominant with the other pillars taking a position of varying dominance depending on the specific role and its requirements (NLIAH 2010). Using the pillars to support our understanding of advanced practice can also demonstrate where this level of practice sits with non-medical consultant practice, which is placed at level eight on the career framework; here, all four pillars would be at their highest level. Non-medical consultant practice and advanced practice are distinctly different roles with consultant practice defined by the breadth of its responsibilities. As well as being expert clinicians, consultant practitioners are expected to lead at a highly strategic level, advancing clinical practice well beyond the scope of their own organisation through high quality research, education and evaluation (Hardy & Nightingale 2014).

# The issues for organisations

Healthcare and how it is delivered will quite rightly always evolve. It is driven by political and societal forces. The constant direction of evolution since the inception of the NHS though has been of increasing demand and complexity. The costs of providing healthcare have also risen, reflecting this; and the public health agenda and principles of prudent healthcare (Welsh Government 2016) encourage a more client-centred and community-focused delivery of services. There is always pressure to look at other ways of delivering healthcare and to re-evaluate how we utilise the workforce to achieve this. In the 1990s we saw increasing professionalisation of the workforce as a result of increased funding for professional education and therefore more availability of registered staff; the post-registration career frameworks have also served to support an increase in opportunities for structured post-registration education. With recent measures of austerity we are now seeing a change in the shape of the workforce. The 'Christmas tree' shape is the analogy applied: at the top of the tree, the leanest part represents the most highly skilled staff; the bottom and most abundant part of the tree represents the support workforce – those without professional registration but with skills and competencies to deliver their roles. Those highly skilled staff at the top of the tree are a very expensive resource and as such they must be used wisely and where they can have the most demonstrable impact. They will have a major role in influencing practice and service delivery and shaping pathways of care. Advanced practice provides organisations with a real opportunity to use their most skilled workforce in a creative way, utilising the skills of those practitioners to develop and sustain innovative working practices that provide services users with streamlined, efficient and effective care pathways. They are a valuable resource and the organisations need to feel able to give them the freedom to practise while governance of the workforce at every level remains an important issue.

Organisations face challenges in establishing advanced practitioner posts. The recent activity to determine consistency around what advanced practice is, through the *Scottish Toolkit,* the *Framework in Wales* and the work completed in the authorities and regions within England, has at least provided a structure to support organisations in achieving this (Health Education East Midlands 2014, Scottish Government 2008, NLIAH 2010).

However, there is evidence that the potential of advanced practice is being rather slowly understood and embraced. The frameworks have not been fully implemented and many organisations do not demonstrate a coordinated approach to establishing, developing, governing and monitoring the impact of this advanced workforce (Welsh Government NHS Workforce Education and Development Service 2013). Organisations need to utilise the workforce planning process to identify how and where the advanced practice roles are required. Achieving 'sign-up' in this process from stakeholders can be problematic as these roles challenge traditional models and professional boundaries. The nursing profession has possibly struggled more with this issue than the allied health professions. There is some evidence that occupational therapists have tended to extend their practice into the realms of other non-medical roles, whereas nursing has tended to extend into the domain of doctors who have perhaps been a little slower to embrace these new ways of working (Pierce & Belling 2011). In the 2013 review on the utilisation of the NHS Wales Advanced Practice Framework (NLIAH 2010, Welsh Government NHS Workforce Education and Development Service 2013), the Welsh Government identified that very often advanced practitioners were faced with barriers and frustration due to lack of support from their organisation around their roles. This was manifested in issues such as slow development of or agreement to protocols which would support the role, restrictions on their practice despite them having the necessary training and skills in place, and lack of understanding or entrenched attitudes to the role thus limiting practice (Welsh Government NHS Workforce Education and Development Service 2013). Organisations need to demonstrate corporate support of these roles if they want them to contribute effectively to organisational improvement through better engagement and promotion of their contribution to service and workforce challenges; the workforce needs the support of their organisation to practise effectively (Welsh Government NHS Workforce Education and Development Service 2013).

In addition to strategically planning the development of this workforce, organisations face the challenge of the hangover of years of ambiguity where a flotilla of roles suggesting a level of skill development above registration level have been allowed to spring up. Many of these roles may not meet the criteria to be considered advanced practice roles. There are examples of practitioners adopting the title 'advanced practitioner' where they are not operating at this level or examples of where they are operating above and beyond their remit with little control or accountability (Welsh Government NHS Workforce Education and Development Service 2013). Organisations need a systematic and fair process of reviewing their existing 'advanced' workforce and dealing with this. Some organisations have collaborated with the health schools in their local university to address this through a portfolio of evidence mapped against the four pillars and assessed against Masters level criteria. This is a collaborative process between senior clinicians and managers in the health organisation and academic staff within the university to give some rigour and objectivity to the process and it is one solution. This process of dealing with the existing workforce will involve workforce departments and some difficult conversations but it very much relies upon a clear and coordinated approach within the organisation for the implementation of this level of practice, including ongoing governance around skill development, maintenance and impact assessment.

Organisations are responsible for the governance of advanced practitioners and robust mechanisms for this are essential for patient safety, workforce development, organisational assurance, as well as acceptance of these roles and acknowledgement of the contribution they make. The organisation must approach this in a coordinated and robust way. For the individual practitioner they need to be supported to be explicit about their skills and learning needs and their practice needs to be transparent. Appropriate supervision and mentorship and robust application of the appraisal process will be important tools in achieving this. In Wales, a portfolio approach has been adopted where the practitioner is required to evidence their advanced level of practice against the four pillars; they are required to carry out a self-assessment and provide forms of evidence to support and validate this self-assessment. In addition, they are required to gather 360-degree feedback to provide a comprehensive review of the role and their practice within it. This portfolio is reviewed in the annual appraisal process where evidence is reviewed by appropriate clinicians, the line manager and academic staff (NLIAH 2011). Within my own occupational therapy service, in order to pre-empt issues for our advanced practitioners, we have stated that the appraisal process should specifically review the following points:

- What objective outcomes are expected of the advanced practitioner role? (These should reflect organisational objectives and timescales.)
- What are the barriers and facilitators to the advanced practitioner role?
- What strategies are required to maximise role facilitators and minimise role barriers?
- What resources and support are required for role development?
- Ensuring that the lines of reporting and accountability are clear and still appropriate
- Metrics which capture the impact and benefits of the role.

A 'novice advanced practitioner', someone new to their advanced practice role, is likely to need additional support to meet the demands of their full post outline. Their ongoing development will need to be supported, most likely through a package of support including academic, skill-based and professional mentorship, because it is unlikely that the development demands of a role can be met from one source. The organisation needs to have a system in place for supporting the education and training needs of advanced practitioners, and they will need to establish relationships with the university system to address these needs through a coordinated education and training strategy.

Succession planning for these roles is also very important for organisations to consider. The skill set of advanced practitioners will be unique and high level. If functioning to their potential they will be vital to the work of the organisation and succession planning should be a high priority for the organisation if its business is not to be interrupted should the advanced practitioner leave for any reason. This cannot be left to chance.

# The issues for the profession

The nebulous nature of advanced practice, the fact that it has developed in a very ad hoc fashion and the lack of consensus on so many aspects of it, have inevitably led to a debate about its regulation by the professional regulatory bodies. The concern of these bodies is primarily that of patient safety, achieved through governing the fitness to practise of those professions registered through them. In its report published in 2009 (CHRE 2009), the Council for Healthcare Regulatory Excellence found that the term 'advanced practice' was being applied inconsistently between different healthcare professional groups and that this had led to confusion about the scope and competence required at an advanced level of practice. It identified the need for a nationally agreed set of standards for advanced level practice to support governance arrangements around this area of clinical practice. In its report, the Council concluded that advanced practice was not a regulatory issue, highlighting that it was the responsibility of employers to ensure that their employees are fit to fulfil the roles and duties outlined in their job description and to ensure robust governance arrangements are in place to manage risk and patient safety. They also highlighted that practitioners have a role and responsibility in ensuring that they have the necessary skills and knowledge to fulfil their role safely and effectively and that this is already covered in the individual's accountability to the regulatory body.

Professional and regulatory bodies are only concerned with fitness to practise at the level of performance required for registration. The view is that advanced practice should be monitored through some sort of separate mechanism, such as an entry on a register for advanced practice (CHRE 2009). Such registers need to sit within the organisations, ideally linked to their electronic staff record, with clear lines of responsibility for ensuring the criteria for advanced practice are met (NLIAH 2010). The register could also include detail of the Masters level education supporting the role and ongoing appraisal records.

Advanced practice is a real opportunity for occupational therapists. We are very well placed to take roles at this level of practice. We are by our nature autonomous, creative, flexible, intelligent, capable and solution-focused, all great qualities to take into an advanced practice role. We have already seen how the underpinning principles sit comfortably with our professional philosophy. In addition to these qualities we have connections across service areas including social care and the third sector because of our professional network and the extent of this network is unique. These relationships facilitate new ways of working. Occupational therapists are also very good at justifying and articulating what it is that we do and this is important in making the contribution of an advanced practice role explicit. Where we have occupational therapists in advanced practitioner roles we need to be clear about what parts of the role are core occupational therapy and what parts sit beyond that. It is in this way that we will protect the place of occupational therapy practice in these services as changes occur in the future and post holders come and go. An ongoing struggle for occupational therapy will be to ensure that the focus of occupation and its value is retained within current posts and practice; this is an important tenet to maintain (Cox *et al.* 2012).

Professional maturity is a key component of developing areas of advanced practice. This is achieved by many factors and post-qualifying education has a role to play. Professional maturity provides a firm and confident base. From this stance we are able to have the confidence to look creatively at new ways of doing things, on occasions pushing professional boundaries, developing emerging areas of practice, and working with others inter-professionally in new and exciting ways, with the development of effective and meaningful patient pathways as the core drivers for this. Post-qualifying education provides us with the skills to use evidence and demonstrate the value of the new ways of working as well as promoting these beyond our own area through the sharing of academic literature and debate.

Advanced practice is not a linear route of professional development. To have successful advanced level practice we all need to look up and out beyond our professional boundaries into areas that have traditionally sat with other professional groups. We cannot achieve this in isolation or by thinking about advanced practice within our own professional group. Advanced level practice and advanced practitioner posts need to be developed from a service perspective as a route to providing solutions – as a professional group we need to ensure that we are at the table with our colleagues from other professional backgrounds. With the erosion of professional leadership structures this is a challenge in its own right, but we need to actively seek involvement in workforce development as that way we can shape it to be occupationally focused (Cox *et al.* 2012). The issue for occupational therapists, and all allied health professionals, is that historically we have not had equal opportunities for choices of appropriate Masters programmes. More importantly, access to funding and study leave to support our involvement on these programmes has certainly been less forthcoming for allied health professionals than it has for some professional groups.

As occupational therapists we need to monitor the progress of advanced level practice within our profession, particularly those posts occupying a predominantly clinical domain. We need to capture the impact of occupational therapists in those roles and build an evidence base around this which we can share across the occupational therapy community. At present there are very few published articles demonstrating the impact of occupational therapy practitioners in advanced practice roles (Saxon *et al.* 2014).

# Conclusion

Advanced practice has the potential to provide some real solutions to the challenges of the modern healthcare climate. It provides the flexibility to extend roles beyond their usual professional boundaries but, much more significantly, it is an opportunity to develop new and innovative ways of working, developed and shaped in response to the needs of the people who use our services. It is a chance to use very skilled staff effectively and efficiently to provide people with the care and intervention that they need in a rationalised way. Occupational therapists are inherently creative and flexible, and they are collegial in their working practices which have always placed the service users at the centre. They benefit from the uniqueness of their professional network which extends across health, social care and the third sector and for all these reasons they are very well placed to take on the opportunities of advanced practice. These roles are not about diluting the core skills of occupational therapy; an occupational focus will always be central to an occupational therapist working in an advanced practitioner role, and we must be mindful of the potential to fall into 'the generic trap' which ultimately can weaken our professional standing and the opportunities for those who follow us.

# Useful resources

- National Leadership and Innovation Agency for Healthcare (2010). Framework for Advanced Nursing, Midwifery and Allied Health Professional Practice in Wales. http:www.wales.nhs.uk

- National Leadership and Innovation Agency for Healthcare (2011). Advanced Practice: The Portfolio. http:www.wales.nhs.uk

- Scottish Government (2008). Supporting the Development of Advanced Nursing Practice – A Toolkit Approach. http:www.advancepractice.scot.nhs.uk

# References

Benner, P. (1984). *From Novice to Expert: Excellence and Power in Clinical Nursing Practice.* Menlo Park, California: Addison-Wesley Publishing Company.

Canadian Association of Occupational Therapists (2016). *What is Occupational Therapy? Occupational Therapy Values and Beliefs.* http://www.caot.ca (last accessed: 8.2.2016).

Collaborating Centre for Values-based Practice in Health and Social Care (2016). *Values-based Practice.* http://www.valuesbasedpractice.org (last accessed 3.2.2016).

Comans, T.A., Clark, M.J., Cartmill, L., Ash, S. & Sheppard, L.A. (2011). How do Allied Health Professionals evaluate new models of care? What are we measuring and why? *Journal of Healthcare Quality* **33** (4), 19–27.

Council for Healthcare Regulatory Excellence (2009). *Advanced Practice: Report to the four UK Health Departments, (Unique ID 17/2008).* http://www.advancedpractice.scot.nhs.uk (last accessed: 8.2.2016).

Cox, C.L., Hill, M.C. & Lack, V.M. (eds) (2012). *Advanced Practice in Healthcare Skills for Nurses and Allied Healthcare.* Abingdon: Routledge.

Department of Health (2007). *Agenda for Change.* http://www.nationalarchives.gov.uk/webarchive (last accessed: 31.10.2016)

Department of Health (2000). *Meeting the Challenge: A Strategy for the Allied Health Professions.* http://webarchive.nationalarchives.gov.uk/+/www.dh.gov.uk/assetRoot/04/05/51/80/04055180.pdf (last accessed: 31.10.2016)

Department of Health (2010). *Advanced Level Nursing: A Position Statement.* London: TSO.

Hardy, M. & Nightingale, J. (2014). Conceptualizing the transition from advanced to consultant practitioner: career promotion or significant life event? *Journal of Medical Imaging and Radiation Sciences* **45**, 356–364.

Health Education East Midlands (2014). *East Midlands Advanced Clinical Practice Framework.* https://www.hee.nhs.uk (last accessed: 15.1.2016).

McGee, P. (ed.) (2009). *Advanced Practice in Nursing and the Allied Health Professions*, 3rd edn. West Sussex: Wiley-Blackwell.

National Leadership and Innovation Agency for Healthcare (2010). *Framework for Advanced Nursing, Midwifery and Allied Health Professional Practice in Wales.* http://www.wales.nhs.uk (last accessed: 8.2.2016).

National Leadership and Innovation Agency for Healthcare (2011). *Advanced Practice: The Portfolio.* http://www.wales.nhs.uk (last accessed: 8.2.2016).

NHS Education for Scotland (2016). *Post Registration Career Development Framework for Nurses, Midwives and Allied Health Professionals.* http://www.careerframework.nes.scot.nhs.uk (last accessed: 3.2.2016).

Pierce, E. & Belling, R. (2011). Advanced practitioner roles: relevance and sustainability in a 'liberated' NHS. *International Practice Development Journal* **1** (2), 1–12.

Saxon, R.L., Gray, M.A. & Oprescu, F.I. (2014). Extended roles for allied health professionals: an updated systematic review of the evidence. *Journal of Multidisciplinary Healthcare* **7**, 479–488.

Schon, D. (1991). *The Reflective Practitioner.* Aldershot: Ashgate Publishing Ltd

Scottish Government (2008). *Supporting the Development of Advanced Nursing Practice – A Toolkit Approach.* http://www.advancedpractice.scot.nhs.uk/media/1371/supporting%20the%20development%20of%20advanced%20nursing%20practice.pdf (last accessed: 31.10.2016)

Skills for Health (2010). *Key Elements of the Career Framework.* http://www.skillsforhealth.org.uk (last accessed: 8.2.2016).

Welsh Government (2016). *Making Prudent Healthcare Happen.* http://www.prudenthealthcare.org.uk (last accessed: 8.2.2016).

Welsh Government Workforce Education and Development Service (2013). *Report: Review of the Utilisation of the NHS Wales Advanced Practice Framework.* http://www.weds.wales.nhs.uk (last accessed: 8.2.2016).

# Chapter 22

# Research roles for occupational therapists

Lesley Haley

## Introduction

> Research knowledge, skills and abilities are essential, not just desirable competences that all ... occupational therapists need to gain, develop and apply to their practice. (COT 2016, p. 1).

This chapter examines how occupational therapists can develop research skills and participate in research. It is a personal reflection on the current research environment, as seen through the lens of a Health Care Professions Council (HCPC) registered occupational therapist working as a Clinical Studies Officer full-time in an NHS mental health research context. The discussion pertains to the mental health NHS environment in England as it stood in late 2015. Occupational therapy colleagues from the current devolved nations, who are interested in research, may find some of the principles outlined in this chapter useful but they are strongly encouraged to explore the research landscape in their own healthcare environments.

The issues explored in this chapter are relevant to occupational therapists planning to develop research skills whilst maintaining their current occupational therapy clinical role, as well as those planning to move into a more research-specific role. The complementary relationship between occupational therapy core skills and research skills is explored, and the ever-changing research environment is examined. Engaging in occupational therapy-specific research will also be discussed.

Starting out in research can be bewildering, so this chapter suggests ideas for both getting started, and continuing, on the research journey. These suggestions may also encourage occupational therapy colleagues who have previously found research difficult or off-putting to re-engage with the research process. Participation in research by many more occupational therapists, irrespective of clinical speciality or role, would benefit the profession, and ultimately service users.

## Key points

- All occupational therapists in any field or organisation might consider gaining experience contributing to research; there are many roles and opportunities available.

- Development of research, enquiry and critical skills brings a deeper appreciation and understanding to the practitioner.

- The profession of occupational therapy would benefit from robust research evidence to demonstrate the effectiveness of the work of occupational therapists.

# Why get involved in research?

The Health Research Authority (HRA) defines research as an 'attempt to derive generalizable new knowledge including studies that aim to generate hypotheses as well as studies that aim to test them' (HRA 2013, p. 3), and therefore differs from service evaluation or audit, in which many occupational therapists may already be involved.

Within the constantly evolving NHS, it can be difficult for occupational therapists to see how research can be incorporated into everyday practice, where research may be viewed as a peripheral activity to their service demands. Service users, however, want the opportunity to be involved in research. The Clinical Research Network (CRN) commissioned research in 2014 which showed that 89 per cent of those asked would be willing to take part in clinical research (NIHR CRN 2015).

Occupational therapists working within an extended role have the opportunity to explore the efficacy of any role or new treatment through research, and demonstrate the profession's worth in that role. In addition, with extended roles, there is a huge opportunity to embed a research culture in emerging roles for occupational therapists. Engaging in research can therefore benefit service users, foster an occupational therapist's personal development, and develop the profession's evidence base.

# Getting involved in research

Despite the wealth of local, national, professional, academic and virtual research environments in which to engage in research, it can, paradoxically, be difficult to get started in research. The first crucial step is, therefore, exploring opportunities within the research landscape.

To actively participate in many different levels of research, it is useful to understand the research context within mental health in NHS England, and the different research roles open to occupational therapists. The research opportunity landscape is constantly in flux, both at a local and a national level; it is acknowledged that the research environment in the current devolved nations is not addressed, and it is recommended that occupational therapists contact the relevant College/ Association of Occupational Therapists for each nation, as well as looking for relevant research information on the COT website.

Most NHS Trusts have a Research & Development/Innovation department (R&D), one of the roles of which will be to support research within the Trust (e.g. clinicians who are employed by the Trust and are engaged also in research), and research which is organised by external researchers but recruiting into the Trust (e.g. universities, the life sciences industry or the Clinical Research Networks).

Since 2008 the majority of England has been served by the Clinical Research Network. In 2014 the CRN restructured to cover the whole of England. The Network is part of the National Institute for Health Research (NIHR) wider research system which coordinates and funds research throughout England. The CRN provides researchers with the practical support they need to make clinical studies happen in the NHS, so that more research takes place across England, and more patients can take part. This practical support includes: reducing the 'red tape' around setting up a study; enhancing NHS resources, by funding the people and facilities needed to carry out research 'on the ground'; helping researchers to identify suitable NHS sites, and recruiting patients to take part in research studies; advising researchers on how to make their study 'work' in the NHS environment. Within the CRN, clinical specialities are grouped into 'clusters', with mental health, learning disabilities, neurodegenerative disorders and dementias under the same cluster umbrella. The CRN collaborates with NHS Trust R&D departments, university study teams and partners in the life sciences industry (NIHR CRN, personal communication January 2016).

A first step for an occupational therapist working within a Trust could be to contact their local R&D department or CRN office and ask what research projects are recruiting in their Trust. The research may or may not be occupational therapy profession specific, and this will be explored further in the chapter. Occupational therapists (irrespective of their role) can become involved in CRN research by referring service users into CRN-promoted research, becoming participants themselves, and promoting specific research studies within their working environment.

Another research environment is the occupational therapy profession-specific environment. Again, one of the most useful research contacts for occupational therapists is the College of Occupational Therapists (COT). Access to the Research and UK Occupational Therapy Research Foundation (UKOTRF) webpage of the COT website provides a multitude of resources such as a regular Research Bulletin, research publications, access to research awards, and support for research-active occupational therapists. The UKOTRF can provide funding to support COT members' research activities and research capacity building, and includes a range of grants available. As occupational therapists increase the breadth and depth of their research activity, articles describing their experiences have appeared in publications such as *OT News*, which offer a personal insight into their journey.

The Council of Allied Health Professions Research (CAHPR), (created in 2014 from the previous Research Forum for Allied Health Professionals and Allied Health Professions Research Networks), aims to support the development of individuals interested in research. For occupational therapists wishing to start the research journey, there are hubs throughout the UK, each providing research advice and support for new and experienced researchers, clinicians, managers, consultants and academics from all Allied Health Professions (AHPs). This is an ideal forum for occupational therapists to meet research-interested peers locally, and perhaps even representatives/contacts from local universities, local NHS Trusts and the Clinical Research Network.

Both the local and national organisations will have websites and social media where the most up-to-date and relevant information can be found. However, the research environment also encompasses online health research communities, for people both conducting and participating in research. At the time of writing, for example, there is the NIHR's 'Contact, Help, Advice and Information Network' (CHAIN) for people working in health and social care to exchange ideas and share knowledge. There are other online communities of researchers designed to contact and collaborate with peers, and taking advice from COT and CAHPR will steer the occupational therapist starting in research towards the most current online community.

Health research roles currently include a myriad of terms – for example, Research Assistant, Clinical Studies Officer, Clinical Trials Officer and Research Facilitator. Often these roles are not profession-specific, and therefore occupational therapists have the transferable knowledge and skills to apply for them. These roles often involve working on several research studies simultaneously, but these studies will not always be occupational therapy-specific. An element of engaging in research can be embedded in other job roles and descriptions, such as the Consultant Occupational Therapist role, and occupational therapy managerial roles within NHS Trusts.

For occupational therapists starting out in research and still working in a clinical role, the Clinical Academic Careers Pathway Capability Framework for Nurses, Midwives and Allied Health Professionals (Association of UK University Hospitals 2014) sets out indicative role responsibilities, including clinical and research capabilities, with respect to early, mid- and senior career roles across the pathway. The document is designed to be used flexibly as individuals may enter the pathway at different clinical and academic levels.

To bridge the gap between working as a clinician in the NHS and getting developing research experience, the Clinical Academic Studentships (in 2015 supported by the Health Education England/National Institute Health Research) are designed to provide a developmental pathway to increase research expertise and research capacity, by having research opportunities at intern, masters and doctoral levels. For occupational therapists with no research experience, the paid internship level may offer the opportunity to gain research experience, and contribute to the occupational therapy knowledge base by undertaking a small scale research project with supervised support, whilst still maintaining their clinical role. For occupational therapists working in extended roles, this may offer a way of defining their added value in the role, but for all occupational therapists it can be a crucial first step contributing towards the occupational therapy knowledge base as well as a stepping stone towards the next level of engaging in research. Thus the scheme enables occupational therapists to combine their clinical role in the NHS whilst building up research capacity and expertise, personally, professionally and within their clinical work place. Current information will be displayed on the relevant websites for the above organisations. See Box 22.1 for an account by Jane Clewes of her research journey on the Clinical Academic scheme.

## Box 22.1: Account by Jane Clewes of her research journey on the Clinical Academic scheme

I work as a clinician in mental health services in the West Midlands. I submitted an application to do the MClinRes via the NIHR scheme a few years ago. This involved me first gaining the permission of my managers. As the only occupational therapist in a CMHT my managers were not keen for me to do the part-time course (comprising two days per week out for two years) but would have been happy if I did the full-time route (full-time for one year). The NIHR provide back-fill funding so that services do not have to suffer. My managers had the impression that they would be unable to find an occupational therapist to back-fill my work unless on a full-time basis. As it happened, the full-time places for the forthcoming intake were all full; I personally preferred the part-time route anyway. I discussed a possible three-way swap with occupational therapy colleagues in the same Trust in mental health – I knew that these individuals were ready for a change in post – and managed to gain agreement; thus I could be released to apply for the MClinRes course.

The application for a place on the course itself comprised a written submission and then I was invited for interview after being shortlisted. The written submission was straightforward with details of past work experience, Continuing Professional Development (CPD), future career aspirations, research experience, and reasons why you wanted to undertake the course. I was asked to prepare a short presentation for the interview about an idea I had for investigation. I had at the time become worried by the sustained drive to get services to focus on Cognitive Behavioural Therapy (CBT) where everyone around me seemed to be asserting that CBT was the one element in service users' recovery which worked. It seemed to me that CBT could even cure gout! I knew from experience that even though our group therapies were called 'CBT', that it wasn't necessarily just the CBT which was the effective ingredient but the tea break chat, the group process, the interpersonal dynamics, etc. In fact, when I asked many service users what CBT stood for and what it was, they were unable to tell me despite numerous handouts and worksheets and group exercises. So I got on my soap box and presented this, backed up with examples of the published studies which purported to be the 'evidence' in the Evidence Based Practice (EBP) which Lord Layard (Pollock 2009) had put forward as his reasoning around the need for Improving Access to Psychological Therapies (IAPT). This must have resonated with the panel as they offered me a place on the course.

So I started work in my 'swapped' post on the inpatient wards for three days per week and started the course on the part-time route. My employer did not seek to find a temporary occupational therapist to back-fill my two days per week out of the workplace. They may have been under the impression that they were making a saving, but the NIHR do not pay the employer anything unless someone is actually employed for that specific post. Having newly moved to the post I didn't have the pressure to continue a level of and caseload of work which I had been doing prior to starting the course; many of the other students on the course had difficulties with pressures from their workplaces to continue with what was really five days' work whilst they were supposed to be working three days per week. I know that this would have applied to me if I had remained at the CMHT where I was an occupational therapist/care coordinator so felt advantaged to be in the position of establishing a three-day only work routine from scratch.

The course I did was provided from the University of Manchester. Other universities are used in different years; this is to help people from different parts of the country to access the scheme. All course costs were covered by the NIHR and they also paid my going salary for the time out (my employer continued to pay me for full time as the NIHR gave them my salary for the two days per week). I had to pay for travel, books, stationery, etc. There were a few students on the course who lived over 100 miles away from the university and the NIHR paid their travel and overnight hotel expenses.

It was of benefit to me that it was the part-time course which I was on as I hadn't firmed up an idea for my research study until well into the first of the two years of the course. Time management is essential as securing the various permissions (university ethics department, own employing Trust Research and Development department, and the National Research Ethics Committee (NREC)) can take a long time and you can't begin gathering data for a study until these permissions are gained. It is possible, however, to choose a research question where ethics permissions are not required; something such as a systematic review would not need to go through ethics. Some of the students on the course had already worked up a study question and written a research protocol prior to beginning the course, and this was necessary for timetabling reasons if doing the full-time one-year course.

In order to undertake research using people within health services as subjects, the Good Clinical Practice (GCP) basic course has to be passed. The NIHR coordinates these and they run regularly in many localities throughout the UK – usually just one day of workshop and lectures with a brief assessment at the end of the day. The GCP certificate accredits you to practise research within health services for a couple of years and then it is renewable through reassessment.

The MClinRes can in some instances be used as an alternative to the first year of a PhD. There are time limits on doing this. An example of this is the University of Derby's New Route PhD.

I found the course to be structured and guided. The modules used on-line tools such as tasks for the student group each week and computer spaces to 'chat'. There was guided reading and easy access on-line to the library. I made the effort to produce 'outputs' from my research project (presenting at conferences and writing articles for publication).

I would highly recommend the course to anyone who wants to develop their thinking skills. It isn't just for those who want to go into research careers. I have used the new skills in soft ways to enhance my work on an everyday basis. It has knock-on effects for my colleagues who use me as a resource as well as listen to me when I discuss our work. I consider the course was a 'gift' to me as I was able to maintain my level of income rather than having to take a cut in pay. It opens doors for you if you want to progress with teaching and research.

Some occupational therapists access post-graduate university education as part of engaging in research, both in occupational therapy and non-occupational therapy-specific courses and qualifications. For those wishing to get more involved in research, Box 22.2 shows some initial routes for engagement with research, which includes activities such as making contact with R&D departments and their local Clinical Research Network. These research activities are easily integrated into everyday practice, such as giving service users information about research projects, recruiting in the occupational therapist's Trust, putting up posters promoting research studies, integrating research promotion into clinical pathways, starting up journal clubs and taking part in NIHR campaigns.

## Box 22.2: Ideas to integrate research activities into clinical practice

- Contact your Trust's R&D to see what research is taking part in the Trust
- Contact your local Clinical Research to find out more about research studies and training
- Join the College of Occupational Therapists' Specialist Section/COT research section and subscribe to the COT Research Bulletin
- Engage with the Council for Allied Health Professions Research
- Find a research-active mentor (ask your Trust's R&D)
- Enrol in a research methods course, or other course with a research component to it
- Develop a journal club
- Network at conferences

- Ask to observe your local ethics committee in action
- Find out what research is going on in your Trust and contact the Principal Investigator for that study in your Trust to see how you can help, such as referring service users into the study or collecting data. Become a participant, promote research in your clinical area, invite your service users to take part in research
- Become an NIHR research reviewer or Cochrane reviewer – see the NIHR website for details.

Box 22.3 represents a more formal engagement with research, from the concept of a Research Champion (an occupational therapist who acts as the team research focus integrating research activities into the clinical team), 'Research Ready Teams' (where the whole team has specific role in engaging and recruiting to discrete research projects), to more research-orientated roles, such as 'Local Collaborator' and 'Principal Investigator'.

## Box 22.3: Further ideas to engage in more formal research activities

- Find out more about the Clinical Academic Scheme
- Undertake a course with a research component, e.g. Masters in Research
- Become a Local Collaborator for a research study
- Become a Principal Investigator for a research study
- Explore the role of a research assistant
- Do the Good Clinical Practice (GCP) training – this is research-specific training
- Subscribe to NHS and academic job websites to scope the variety of opportunities and the skills/training needed.

# What occupational therapy core skills are used in research?

Occupational therapy core skills can be seen as a bedrock for developing skills needed for research. By embedding research skills at the core of every occupational therapist's role, occupational therapists can build on their skills. The skills developed and enhanced by engaging in research can be transferred easily to roles emerging in mental health fields where occupational therapists have not worked in the past.

Creek (2003) identified the core skills of occupational therapy as: collaboration, assessment, enablement, problem solving and using activity as a therapeutic tool. Core skills such as these are fundamental in delivering high quality research for service user benefit. Occupational therapists can therefore use their core skills to engage in all aspects of the research, and, in addition, may well find that these core skills are enhanced by the rigour demanded by the research process.

Collaboration between the participant and the researcher is key to successfully recruiting participants, keeping them engaged in the research process, and for maintaining the participant's safety. Recruitment is fundamental to the scientific credibility of the research; for without the recruitment and retention of participants within study targets, a research study will not fully meet its core objectives. In addition, a major collaborative relationship exists between those running the study (often university-based) and the clinical team from which participants are recruited. Balancing the needs and objectives of different organisations and team members requires tact, diplomacy and understanding of the needs of all the stakeholders involved.

Research also relies on accurate and clear assessment, often using a range of standardised assessment tools, some of which may be specific to a particular profession or clinical speciality. Study teams will often give in-depth training on these assessments to occupational therapists participating in research, and if in line with the professional and practice guidelines, these particular assessment skills can transfer to the clinical setting.

The occupational therapist's core skill of assessing the individual's occupational performance and the environment can be crucial to enable participants to access and engage fully in the research process. For example, ensuring that a participant's needs are accounted for in terms of location, timing and how the research process is undertaken (while still rigorously adhering to study guidelines) is a key skill in ensuring high quality research; it is also important to ensure that everyone eligible for a study is supported to participate, whatever their individual needs.

For some service users, becoming involved in research can provide further opportunities in terms of their occupational performance needs and aspirations. Increasingly, service user and carer groups contribute to research design, advising on participant information and recruitment and retention, and generating research ideas from service users' perspectives. Organisations such as INVOLVE, funded by the NIHR to support public involvement in NHS, public health and social care research, provide a range of opportunities for interested service users. Giving service users and carers the opportunity to engage in research, in whatever role feels comfortable for them, can be part of the therapeutic engagement in occupation in its broadest sense. If occupational therapists are involved in research, then they, therefore, introduce research participation as a meaningful option for some service users to explore their occupational fulfilment through participating in the breadth and diversity of roles in healthcare research. However, in research as well as any clinical role, the occupational therapist must always acknowledge and balance conflicts of professional power, legal requirements, social pressure and service users' rights (Creek 2003).

As occupational therapy is a complex intervention (Creek 2003), the occupational therapist's professional skills enable them to manage the complexities of healthcare research. Creek (2003, p. 18) illustrates that in health promotion, for example, the occupational therapist's skills and knowledge are translated into action targeted at particular groups of people. It can be argued that this is also the case for occupational therapists engaged in research activities.

# Maintaining occupational therapy professional identity and continuing professional development

Being the only occupational therapist in a multi-professional research environment brings its own issues, especially if one is involved in non-occupational therapy-specific research. Professional identity can be difficult to maintain when research has myriad terms for research activity roles. However, there are many ways in which occupational therapists working in research can maintain their professional identity. Connecting with the established occupational therapy community described above, such as specialist sections, the AHP research network, and attending occupational therapy conferences, can help consolidate professional identity within a new role in research. The COT *Code of Ethics* 'is also pertinent to occupational therapists who are managers, educators and researchers' (COT 2015).

Aligned with professional identify is Continuing Professional Development (CPD). Demonstrating competency in research meshes together other competency frameworks which occupational therapists in NHS clinical practice may encounter. These will include their own employer's appraisal framework, NHS Knowledge Skills Framework (KSF), and Health and Care Professions Council (HCPC) registration, as well as guidance from COT. These are useful to capture strengths and emerging developmental needs, and cover a wide variety of core skills for running research in the NHS. The KSF has research roles and competency dimensions which, although not occupational therapy-specific, nevertheless capture the transferable skills and unique contributions of occupational therapists to the research environment, and to the profession. By judicial use of these multiple frameworks, it is possible to map out the skills, development needs, and the competencies of occupational therapists working in research.

Health Care Professions Council registration can be maintained in a research role by engaging in occupational therapy conferences and occupational therapy-specific research, specialist sections, and taking occupational therapy students in extended role placements, for example. The COT also has a vibrant research section with excellent advice on engaging research, and is an extremely useful way of maintaining professional links. Keeping the professional portfolio updated is crucial to demonstrate competency and maintain HCPC registration, especially in extended roles.

Some research studies require administration of assessments or procedures that are not usually part of current occupational therapy clinical practice. Often the transferable skills gained by this training can be credited towards continued professional development and enhance occupational therapy clinical practice. However, the occupational therapist is strongly advised to check the COT

*Code of Ethics*, the HCPC requirements, and their insurance policies to make sure that their research role and CPD activities fit the current scope and definition of occupational therapy, especially if working in non-occupational therapy-specific research (Pearman 2015). The COT *Code of Ethics and Professional Conduct* advises that:

> [i]f you are seeking to work in areas with which you are unfamiliar or in which your experience has not been recent, or if you take on a more diverse role, you must ensure that you have adequate skills and knowledge for safe and competent practice and that you have access to appropriate support.
>
> (COT 2015, section 5.1.7)

The Code also states that occupational therapists:

> [s]hould maintain an awareness of current policy, guidelines, research and best available evidence, and should incorporate this into your work where appropriate.
>
> (COT 2015, section 2.2.5)

Competencies can therefore add depth and breadth to the occupational therapist's portfolio of skills that they can bring to extended roles such as research, and demonstrate the 'added value' of occupational therapists in those roles, and for the development of the profession.

# Research-specific standards

Any occupational therapist undertaking research should ensure they comply fully with the specific sets of research guidelines and standards called 'Good Clinical Practice' (GCP). It is essential for all healthcare researchers to demonstrate competency, and a legal requirement for those working in Clinical Trials of Investigative Medicinal Products (CTIMP). These GCP standards cover research ethics, informed consent, setting up, running and conducting research in the NHS. Courses can currently be accessed via local CRNs, or contact NHS Trust R&D departments for more details.

In early 2016, the consultation period for the draft *UK Policy Framework for Health and Social Care Research 2015* ended (HRA 2015). This will replace the *Research Governance Framework* (DoH 2005). *The Medicines for Human Use (Clinical trials) Regulations* (UK Parliament 2004) is also essential reading.

Just as the Data Protection Act (UK Parliament 1998) and Mental Capacity Act (UK Parliament 2005) are relevant in clinical practice, so they are applicable to research. In addition, most NHS research departments have operational guidance for conducting research within their Trust. Every research study will have a protocol (a study specific guidance manual) which outlines exactly how each study is ethically conducted, including how participants are consented ethically.

# Current issues of working in research as an occupational therapist

In the current climate, research delivery in the NHS tends to be very competitive, and work is generally either project-specific or comprises short-term temporary contracts. The NHS currently has an unclear career structure for researchers, and this is something that the Integrated Clinical Academic Framework is addressing.

There is also the inevitable conundrum of needing research experience to get into research, so working through the ideas in Boxes 22.2 and 22.3 could help with getting some of that initial experience and building important research networks.

As in many areas of working life, there are gatekeepers – different professions, different grades, different opinions regarding how research should be conducted, and differing cultures of employing organisations or clinical specialities.

So how will all this research activity influence the occupational therapy evidence base? Health commissioners and policy makers rely on research evidence, which emerges from rigorous research methods (such as randomised controlled trials). In order to demonstrate 'added value', occupational therapists need to aim towards developing skills in these research methods. As a profession, and particularly one that is eager to move into extended roles, demonstrating a rigorous level of evidence for service user benefit and cost-effectiveness is crucial. With this goal in mind, occupational therapists participating in research activities will develop research skills and multi-professional/multi-organisational research networks, and build credibility, which is essential for developing research.

However, much of current NHS healthcare research is not designed to enable demonstration of the efficacy of occupational therapy. If occupational therapists are engaged in research activities that are not directly related to occupational therapy, what is the potential impact on the occupational therapy evidence base? Will there be the unintended consequence of reducing the opportunities for occupational therapists to generate ideas and participate in occupational therapy-specific research?

This transformation towards generating and leading occupational therapy-specific research could emerge if all occupational therapists – irrespective of their current role – network with other occupational therapists across research boundaries. In this way, the skills, networks and confidence built up by all occupational therapists, whether in occupational therapy-focused research or not, are shared. This could take place within the organisations described earlier as part of the research environment.

Irrespective of the role taken by occupational therapists in research, by being part of the research environment and by developing transferable research skills, they will be contributing to the occupational therapy evidence base and wider healthcare research. As occupational therapists spread into non-traditional roles, it is an ideal opportunity to research the impact of occupational therapy and occupational therapists. Perhaps the most positive way forward is for all occupational therapists working in research to encourage and embed research activity in clinical specialities and new roles which are emerging for occupational therapists. This could be encouraged by having research participation as part of the emerging-role job description. Ultimately, it is perhaps only by actively engaging in research that occupational therapists can fully demonstrate their potential and their 'added value'.

# Conclusion

In summary, this chapter has explored the mental health research environment in the NHS in England, and has proposed ideas for getting started in research and to build up research experience. Maintaining skills, professional identity and demonstrating competence have been discussed. The chapter has then broadened out to explore contemporary issues such as the potential pitfalls and benefits of working in research for the occupational therapist. To conclude, by participating in research, occupational therapists who are working in emerging areas are uniquely placed to demonstrate their 'added value'.

## Box 22.4: Reflection

Using Boxes 22.2 and 22.3:

- What research activities do you currently do?
- Where would you like to be in one year's time? Use the ideas in Box 22.2 to start/ expand your engagement in research activities.
- Where would you like to be in five years' time? Use the ideas in Box 22.3 to help you move into more research opportunities.

# Useful resources

- https://www.gov.uk/government/publications/research
- National Institute for Health Research (NIHR) http://www.nihr.ac.uk
- Public involvement in the NHS including research: INVOLVE http://www.invo.org.uk

# References

Association of UK University Hospitals (2014). *Clinical Academic Careers Pathway Capability Framework for Nurses, Midwives and Allied Health Professionals.* http://www.aukuh.org.uk (last accessed: 23.1.2016).

College of Occupational Therapists (2015). *Code of Ethics and Professional Conduct.* Revised edn. London: COT.

College of Occupational Therapists (2016). *Research Guide: Capabilities, Career Planning and Funding Opportunities.* London: COT.

Creek, J. (2003) *Occupational Therapy Defined as Complex Intervention.* London: COT.

Department of Health (2005). *Research Governance Framework for Health and Social Care,* 2nd edn. London: TSO.

Health Research Authority (2013). *Defining Research*, revised April 2013. HRA. http://www.hra.nhs.uk (last accessed: 23.1.2016).

Health Research Authority (2015). *Draft UK Policy Framework for Health and Social Care Research – for comment.* London: NHS, HRA.

National Institute Health Research – Clinical Research Network (2015). https://www.crn.nihr.ac.uk (last accessed: 22.12.2015).

Pearman, H. (2015). Defining the scope of occupational therapy. *OT News* **23** (3), 25.

Pollock, L. (2009). *Fit for Purpose: a Push for General Mental Fitness, Combined with Easier Access to Treatments, Could Make a Real Difference to Mental Health Levels in the UK.* https://www.theguardian.com/society/2009/feb/18/mental-health3

United Kingdom Parliament (1998). Data Protection Act. London: TSO.

United Kingdom Parliament (2004). *Statutory Instruments No. 1031: Medicines: The Medicines for Human Use (Clinical Trials) Regulations.* London: TSO.

United Kingdom Parliament (2005). *Mental Capacity Act.* London: TSO.

# Afterword

## Jane Clewes

One of the five themes identified in the half-way review of *Recovering Ordinary Lives* (Smyth 2012) was 'new forms of employment for occupational therapists' (COT 2014). These themes were then incorporated into the College of Occupational Therapists' action plan (Smyth, G., personal communication by email, 10 October 2014). The identification of this as a theme is not surprising, given recent changes to policy and legislation in British healthcare provision such as *New Ways of Working* (DoH 2007), genericism (e.g. with CPA and care-coordination), evidence-based practice (e.g. increase of CBT provision, Marzillier & Hall 2009), matrix management (where practitioners are no longer necessarily line-managed by their own profession, e.g. Øvretveit 1986), the revised Mental Health Act (UK Parliament 2007) and the proposed changes to the Deprivation of Liberty Safeguards (Law Commission proposals 2015), high pressure on beds (Lockart 2016), and more. Occupational therapy, as does any profession, wants to survive (Illich *et al.* 1977). Anne Lawson-Porter and Julia Skelton (2009) ask '[w]ill your *service* survive?' (my italics) (p. 47). Individual occupational therapists are people seeking paid employment, recognition and career progression, and therefore have a *personal* interest in retention of suitable job opportunities for their futures. Seeking new areas of practice and new forms of employment for occupational therapists could prove useful as a survival strategy on all these levels. In reflection of newly emerging roles, occupational therapy courses at universities are increasingly seeking emerging-role placements for fieldwork practice (e.g. Bingham *et al.* 2012).

This book was intended to form a celebration of new forms of employment for occupational therapists. It set out to share ideas and information on ways to pursue novel roles, and inspire occupational therapists to utilise their unique skills and wealth of experience in new ways. It could be said that occupational therapists are faced with a number of hurdles over and above those of other disciplines: for example, even though new policy presents opportunities, being 'a relatively small profession, occupational therapists do not occupy enough executive posts in the NHS to be influential in issues of policy and market orientation' (Pollard & Sakellariou 2012, p. 34). Against such disadvantage, we may face extinction. Through a process of mutation and 'passing' (Hostert 2007), I have found personal satisfaction in recent years working in non-traditional roles which are open to occupational therapists: that of 'mental health professional' within a liaison psychiatry RAID team, and as a full-time Best Interests Assessor. Other occupational therapists find new avenues where they retain their label of occupational therapist, forging onward to offer an occupational therapy contribution to developing services including non-traditional ones, demonstrating effective clinical outcomes, and contributing to overall healthcare service development.

It is hoped that this book proves supportive and helpful to occupational therapists in assisting their practice to be considered and effective, to secure the outcomes of occupational therapy for the health benefits and quality of life of the general population.

# References

Bingham, H., Reynolds, L. & Smith, R. (2012). Trialling non-traditional placements. *OT News* **20** (10), 25.

College of Occupational Therapists (2014). Recovering Ordinary Lives: the successes, challenges and future. *OT News* **22** (9), 22–23.

Department of Health (2007). *Mental Health: New Ways of Working for Everyone: Developing and Sustaining a Capable and Flexible Workforce.* London: DoH.

Hostert, A.C. (2007). *Passing: a Strategy to Dissolve Identities and Remap Differences.* Madison, Teaneck: Fairleigh Dickinson University Press.

Illich, I., Zola, I.K., McNight, J., Caplan, J. & Shaken, H. (1977). *Disabling Professions.* London: Marion Boyers.

Law Commission (2015). *Mental Capacity and Deprivation of Liberty Consultation Paper.* http://lawcom.gov.uk (last accessed: 19.2.2016).

Lawson-Porter, A. & Skelton, J. (2009). Transforming Community Services (TCS): Will your service survive? *OT News* **17** (3), 47.

Lockart, L. (2016). *Number of Beds Cut while Involuntary Admissions Soar.* http://www.mentalhealthy.co.uk (last accessed: 23.2.2016).

Marzillier, J. & Hall, J. (2009). The challenge of the Layard Initiative. *The Psychologist* **22** (5), 396–399.

Øvretveit, J. (1986). *Organisation of Multidisciplinary Community Teams: A Health Services Centre Working Paper.* Brunel University of West London: Brunel Institute of Organisation and Social Studies.

Pollard, N. & Sakellariou, D. (eds) (2012). *Politics of Occupation-centred Practice: Reflections on Occupational Engagement across Cultures.* Chichester: Wiley-Blackwell.

Smyth, G. (2012). Recovering Ordinary Lives: five years on. *OT News* **20** (8), 24.

United Kingdom Parliament (1983/2007). *Mental Health Act.* London: TSO.

# A note about occupational therapists' professional registration when working in a non-traditional/extended role

## Extended roles for occupational therapists and the HCPC

When taking up a post which is not specifically that of an occupational therapist, such as a management position, lecturer, or a full time generic or extended role, the position is likely to require you to retain your clinical/professional registration. Your HCPC-registration is your licence to practise, but because your qualification is as an occupational therapist, it demands that to retain registration you must satisfy the requirements of the HCPC. There is good provision in policy for those with generic and extended roles to meet these requirements.

A sample of CPD portfolios is taken for audit by the HCPC regularly. If the occupational therapist is working in a non-traditional role and they are called to submit, they would simply write a 500-word description of the role and provide CPD relevant to this, as well as providing evidence of a range of different CPD experiences.

## Sources of information and guidance regarding registration, include:

- College of Occupational Therapists (2015). *Scope for Occupational Therapy, Essential Briefing*. London: COT.
- Health and Care Professions Council (2013). *Standards of Proficiency – Occupational Therapists*. London: HCPC.

**See websites:**

- http://www.cot.co.uk
- http://www.hcpc-uk.org.uk

# Index